Updates on Interstitial Lung Disease

Updates on Interstitial Lung Disease

Guest Editors

Atul C. Mehta
Sameep Sehgal

MDPI

Basel • Beijing • Wuhan • Barcelona • Belgrade • Novi Sad • Cluj • Manchester

Guest Editors
Atul C. Mehta
Department of
Pulmonary Medicine
Cleveland Clinic
Cleveland, OH
USA

Sameep Sehgal
Department of
Pulmonary Medicine
Cleveland Clinic
Cleveland, OH
USA

Editorial Office
MDPI AG
Grosspeteranlage 5
4052 Basel, Switzerland

This is a reprint of the Special Issue, published open access by the journal *Journal of Clinical Medicine* (ISSN 2077-0383), freely accessible at: https://www.mdpi.com/journal/jcm/special_issues/695V200824.

For citation purposes, cite each article independently as indicated on the article page online and as indicated below:

Lastname, A.A.; Lastname, B.B. Article Title. *Journal Name* **Year**, *Volume Number*, Page Range.

ISBN 978-3-7258-6846-9 (Hbk)
ISBN 978-3-7258-6847-6 (PDF)
https://doi.org/10.3390/books978-3-7258-6847-6

Contents

About the Editors

Atul C. Mehta

Atul C. Mehta is a Professor of Medicine at the Cleveland Clinic Lerner College of Medicine and holds the position of Buoncore Family Endowed Chair in Lung Transplantation. He is internationally recognized for his expertise in interventional pulmonology, lung transplantation, diagnostic and therapeutic bronchoscopy, and interstitial lung diseases. Throughout his distinguished career spanning over three decades, Dr. Mehta has published more than 500 peer-reviewed papers and over 100 book chapters; he has also edited 16 books, including authored works in diagnostic and therapeutic bronchology. He is a founding member and former President of the American Association for Bronchology, and serves on editorial boards for several journals.

Sameep Sehgal

Sameep Sehgal, MD, is an Associate Professor of Medicine at Cleveland Clinic Lerner College of Medicine and Pulmonary Physician at the Cleveland Clinic, with clinical and academic expertise spanning rheumatic lung diseases, interstitial lung disease (ILD), and lung transplantation. His research interests include pulmonary manifestations of systemic autoimmune rheumatic diseases and lung transplantation.

Journal of
Clinical Medicine

MDPI

Editorial

Interstitial Lung Disease in 2025—Progress, Challenges, and Hope Ahead

Sameep Sehgal * and Atul Mehta

Department of Pulmonary Medicine, Integrated Hospital Institute, Cleveland Clinic, Cleveland, OH 44195, USA; mehtaa1@ccf.org
* Correspondence: sehgals@ccf.org

Interstitial lung disease (ILD) remains one of the most challenging conditions in respiratory medicine, with outcomes often as poor as those seen in advanced malignancies. Despite a decade of progress in diagnostics and management, ILD continues to be a relentlessly progressive disorder for many patients. Mortality remains high, and the burden on patients, caregivers, and health systems is immense; as such, ILD remains a focus of intensive research and clinical innovation.

The defining feature of ILD is its heterogeneity. The term "ILD" encompasses a spectrum of fibrosing and inflammatory lung disorders, ranging from idiopathic pulmonary fibrosis (IPF) to connective tissue disease-associated ILD, hypersensitivity pneumonitis, and rarer entities such as pleuroparenchymal fibroelastosis. Each subtype presents unique clinical, radiological, and histopathological characteristics, underscoring the need for personalized approaches to diagnosis and care. A "one-size-fits-all" strategy is not adequate; individualized management anchored in disease phenotyping and patients' personal values should be the standard of care.

Our understanding of ILD has evolved, leading to refinements in nomenclature and diagnostic criteria. The updated 2025 guidelines provide new terminology and frameworks that reflect current knowledge of disease biology and progression [1]. Clinicians now have access to emerging blood-based biomarkers, genomic assays, and advanced imaging tools that may improve early detection and prognostication. While many remain investigational, such tools bring us closer to the use of precision medicine in ILD. These advances also facilitate better stratification in clinical trials, ensuring that novel therapies are tested in the patients most likely to benefit from them. Despite these advances, the role of the multidisciplinary team (MDT) remains central in reaching accurate diagnoses, ensuring nuanced decision-making in a field where subtle distinctions can profoundly influence management [2].

Therapeutically, the last transformative breakthrough in ILD came in 2014 with the introduction of antifibrotic agents, which slowed IPF disease progression for the first time and later demonstrated benefits across a broader spectrum of progressive fibrosing ILD [3,4]. Yet antifibrotics remain imperfect solutions: they mitigate but do not halt fibrosis, and they do not reverse established disease. Encouragingly, the therapeutic pipeline has accelerated. Multiple phase 2 and 3 trials are investigating agents that target novel pathways, including anti-inflammatory, anti-fibrotic, and regenerative strategies. Early data are promising, fueling cautious optimism that the next decade will deliver therapies capable of altering the natural history of these devastating disorders [5]. Nerandomilast, a PDE4B inhibitor, recently reached its primary endpoint in a phase three trial, marking the first positive trial of a novel agent since antifibrotics [6].

This thematic issue of the *Journal of Clinical Medicine* brings together a collection of original research studies and state-of-the-art reviews that reflect both pragmatic aspects of day-to-day ILD care and the frontiers of discovery. Topics range from optimal strategies for symptom management and supportive care to advances in molecular diagnostics and emerging therapeutic modalities. Together, these contributions underscore both the progress achieved and the urgent unmet needs that remain.

As we look ahead, the ILD field stands at a critical juncture. With refined diagnostic tools, deeper biological insights, and a rich therapeutic pipeline, there is reason to hope that patient outcomes will improve in the years to come.

Conflicts of Interest: The authors declare no conflict of interest.

References

1. Ryerson, C.J.; Adegunsoye, A.; Piciucchi, S.; Hariri, L.P.; Khor, Y.H.; Wijsenbeek, M.S.; Wells, A.U.; Sharma, A.; Cooper, W.A.; Antoniou, K.; et al. Update of the International Multidisciplinary Classification of the Interstitial Pneumonias: An ERS/ATS Statement. *Eur. Respir. J.* **2025**, 2500158. [CrossRef] [PubMed]
2. Tharwani, A.; Ribeiro Neto, M.L. Updates in Diagnostic Tools for ILD. *J. Clin. Med.* **2025**, *14*, 2924. [CrossRef] [PubMed] [PubMed Central]
3. Richeldi, L.; du Bois, R.M.; Raghu, G.; Azuma, A.; Brown, K.K.; Costabel, U.; Cottin, V.; Flaherty, K.R.; Hansell, D.M.; Inoue, Y.; et al. INPULSIS Trial Investigators. Efficacy and safety of nintedanib in idiopathic pulmonary fibrosis. *N. Engl. J. Med.* **2014**, *370*, 2071–2082. [CrossRef] [PubMed]
4. King, T.E., Jr.; Bradford, W.Z.; Castro-Bernardini, S.; Fagan, E.A.; Glaspole, I.; Glassberg, M.K.; Gorina, E.; Hopkins, P.M.; Kardatzke, D.; Lancaster, L.; et al. ASCEND Study Group. A phase 3 trial of pirfenidone in patients with idiopathic pulmonary fibrosis. *N. Engl. J. Med.* **2014**, *370*, 2083–2092, Erratum in *N. Engl. J. Med.* **2014**, *371*, 1172. [CrossRef] [PubMed]
5. Moua, T.; Baqir, M.; Ryu, J.H. What Is on the Horizon for Treatments in Idiopathic Pulmonary Fibrosis? *J. Clin. Med.* **2024**, *13*, 6304. [CrossRef] [PubMed] [PubMed Central]
6. Richeldi, L.; Azuma, A.; Cottin, V.; Kreuter, M.; Maher, T.M.; Martinez, F.J.; Oldham, J.M.; Valenzuela, C.; Clerisme-Beaty, E.; Gordat, M.; et al. FIBRONEER-IPF Trial Investigators. Nerandomilast in Patients with Idiopathic Pulmonary Fibrosis. *N. Engl. J. Med.* **2025**, *392*, 2193–2202. [CrossRef] [PubMed]

Journal of
Clinical Medicine

MDPI

Review

What Is on the Horizon for Treatments in Idiopathic Pulmonary Fibrosis?

Teng Moua *, Misbah Baqir and Jay H. Ryu

Division of Pulmonary and Critical Care Medicine, Mayo Clinic, 200 First St SW, Rochester, MN 55905, USA; baqir.misbah@mayo.edu (M.B.); ryu.jay@mayo.edu (J.H.R.)
* Correspondence: moua.teng@mayo.edu

Abstract: Idiopathic pulmonary fibrosis (IPF) is a progressive and often fatal lung disease most commonly encountered in older individuals. Several decades of research have contributed to a better understanding of its pathogenesis, though only two drugs thus far have shown treatment efficacy, i.e., by slowing the decline of lung function. The pathogenesis of IPF remains incompletely understood and involves multiple complex interactions and mechanisms working in tandem or separately to result in unchecked deposition of extracellular matrix components and collagen characteristic of the disease. These mechanisms include aberrant response to injury in the alveolar epithelium, inappropriate communication between epithelial cells and mesenchymal cells, imbalances between oxidative injury and tissue repair, recruitment of inflammatory pathways that induce fibrosis, and cell senescence leading to sustained activation and proliferation of fibroblasts and myofibroblasts. Targeted approaches to each of these mechanistic pathways have led to recent clinical studies evaluating the safety and efficacy of several agents. This review highlights selected concepts in the pathogenesis of IPF as a rationale for understanding current or future therapeutic approaches, followed by a review of several selected agents and their recent or active clinical studies. Current novel therapies include approaches to attenuating or modifying specific cellular or signaling processes in the fibrotic pathway, modifying inflammatory and metabolic derangements, and minimizing inappropriate cell senescence.

Keywords: therapeutics; treatment; idiopathic pulmonary fibrosis; lung fibrosis

1. Introduction

Idiopathic pulmonary fibrosis (IPF) is a progressive and often fatal disease characterized by the accumulation of fibrotic tissue in the lung [1]. While two antifibrotic medications (nintedanib and pirfenidone) [2,3] have been shown to slow disease progression and are currently in use, a significant need remains for more effective agents that may prevent loss of lung function and even reverse fibrosis. Adverse effects and long-term adherence remain difficult and may confound real-world effectiveness, despite long-term use demonstrating sustained lung function benefit, decreased exacerbation rate, or better mortality outcomes in certain studies [4,5]. Over the past two and a half decades, multiple clinical trials have assessed the efficacy of various agents, including azathioprine in combination with prednisone (anti-inflammatory) [6], interferon-γ (immune response regulator) [7], etanercept (tumor necrosis factor-receptor (TNF-α) inhibitor) [8], macitentan [9], bosentan [10], and ambrisentan [11] (endothelin receptor antagonists), sildenafil (phosphodiesterase-5 inhibitor) [12], imatinib mesylate (tyrosine kinase inhibitor) [13], N-acetylcysteine (anti-oxidant) [14], warfarin (anti-coagulant) [15], ziritaxestat (autotaxin inhibitor) [16], simtuzumab (lysyl oxidase inhibitor) [17], and pamrevlumab (human monoclonal antibody against connective tissue growth factor (CTGF)) [18], all with little-to-no impact on lung function or other secondary outcomes. Recent research has focused on additional molecular targets in the cell signaling of fibrotic pathways [19,20], oxidative stress and inflammatory responses [21], and cell senescence [22,23], with the potential combination of currently established and novel therapies for synergistic effect. The first section of this review broadly highlights concepts in the pathogenesis of IPF that underlie current therapeutic approaches. The second section provides updates on recently tested medications based on these concepts for a better understanding of current drug rationale and future therapeutic directions.

2. Selective Overview of IPF Pathogenesis

IPF is characterized by the inappropriate or unchecked deposition of collagen and extra-cellular matrix (ECM) in lung tissue. This is the result of dysregulated host responses at the alveolar epithelium [24], excessive proliferation and propagation of pro-fibrotic cells either by sustained cytokine or chemokine-driven processes and inappropriate cell senescence [23,25], and imbalances between propagating and degrading fibrotic response [26]. Abnormal cell repair or recovery from oxidative stress or inflammation also contribute to pro-fibrotic processes [27]. An overview of selected pathologic mechanisms is provided in Table 1.

2.1. Abnormalities at the Alveolar Epithelium and Alveolar Epithelial Cells

Injury to the alveolar epithelium has long been a point of interest as an initial trigger of parenchymal fibrosis [24,28]. Alveolar epithelial cells (AECs) produce surfactant and play central roles in maintaining alveolar integrity and directing cell repair after injury [29]. Damage to type II AECs leads to the release of pro-fibrotic mediators, particularly transforming growth factor-beta (TGF-β) [30–32], responsible for multiple downstream fibrotic effects. Epithelial-mesenchymal transition (EMT), characterized by the transformation of epithelial cells to mesenchymal phenotypes [33], is another mechanism by which AECs contribute to lung fibrosis [34–36]. TGF-β signaling is a driver of EMT and leads to fibroblast imitation and activation [37,38]. AECs are also susceptible to oxidative damage from environmental or inflammatory mediators [39,40]. Prior studies have demonstrated oxidative stress may induce cellular senescence in AECs [41], impairing their regenerative capacity and promoting a pro-fibrotic environment [42]. The accumulation of senescent AECs has been associated with mitochondrial dysfunction [43]. Lastly, AECs secrete various cytokines and chemokines that influence the behavior of macrophages [44], promoting their activation and contribution to an inflammatory milieu that promotes fibrotic response.

2.2. TGF-β, Fibroblasts, and Myofibroblasts

TGF-β is a multifaceted cytokine involved in various cellular processes in the lung, including EMT, fibroblast activation, and ECM deposition [45]. It is primarily secreted by AECs [30] and activated macrophages [46,47], with its dysregulation leading to unchecked activation of fibroblasts and myofibroblasts. TGF-β also activates various downstream pathways including Smad signaling which mediate transcriptional responses involved in fibroblast proliferation and differentiation [48,49]. Interaction between TGF-β and other fibroblast growth factor pathways has been shown to influence fibroblast activation and ECM production [50].

Fibroblasts and myofibroblasts are mesenchymal cells directly involved in the deposition of ECM and collagen in the lung parenchyma. Fibroblasts may proliferate from inappropriate cytokine-driven activation or cell senescence [23]. The role of extracellular vesicles (EVs) in mediating fibroblast dysfunction is an emerging area of research [51,52]. EVs are lipid-bound vesicles secreted by cells into the extracellular space and are derived from various cell types, including macrophages and epithelial cells [53]. Fibroblasts exposed to EVs containing fibronectin exhibit increased migratory capacity and invasive behavior [54]. Increased stiffness of the lung may also promote fibroblast activation and myofibroblast differentiation through mechanotransduction pathways [55,56].

2.3. Cellular Mediators of Fibrosis

Cyclic adenosine monophosphate (cAMP) is a hydrophilic intracellular secondary messenger molecule involved in the regulation of multiple cellular processes [57]. Loss or dysregulation of cAMP signaling has been associated with the development or progression of fibrosis through fibroblast activation, inflammation, and ECM remodeling [58]. cAMP primarily exerts its effects via the activation of protein kinase A and other intracellular pathways which better regulate fibroblast function and reduce ECM deposition [59]. Attenuation of fibrosis has also been linked to decreased TGF-β signaling, where increased cAMP signaling has been shown to inhibit TGF-β production and activation [60]. Elevated cAMP levels have also been shown to inhibit the production of pro-inflammatory cytokines and chemokines, reducing inflammation in the lung and potentially attenuating pro-fibrotic pathways [61,62]. Phosphodiesterase 4 (PDE4) inhibitors, which increase intracellular cAMP levels, have been shown to decrease fibroblast proliferation and myofibroblast differentiation [63].

Lysophosphatidic acid (LPA) is a bioactive lipid mediator involved in various cellular processes including cell proliferation, migration, and survival [64]. It is synthesized by autotaxin, an enzyme that catalyzes the hydrolysis of lysophosphatidylcholine to LPA, the latter serving as the primary ligand for lysophosphatidic acid receptor 1 (LPAR1) [65]. The activation of LPAR1 is associated with several intracellular signaling pathways in fibrosis including those promoting cytoskeletal rearrangements, and fibroblast migration and proliferation [66,67]. LPAR1 also activates TGF-β and other pro-fibrotic mediators [68], with LPAR1 signaling involved in the recruitment and activation of inflammatory macrophages [69].

Integrins are transmembrane glycoprotein receptors that serve as mediators of cell adhesion, communication, and membrane integrity. Interplay between integrins and TGF-β has been associated with aberrant induction of pro-fibrotic pathways [70]. Integrin αVβ6, found predominantly in epithelial cells, induces TGF-β activation after cell injury [71], while integrin α3β1 has been associated with EMT and myofibroblast proliferation in murine models of bleomycin-induce fibrosis [72].

2.4. Dysregulation of Extra-Cellular Matrix

Dysregulation of ECM homeostasis with an imbalance between synthesis and degradation of ECM components may result in inappropriate accumulation of fibrotic tissue [73,74]. Collagen (types I and III) is an essential protein in the ECM of lung tissue and is deposited by activated fibroblasts and myofibroblasts derived from resident or circulating fibrocytes, and epithelial cells undergoing EMT [75,76]. Excessive accumulation of collagen leads to the thickening of alveolar walls and the formation of fibroblast foci. Other ECM proteins and cytokines, including fibronectin and connective tissue growth factor (CTGF), have been associated with the formation of fibrotic tissue. Fibronectin is an adhesive glycoprotein crucial for cell adhesion, migration, and ECM organization, while CTGF is induced by TGF-β [77] and further promotes fibroblast proliferation and ECM production. ECM may also contribute to fibroblast proliferation through mechanotransduction pathways [78] and increased cell senescence [79].

The role of matrix metalloproteinases (MMPs) in ECM remodeling has been associated with disease progression in IPF. MMPs are enzymes responsible for the breakdown of ECM components, with their dysregulation leading to imbalances between ECM synthesis and degradation [80,81]. Elevated levels of MMPs in serum and bronchoalveolar lavage fluid (BAL) have been correlated with disease severity and progression [82–84]. In one study, BAL MMP-7 (matrilysin) levels were similarly elevated in IPF and non-IPF interstitial lung diseases with IPF distinguished by MMP-7 immunoreactivity in areas of parenchymal fibrosis compared to areas of acute inflammation in non-IPF diseases [84]. TGF-β is a key regulator of MMP expression in mice models of lung fibrosis, in particular limiting the activity of MMP-2 and MMP-9, which contributes to the aberrant accumulation of ECM proteins [85,86]. MMP-9 has also been shown to induce TGF-β production in human airway epithelium in one in vivo study [87], while MMP-12 acts as a downstream mediator of TGF-β-induced inflammation and fibrosis [88]. Its expression appears upregulated in response to TGF-β [89], though subsequent MMP-12 negative mice models did not demonstrate attenuated fibrotic responses to bleomycin lung injury [90]. Hyaluronan (HA) is a major component of the ECM in most organs. It is a glycosaminoglycan previously believed to be inert, but may play a regulatory role in the ECM of lung submucosa and alveoli [91]. HA is broken down by lysosomal enzymes known as hyaluronidases with prior studies demonstrating elevated levels of HA in the BAL of patients with IPF compared to controls [92,93]. Higher BAL levels of HA were also associated with worse clinical disease or progression [92]. Prior studies suggest HA-directed pathways may promote fibroblast proliferation and invasion [94,95], with HA synthases also driving fibroblast senescence [96].

2.5. Oxidative Stress, Mitochondria, and Macrophages

Imbalances between reactive oxygen species (ROS) production and antioxidants resulting in excessive oxidative injury have been recognized as a significant contributor to pro-fibrotic pathways [27]. Oxidative injury commonly damages epithelial cells and enhances TGF-β signaling [97]. Environmental triggers such as cigarette smoke [40] or cyclic mechanical stretch as seen with mechanical ventilation [98] have been associated with oxidative injury. Mitochondrial dysfunction is increasingly recognized as a contributor to profibrotic pathways [99]. While involved in the regulation of apoptosis [43], oxidative stress, and cellular metabolism, mitochondria also produce ROS as byproducts of oxidative phosphorylation [100].

Recent studies have highlighted the role of macrophage polarization and pro-inflammatory responses in IPF. In this setting, macrophages are categorized as either M1 (pro-inflammatory) or M2 (anti-inflammatory or profibrotic) [101]. M1 macrophages are typically activated in response to pathogens and tissue damage, releasing pro-inflammatory cytokines that may further exacerbate lung injury. M2 macrophages are associated with tissue repair and remodeling but promote fibrosis through activating the secretion of growth factors and ECM components by AECs and fibroblasts [102]. An imbalance between these two phenotypes may play a role in cellular responses to lung injury with activated macrophages also secreting TGF-β [47]. Lastly, macrophages also produce ROS [103] and increase inflammatory responses associated with fibrosis through activation of AIM2 inflammasomes [104].

2.6. Cell Senescence

Cell senescence in IPF is characterized by irreversible cell cycle arrest and secretion of pro-inflammatory factors, collectively known as the senescence-associated secretory phenotype [105,106]. This phenomenon affects various cells in the lung, including AECs [107], fibroblasts [23], and macrophages [108], all with particular roles in the progression and severity of fibrosis. Prior studies have also highlighted the role of specific signaling pathways in mediating the effects of cellular senescence in lung fibrosis [107,109]. β-catenin/p53 pathways have been shown to induce senescence in A549 cells (an AEC model) in response to various stressors [110]. Senescent AECs also exhibit increased expression of p16INK4a and p21WAF1/CIP1 markers, which have been associated with cell cycle arrest [111]. TGF-β signaling is a significant contributor to AEC senescence [112,113], promoting their transition to myofibroblast-like phenotypes and enhancing their fibrotic response.

Table 1. Selected mechanisms of fibrosis in idiopathic pulmonary fibrosis.

Mechanism Type	Summary	Key References
Alveolar epithelial injury and dysregulation	Damage to the alveolar epithelium and type II alveolar epithelial cells (AECs) may lead to aberrant pro-fibrotic responses, including excessive release of TGF-β, epithelial-mesenchymal transition (EMT), and inappropriate senescence of AECs	[24,28,31,33,35,42]

Table 1. *Cont.*

Mechanism Type	Summary	Key References
TGF-β, Fibroblasts and Myofibroblast dysfunction	Aberrant and sustained release of TGF-β may promote fibroblast and myofibroblast activation resulting in excessive extra-cellular matrix (ECM) deposition	[23,30,45,56]
Cellular Mediators of Fibrosis	Intracellular and extracellular mechanisms of fibrosis involve multiple pathways, including intracellular messenger molecule cyclic adenosine monophosphate (cAMP), lipid mediator lysophosphatidic acid (LPA), and cellular integrins or transmembrane glycoproteins, serving key roles in aspects of TGF-β release, fibroblast activation, proliferation, or migration, and inflammation.	[58,59,61,65,67,70]
Dysregulation of Extra-cellular matrix	Abnormal ECM homeostasis is characterized by an imbalance between fibroblast and myofibroblast activity with aberrant ECM deposition and dysregulated matrix metalloproteinases, which are ineffective in the breaking down of ECM.	[74,79,81,85,94,96]
Oxidative Stress, Mitochondria, and Macrophages	Oxidative stress is a common trigger of AEC injury and may result from mitochondrial dysfunction, which is involved in the creation of reactive oxygen species through oxidative phosphorylation. Macrophage polarization is involved in promoting inflammatory and anti-inflammatory (or pro-fibrotic) pathways, leading to aberrant AEC and fibroblast responses to injury.	[97,99,101]
Cell Senescence	Inappropriate cell cycle arrest and its related pro-inflammatory phenotype may involve AECs, fibroblasts, and macrophages, resulting in persistent and inappropriate fibrotic responses to cell injury and repair.	[23,25,42,107–109]

3. Potential Medical Therapies for IPF

Novel approaches targeting mechanisms of fibrosis, as outlined above, form the basis of recent clinical studies in IPF. This section highlights selected agents being evaluated in ongoing or recently completed Phase I or higher comparative trials in the last few years (Table 2), with a focus on drug mechanism, safety profile, and potential efficacy.

Table 2. Selected study agents and their mechanisms in the treatment of IPF.

NCT Number	Phase	Drug/Intervention	Mechanism Class
NCT05032066	2	HZN-825	LAPR1 receptor modulator, LPA pathway for fibrosis
NCT05321069	3	BI 1015550 (nerandomilast)	PDE4 inhibitor, fibrotic pathway reduction
NCT04312594	2	Jaktinib	JAK inhibitor, blocks JAK-induced pro-fibrotic cytokines, also anti-inflammatory
NCT05483907	2	BBT-877	autotaxin inhibitor, LPA pathway for fibrosis
NCT04598919	1	saracatinib	tyrosine kinase inhibitor, blocks TGF-β-induced Src kinase activation
NCT05255991	3	inhaled treprostinil	prostacyclin analogue, cAMP inhibition which has antifibrotic properties
NCT05515627	1	atezolizumab	immune checkpoint inhibitor, PDL-1 inhibitor for cell cycle
NCT06097260	2	bexotegrast (PLN-74809)	integrin inhibitor, blocks TGF-beta pathway
NCT06003426	3	BMS-986278	LPA receptor antagonist
NCT06132256	2	axatilimab	targets colony stimulating factor-1 receptor, or CSF-1R, anti-macrophage and monocyte therapy
NCT05722964	2	SHR-1906	monoclonal antibody against CTGF
NCT03865927	2	GKT137831 (setanaxib)	NADPH oxidase inhibitor

Table 2. *Cont.*

NCT Number	Phase	Drug/Intervention	Mechanism Class
NCT06331624	2	Tazarotene (GRI-0621)	retinoic acid receptors binder, promotes apoptosis or stopping cell proliferation, iNKT inhibitor
NCT05828953	2 to 3	Anlotinib	tyrosine kinase inhibitor of TGF-β pathway, antifibrotic properties

Abbreviations: cAMP = cyclic adenosine monophosphate, CTGF = connective tissue growth factor, iNKT = invariant natural killer T-cell, LPA = lysophosphatidic acid, LAPR1 = lysophosphatidic acid receptor 1, NADPH = nicotinamide adenine dinucleotide phosphate, PDE4 = phosphodiesterase 4, PDL-1 = programmed death-ligand 1, TGF-β = transforming growth factor beta.

3.1. Molecular Targets of Fibrotic Pathways

3.1.1. BI 1015550 (Nerandomilast)

BI 1015550 is an oral phosphodiesterase 4EB (PDE4B) inhibitor that selectively targets the PDE4B subtype, a regulator of intracellular signaling pathways associated with inflammation and fibrosis [114]. Inhibition of PDE4B is associated with increased cAMP levels, a secondary messenger known to exert anti-inflammatory and antifibrotic effects [61].

Recent clinical trials have explored the efficacy and safety of BI 1015550 in patients with both IPF and non-IPF progressive fibrotic disease. FIBRONEER is a phase III, double-blind, randomized, placebo-controlled study, aiming to evaluate the effects of BI 1015550 over 52 weeks in those with or without concomitant antifibrotic therapies (NCT05321069). Results from a phase II trial indicate BI 1015550 may stabilize lung function as measured by forced vital capacity (FVC) at 12 weeks [115]. In addition to its antifibrotic effects, BI 1015550 may also exert immunomodulatory effects that attenuate fibrotic processes in the lung [116,117]. Studies have shown that PDE4 inhibitors reduce the production of pro-inflammatory cytokines, including TNF-α and interleukin-4 [118,119], which are implicated in the pathogenesis of IPF. The safety profile of BI 1015550 appears to suggest minimal or tolerable adverse effects. In phase I studies, the drug was relatively well tolerated among healthy subjects with adverse effects reported in 50% and 90% of those on selected dosing, dominated by diarrhea and headaches [120]. Adverse effects in the phase II study were reported in 65% and 73% of those on and not on background antifibrotics, respectively, again dominated by diarrhea or loose stools [115].

3.1.2. Inhaled Treprostinil

Treprostinil is a stable analogue of prostacyclin, a potent vasodilator involved in the regulation of vascular tone and inhibition of platelet aggregation. Activation of prostacyclin receptors by treprostinil leads to increased intracellular cAMP, associated with the inhibition of fibroblast proliferation and ECM deposition [59]. It is administered specifically in this setting using a specialized device for inhalation, typically four times a day. This allows the drug to act directly on the lungs, which can have fewer systemic adverse effects.

Inhaled treprostinil has been shown to attenuate fibrotic responses in various pre-clinical models, including those induced by bleomycin [121,122]. Treprostinil's efficacy in IPF is further supported by its ability to reconstitute mitochondrial organization and structure in cells affected by the disease [123]. Mitochondrial dysfunction is a recognized feature of IPF, leading to imbalances in oxidative damage and repair. Inhaled treprostinil is currently approved for secondary pulmonary hypertension associated with interstitial lung disease [124]. Post-hoc analysis of the INCREASE trial evaluating efficacy of inhaled treprostinil in patients with secondary pulmonary hypertension due to fibrotic interstitial lung disease, found lower incidence of FVC decline [125], six-minute walk distance decline, and cardiopulmonary hospitalizations [126]. Current clinical trials are exploring the efficacy and safety of inhaled treprostinil in patients with IPF targeting FVC endpoints. TETON [127] and TETON-PPF are phase 3 randomized controlled trials assessing the impact of inhaled treprostinil on FVC change at 52 weeks in IPF and progressive pulmonary fibrosis, respectively (NCT05255991 and NCT05943535). The adverse-effect profile of inhaled treprostinil appears to be tolerable, and manageable with supportive medications (cough, throat irritation, and headache). Adverse effects were noted in the majority of treated patients in the INCREASE study though similar in terms of frequency to placebo (93% vs. 91%) (predominantly cough (44%) and headache (28%)) [124].

3.1.3. Anlotinib

Anlotinib is a multi-targeted tyrosine kinase inhibitor originally developed for the treatment of various cancers [128], but has also shown promising antifibrotic effects in preclinical models of both pulmonary and non-pulmonary fibrosis [129]. Anlotinib exerts its antifibrotic effects through the inhibition of several key signaling pathways leading to the attenuation of TGF-β. Anlotinib attenuates TGF-β1 signaling [129] and facilitates apoptosis of myofibroblasts with slowing of EMT pathways in AECs [130]. Anlotinib has also been shown to inhibit glycolysis in myofibroblasts decreasing their activation and proliferation [131]. A current multicenter placebo-controlled phase II to phase III study is ongoing assessing FVC endpoints and safety outcomes at 52 weeks (NCT05828953). Its safety profile is derived from its use as monotherapy in extended stage small-cell lung cancer, highlighted by hypertension, hand-foot syndrome, and fatigue [132].

3.1.4. Saracatinib

Saracatinib, also known as AZD0530, is a dual inhibitor of tyrosine kinases c-Src and Bcr-Abl, originally developed for the treatment of cancer but granted orphan drug designation by the US Food and Drug Administration for testing in IPF [133]. Prior research has demonstrated saracatinib effectively blocks TGF-β-induced Src kinase activation [134] and reduces α-smooth muscle actin expression, a marker of myofibroblast activation [135]. In preclinical studies, saracatinib has shown promise in reducing lung fibrosis in various models, including those induced by bleomycin [136]. The safety profile of saracatinib has been evaluated in early-phase clinical trials for various cancers, suggesting overall tolerance [137]. A current phase I study is ongoing to assess safety and tolerance outcomes in patients with IPF at 24 weeks (NCT04598919).

3.1.5. SHR-1906

SHR-1906 is a fully humanized monoclonal antibody targeting CTGF. CTGF is a key mediator of fibroblast proliferation and ECM deposition with elevated tissue expression and plasma levels seen in IPF correlating with disease severity and progression [77,138,139]. Notably, pamrevlumab, a recombinant monoclonal antibody against CTGF showed early promise in a phase II study with a well-tolerated adverse effect profile [140], but did not meet FVC study endpoints in a large phase III study [18]. SHR-1906 was assessed in healthy participants in a phase I study, demonstrating a favorable safety profile with manageable adverse effects [141]. A phase II study is underway to further assess safety and efficacy over 26 weeks (NCT05722964).

3.1.6. BMS-986278

BMS-986278 is a selective antagonist of LPAR1 involved in the promotion of various fibrotic pathways. Its ligand, LPA, is associated with fibroblast activation, proliferation, and deposition of ECM. In addition to its fibrotic effects, LPA also promotes inflammatory pathways that may contribute to fibrosis. In animal models, treatment with BMS-986278 has been associated with decreased collagen accumulation and improved lung function [142,143]. The safety profile of BMS-986278 has been assessed in early-phase studies, noting minimal adverse effects and general tolerability [144]. A phase II study assessing percent predicted change in FVC over 26 weeks in both IPF and non-IPF progressive ILD was recently completed [145] (NCT06003426). Preliminary findings presented in abstract form suggested decreased rate of FVC decline with or without background antifibrotic use [146].This drug has received Breakthrough Therapy Designation from the US FDA for the treatment of progressive pulmonary fibrosis.

3.1.7. HZN-825 (Fipaxalparant)

HZN-825 is a selective allosteric modulator of LPAR1, the primary receptor for LPA-mediated fibrotic pathways. Dysregulated LPAR1 signaling again has been implicated in the promotion of fibroblast activation and fibrotic responses to lung injury [67]. The safety profile of HZN-825 has been evaluated in healthy participants where it showed favorable tolerances [147]. Adverse events reported were generally mild to moderate. A prior clinical study in patients with diffuse cutaneous scleroderma assessing Rodnan skin thickness scores and safety as primary endpoints suggested general tolerance and improvement in skin scores, though not statistically significant [148]. A multicenter randomized placebo-controlled phase IIb study is ongoing assessing FVC change at 52 weeks in patients with IPF (NCT05032066).

3.1.8. BBT-877

BBT-877 is a novel inhibitor of autotaxin, the primary enzyme involved in the synthesis of LPA. Prior research indicates BBT-877 effectively reduces LPA production in various models of fibrotic injury [149,150], particularly antifibrotic effects in bleomycin-induced fibrosis [151]. In vivo studies have demonstrated BBT-877 does not significantly impair cell viability, even at high concentrations, suggesting a favorable safety profile for potential clinical use [151]. Notably, a prior novel autotaxin inhibitor ziritaxeset showed promise in early phase studies for treatment of IPF but did not meet primary or secondary study endpoints in two large multicenter phase III studies [16]. A phase II study with BBT-877 is ongoing, targeting absolute change in FVC over 24 weeks in patients with IPF (NCT05483907)

3.2. Integrin Inhibition

Bexotegrast or PLN-74809

Bexotegrast is an oral dual inhibitor of integrins αvβ6 and αvβ3, involved in several fibrotic pathways in the lung. Known to activate TGF-β, they play a constitutional role in promoting fibroblast proliferation and differentiation into myofibroblasts [72,152]. Pre-clinical studies have demonstrated bexotegrast may effectively inhibit TGF-β activation and reduce collagen deposition in lung fibroblast cultures and animal models of lung fibrosis [153]. Notably, a prior study assessing the efficacy of a subcutaneous monoclonal antibody inhibitor of αvβ6 failed to meet study endpoints due to early termination [154]. A multicenter phase IIb clinical trial assessing absolute change in FVC over 52 weeks in patients with IPF is ongoing for bexotegrast (NCT06097260).

3.3. Anti-Inflammatory Pathways

3.3.1. Axatilimab

Axatilimab, also known as Niktimvo, is a humanized IgG4 monoclonal antibody that targets colony stimulating factor-1 receptor (CSF-1R), a cell surface protein thought to control the survival and function of monocytes and macrophages [155]. Axatilimab is involved in modulation of macrophage activity, believed to be a contributor in various fibrotic diseases, including IPF. In pre-clinical models, inhibition of signaling through the CSF-1 receptor was shown to reduce the number of disease-mediating macrophages along with their monocyte precursors [156,157]. Axatilimab has been primarily studied in the context of chronic graft-versus-host disease, showing promise in preclinical models and controlled studies for ameliorating fibrotic responses associated with this immune-mediated process [158,159]. A phase II clinical study is ongoing with absolute decline in FVC over 26 weeks as a primary outcome (NCT06132256).

3.3.2. Jaktinib

The JAK-STAT signaling pathway is associated with the regulation of various cytokines and growth factors contributing to fibrosis in IPF [160]. Inhibiting JAK activity may reduce signaling of these profibrotic cytokines, thereby attenuating fibroblast activation and collagen deposition in the lungs. Jaktinib is a Janus kinase (JAK) inhibitor with potential therapeutic applications in various inflammatory and fibrotic diseases [161,162]. Jaktinib may influence immune response in the lungs and attenuate the activity of immune cells which contribute to fibrosis [163,164]. The safety profile of Jaktinib has been evaluated in early-phase clinical trials in myelofibrosis and hepatic fibrosis, where it has demonstrated a favorable tolerance among participants [161,165]. Common adverse effects associated with JAK inhibitors include gastrointestinal disturbances, increased risk of infections, and hematologic abnormalities. A phase II study assessing its anti-inflammatory and antifibrotic effects in IPF is ongoing, targeting FVC% change over 26 weeks (NCT04312594).

3.4. *Oxidative Pathways*

GKT137831 (Setanaxib)

GKT137831 is a selective inhibitor of nicotinamide adenine dinucleotide phosphate (NADPH) oxidases 1 (NOX1) and 4 (NOX4), which reduces the production of ROS and oxidative injury resulting in the activation of fibroblasts by damaged type II AECs. Preclinical studies have demonstrated GKT137831 effectively inhibits NOX1 and NOX4, leading to reduced oxidative stress and subsequent fibrosis in various fibrosis models [166]. GKT137831 has been shown to attenuate fibrosis associated with primary biliary cholangitis as seen in a phase II clinical study [167]. Similar NOX inhibitors have been evaluated in animal models of lung fibrosis, showing reduction in collagen deposition and improved lung function [168]. The compound's ability to modulate TGF-β signaling pathways may be a key mechanism for its antifibrotic effects [169,170]. A current phase II study in patients with IPF is ongoing targeting a surrogate serum marker of oxidative stress at 24 weeks, along with secondary outcomes of FVC change, six-minute walk, and safety profile (NCT03865927).

3.5. *Immune-Mediated or Cell-Cycle Pathways*

3.5.1. Tazarotene (GRI-0621)

Tazarotene, a synthetic retinoid which binds to retinoic acid receptors (RAR) RARβ and RARγ, was first developed for the topical treatment of plaque psoriasis [171]. Retinoids play important roles in regulating gene expression related to cell differentiation, proliferation, and apoptosis [172,173]. Tazarotene has been shown to induce apoptosis in various cell types, including cancer cells, through pathways that involve caspase activation and generation of ROS [174]. Tazarotene may also normalize cellular differentiation and counteract aberrant processes that lead to myofibroblast formation [173,175].

GRI-0621 is an oral formulation of tazarotene being assessed for its inhibitory effect on natural killer T-cells (NKT). Recent research has highlighted the role of type I NKT or invariant NKT (iNKT) cell types in the propagation of fibrosis [176,177]. Aberrant NKT activity or its absence in pre-clinical models of fibrosis have suggested both pro- and inhibitory effects on fibrotic pathways [178]. In a murine bleomycin-induced model of lung fibrosis, manipulation of iNKT-released IFN-γ resulted in ameliorated TGF-β–dependent fibrosis [179]. iNKT also mediates Th2 pathways attenuating the polarization of macrophages towards pro-fibrotic M2 phenotypes [180]. A phase 2a randomized controlled study is ongoing, assessing the efficacy of GRI-0621 in iNKT targeting primary and secondary endpoints of safety and changes in serologic biomarkers of NKT activity at 12 weeks (NCT06331624).

3.5.2. Atezolizumab

Atezolizumab is a monoclonal antibody that inhibits programmed death-ligand 1 (PD-L1), a surface glycoprotein found on immune cells involved in cell proliferation and apoptosis [181]. The PD-1/PD-L1 pathway is crucial in regulating immune responses, particularly in the context of T-cell activation and tolerance [182,183]. Elevated serum levels of PD-1 and PD-L2 have been found in patients with systemic sclerosis and are associated with severity of lung fibrosis [184]. Elevated PD-L1 activity was detected in explanted fibroblasts of patients with IPF [185] while alveolar epithelial cells with increased surface markers of abnormal check-point activity were identified compared to normal donors [186]. Humanized murine mesenchymal stem cells were impacted by PD-1 pathways in ameliorating lung fibrosis [187]. Preclinical studies have indicated that immune checkpoint inhibitors (ICI), including atezolizumab, may modulate fibrotic responses in various models of lung injury [188,189].

An important concern for the use of atezolizumab in patients with chronic lung disease is the known association of ICI with pulmonary toxicity. Grades 1–4 pulmonary toxicity occurred in 16% of all patients treated with ICI or ICI-containing regimens in one large systematic review, with 6% being grades 4 or higher [190]. Described risk factors include underlying lung disease, particularly baseline fibrosis, which has been associated with higher mortality while on ICI therapy [191]. Risk of pneumonitis in real world settings may also be increased with combination therapies and radiation [192]. Incidence of pneumonitis in patients with non-small cell lung carcinoma and underlying interstitial lung disease treated with atezolizumab as monotherapy was 29.4% in one phase II, with the majority grade 3 or higher in terms of severity [193]. An assessment of anti-inflammatory and antifibrotic effects from ICI will need to be weighed against its pulmonary and other organ toxicity, particularly as long-term use may be necessary for managing chronic fibrosing diseases. A current Phase I study is ongoing to assess safety and efficacy of atezolizumab in patients with IPF over 24 weeks (NCT05515627).

4. Conclusions

IPF is a complex disease highlighted by aberrations in alveolar epithelial response to injury, inappropriate cytokine and chemokine-driven proliferation of fibroblasts and myofibroblasts, dysregulation of epithelial and mesenchymal interplay, and abnormal cell senescence. Novel agents targeting these various mechanisms are ongoing with challenges remaining in translating pre-clinical or molecular studies to in vivo or real-world effectiveness. A review of current concepts regarding the pathogenesis of IPF suggests interacting and overlapping pathways with complex up and downstream effects, making the manipulation or control of one pathway or target often insufficient for clinical effect. Current studies are assessing the impact of combination therapy with background use of approved antifibrotics, though future studies are likely needed to additionally engage additive or synergistic effects of multiple drugs as they become available. Lastly, adverse effects are common and will also be additive in the setting of future combination approaches. A multi-faceted approach may have greater therapeutic impact but will need to be tempered with higher risk of treatment-related toxicity. IPF, as currently diagnosed, is likely a heterogeneous entity, an aspect that needs further exploration in the search for optimal therapy.

Funding: This research received no external funding.

Conflicts of Interest: The authors declare no conflict of interest.

Abbreviations

AEC	alveolar epithelial cell
cAMP	cyclic
CSF-1R	colony stimulating factor-1 receptor
CTGF	connective tissue growth factor
ECM	extracellular matrix
EMT	epithelial-mesenchymal transition
EV	extracellular vehicles
FVC	forced vital capacity
HA	hyaluronan
HRCT	high resolution chest CT
ICI	immune check point inhibitor
IPF	idiopathic pulmonary fibrosis
JAK	Janus kinase
LPA	lysophosphatidic acid

LPAR1	lysophosphatidic acid receptor 1
MMP	matrix metalloproteinases
NADPH	nicotinamide adenine dinucleotide phosphate
NKT	natural killer T-cells
NOX	NADPH oxidase
PDE	phosphodiesterase
PD-L1	programmed death-ligand 1
PFT	pulmonary function test
RAR	retinoic acid receptors
ROS	reactive oxygen species
TGF-β	transforming growth factor-beta
TNF-α	tumor necrosis factor-alpha

References

1. Raghu, G.; Remy-Jardin, M.; Richeldi, L.; Thomson, C.C.; Inoue, Y.; Johkoh, T.; Kreuter, M.; Lynch, D.A.; Maher, T.M.; Martinez, F.J.; et al. Idiopathic Pulmonary Fibrosis (an Update) and Progressive Pulmonary Fibrosis in Adults: An Official ATS/ERS/JRS/ALAT Clinical Practice Guideline. *Am. J. Respir. Crit. Care Med.* **2022**, *205*, e18–e47. [CrossRef] [PubMed]
2. King, T.E., Jr.; Bradford, W.Z.; Castro-Bernardini, S.; Fagan, E.A.; Glaspole, I.; Glassberg, M.K.; Gorina, E.; Hopkins, P.M.; Kardatzke, D.; Lancaster, L.; et al. A phase 3 trial of pirfenidone in patients with idiopathic pulmonary fibrosis. *N. Engl. J. Med.* **2014**, *370*, 2083–2092. [CrossRef] [PubMed]
3. Richeldi, L.; du Bois, R.M.; Raghu, G.; Azuma, A.; Brown, K.K.; Costabel, U.; Cottin, V.; Flaherty, K.R.; Hansell, D.M.; Inoue, Y.; et al. Efficacy and safety of nintedanib in idiopathic pulmonary fibrosis. *N. Engl. J. Med.* **2014**, *370*, 2071–2082. [CrossRef] [PubMed]
4. Iommi, M.; Gonnelli, F.; Bonifazi, M.; Faragalli, A.; Mei, F.; Pompili, M.; Carle, F.; Gesuita, R. Understanding Patterns of Adherence to Antifibrotic Treatment in Idiopathic Pulmonary Fibrosis: Insights from an Italian Prospective Cohort Study. *J. Clin. Med.* **2024**, *13*, 2727. [CrossRef] [PubMed]
5. Ruaro, B.; Salotti, A.; Reccardini, N.; Kette, S.; Da Re, B.; Nicolosi, S.; Zuccon, U.; Confalonieri, M.; Mondini, L.; Pozzan, R.; et al. Functional Progression after Dose Suspension or Discontinuation of Nintedanib in Idiopathic Pulmonary Fibrosis: A Real-Life Multicentre Study. *Pharmaceuticals* **2024**, *17*, 119. [CrossRef]
6. Idiopathic Pulmonary Fibrosis Clinical Research, N.; Raghu, G.; Anstrom, K.J.; King, T.E., Jr.; Lasky, J.A.; Martinez, F.J. Prednisone, azathioprine, and N-acetylcysteine for pulmonary fibrosis. *N. Engl. J. Med.* **2012**, *366*, 1968–1977. [CrossRef]
7. Raghu, G.; Brown, K.K.; Bradford, W.Z.; Starko, K.; Noble, P.W.; Schwartz, D.A.; King, T.E., Jr.; Idiopathic Pulmonary Fibrosis Study, G. A placebo-controlled trial of interferon gamma-1b in patients with idiopathic pulmonary fibrosis. *N. Engl. J. Med.* **2004**, *350*, 125–133. [CrossRef]
8. Raghu, G.; Brown, K.K.; Costabel, U.; Cottin, V.; du Bois, R.M.; Lasky, J.A.; Thomeer, M.; Utz, J.P.; Khandker, R.K.; McDermott, L.; et al. Treatment of idiopathic pulmonary fibrosis with etanercept: An exploratory, placebo-controlled trial. *Am. J. Respir. Crit. Care Med.* **2008**, *178*, 948–955. [CrossRef]
9. Raghu, G.; Million-Rousseau, R.; Morganti, A.; Perchenet, L.; Behr, J.; Group, M.S. Macitentan for the treatment of idiopathic pulmonary fibrosis: The randomised controlled MUSIC trial. *Eur. Respir. J.* **2013**, *42*, 1622–1632. [CrossRef]
10. King, T.E., Jr.; Behr, J.; Brown, K.K.; du Bois, R.M.; Lancaster, L.; de Andrade, J.A.; Stahler, G.; Leconte, I.; Roux, S.; Raghu, G. BUILD-1: A randomized placebo-controlled trial of bosentan in idiopathic pulmonary fibrosis. *Am. J. Respir. Crit. Care Med.* **2008**, *177*, 75–81. [CrossRef]
11. Raghu, G.; Behr, J.; Brown, K.K.; Egan, J.J.; Kawut, S.M.; Flaherty, K.R.; Martinez, F.J.; Nathan, S.D.; Wells, A.U.; Collard, H.R.; et al. Treatment of idiopathic pulmonary fibrosis with ambrisentan: A parallel, randomized trial. *Ann. Intern. Med.* **2013**, *158*, 641–649. [CrossRef] [PubMed]
12. Idiopathic Pulmonary Fibrosis Clinical Research, N.; Zisman, D.A.; Schwarz, M.; Anstrom, K.J.; Collard, H.R.; Flaherty, K.R.; Hunninghake, G.W. A controlled trial of sildenafil in advanced idiopathic pulmonary fibrosis. *N. Engl. J. Med.* **2010**, *363*, 620–628. [CrossRef]
13. Daniels, C.E.; Lasky, J.A.; Limper, A.H.; Mieras, K.; Gabor, E.; Schroeder, D.R.; Imatinib, I.P.F.S.I. Imatinib treatment for idiopathic pulmonary fibrosis: Randomized placebo-controlled trial results. *Am. J. Respir. Crit. Care Med.* **2010**, *181*, 604–610. [CrossRef] [PubMed]
14. Demedts, M.; Behr, J.; Buhl, R.; Costabel, U.; Dekhuijzen, R.; Jansen, H.M.; MacNee, W.; Thomeer, M.; Wallaert, B.; Laurent, F.; et al. High-dose acetylcysteine in idiopathic pulmonary fibrosis. *N. Engl. J. Med.* **2005**, *353*, 2229–2242. [CrossRef] [PubMed]
15. Noth, I.; Anstrom, K.J.; Calvert, S.B.; de Andrade, J.; Flaherty, K.R.; Glazer, C.; Kaner, R.J.; Olman, M.A.; Idiopathic Pulmonary Fibrosis Clinical Research, N. A placebo-controlled randomized trial of warfarin in idiopathic pulmonary fibrosis. *Am. J. Respir. Crit. Care Med.* **2012**, *186*, 88–95. [CrossRef] [PubMed]
16. Maher, T.M.; Ford, P.; Brown, K.K.; Costabel, U.; Cottin, V.; Danoff, S.K.; Groenveld, I.; Helmer, E.; Jenkins, R.G.; Milner, J.; et al. Ziritaxestat, a Novel Autotaxin Inhibitor, and Lung Function in Idiopathic Pulmonary Fibrosis: The ISABELA 1 and 2 Randomized Clinical Trials. *JAMA* **2023**, *329*, 1567–1578. [CrossRef]

17. Raghu, G.; Brown, K.K.; Collard, H.R.; Cottin, V.; Gibson, K.F.; Kaner, R.J.; Lederer, D.J.; Martinez, F.J.; Noble, P.W.; Song, J.W.; et al. Efficacy of simtuzumab versus placebo in patients with idiopathic pulmonary fibrosis: A randomised, double-blind, controlled, phase 2 trial. *Lancet Respir. Med.* **2017**, *5*, 22–32. [CrossRef]
18. Raghu, G.; Richeldi, L.; Fernandez Perez, E.R.; De Salvo, M.C.; Silva, R.S.; Song, J.W.; Ogura, T.; Xu, Z.J.; Belloli, E.A.; Zhang, X.; et al. Pamrevlumab for Idiopathic Pulmonary Fibrosis: The ZEPHYRUS-1 Randomized Clinical Trial. *JAMA* **2024**, *332*, 380–389. [CrossRef]
19. Phan, T.H.G.; Paliogiannis, P.; Nasrallah, G.K.; Giordo, R.; Eid, A.H.; Fois, A.G.; Zinellu, A.; Mangoni, A.A.; Pintus, G. Emerging cellular and molecular determinants of idiopathic pulmonary fibrosis. *Cell. Mol. Life Sci.* **2021**, *78*, 2031–2057. [CrossRef]
20. Kim, K.I.; Hossain, R.; Li, X.; Lee, H.J.; Lee, C.J. Searching for Novel Candidate Small Molecules for Ameliorating Idiopathic Pulmonary Fibrosis: A Narrative Review. *Biomol. Ther.* **2023**, *31*, 484–495. [CrossRef]
21. Estornut, C.; Milara, J.; Bayarri, M.A.; Belhadj, N.; Cortijo, J. Targeting Oxidative Stress as a Therapeutic Approach for Idiopathic Pulmonary Fibrosis. *Front. Pharmacol.* **2021**, *12*, 794997. [CrossRef]
22. Aversa, Z.; Atkinson, E.J.; Carmona, E.M.; White, T.A.; Heeren, A.A.; Jachim, S.K.; Zhang, X.; Cummings, S.R.; Chiarella, S.E.; Limper, A.H.; et al. Biomarkers of cellular senescence in idiopathic pulmonary fibrosis. *Respir. Res.* **2023**, *24*, 101. [CrossRef] [PubMed]
23. Lin, Y.; Xu, Z. Fibroblast Senescence in Idiopathic Pulmonary Fibrosis. *Front. Cell Dev. Biol.* **2020**, *8*, 593283. [CrossRef] [PubMed]
24. Chambers, R.C.; Mercer, P.F. Mechanisms of alveolar epithelial injury, repair, and fibrosis. *Ann. Am. Thorac. Soc.* **2015**, *12* (Suppl. S1), S16–S20. [CrossRef] [PubMed]
25. Hansel, C.; Jendrossek, V.; Klein, D. Cellular Senescence in the Lung: The Central Role of Senescent Epithelial Cells. *Int. J. Mol. Sci.* **2020**, *21*, 3279. [CrossRef]
26. Kristensen, J.H.; Karsdal, M.A.; Genovese, F.; Johnson, S.; Svensson, B.; Jacobsen, S.; Hagglund, P.; Leeming, D.J. The role of extracellular matrix quality in pulmonary fibrosis. *Respiration* **2014**, *88*, 487–499. [CrossRef]
27. Cameli, P.; Carleo, A.; Bergantini, L.; Landi, C.; Prasse, A.; Bargagli, E. Oxidant/Antioxidant Disequilibrium in Idiopathic Pulmonary Fibrosis Pathogenesis. *Inflammation* **2020**, *43*, 1–7. [CrossRef]
28. Selman, M.; Pardo, A. The leading role of epithelial cells in the pathogenesis of idiopathic pulmonary fibrosis. *Cell Signal.* **2020**, *66*, 109482. [CrossRef]
29. Ptasinski, V.A.; Stegmayr, J.; Belvisi, M.G.; Wagner, D.E.; Murray, L.A. Targeting Alveolar Repair in Idiopathic Pulmonary Fibrosis. *Am. J. Respir. Cell Mol. Biol.* **2021**, *65*, 347–365. [CrossRef]
30. Kwong, K.Y.; Literat, A.; Zhu, N.L.; Huang, H.H.; Li, C.; Jones, C.A.; Minoo, P. Expression of transforming growth factor beta (TGF-beta1) in human epithelial alveolar cells: A pro-inflammatory mediator independent pathway. *Life Sci.* **2004**, *74*, 2941–2957. [CrossRef]
31. Xu, Y.D.; Hua, J.; Mui, A.; O'Connor, R.; Grotendorst, G.; Khalil, N. Release of biologically active TGF-beta1 by alveolar epithelial cells results in pulmonary fibrosis. *Am. J. Physiol. Lung Cell. Mol. Physiol.* **2003**, *285*, L527–L539. [CrossRef] [PubMed]
32. Sisson, T.H.; Mendez, M.; Choi, K.; Subbotina, N.; Courey, A.; Cunningham, A.; Dave, A.; Engelhardt, J.F.; Liu, X.; White, E.S.; et al. Targeted injury of type II alveolar epithelial cells induces pulmonary fibrosis. *Am. J. Respir. Crit. Care Med.* **2010**, *181*, 254–263. [CrossRef] [PubMed]
33. Kalluri, R.; Weinberg, R.A. The basics of epithelial-mesenchymal transition. *J. Clin. Investig.* **2009**, *119*, 1420–1428. [CrossRef] [PubMed]
34. Willis, B.C.; Liebler, J.M.; Luby-Phelps, K.; Nicholson, A.G.; Crandall, E.D.; du Bois, R.M.; Borok, Z. Induction of epithelial-mesenchymal transition in alveolar epithelial cells by transforming growth factor-beta1: Potential role in idiopathic pulmonary fibrosis. *Am. J. Pathol.* **2005**, *166*, 1321–1332. [CrossRef] [PubMed]
35. Salton, F.; Volpe, M.C.; Confalonieri, M. Epithelial(-)Mesenchymal Transition in the Pathogenesis of Idiopathic Pulmonary Fibrosis. *Medicina* **2019**, *55*, 83. [CrossRef]
36. Hill, C.; Jones, M.G.; Davies, D.E.; Wang, Y. Epithelial-mesenchymal transition contributes to pulmonary fibrosis via aberrant epithelial/fibroblastic cross-talk. *J. Lung Health Dis.* **2019**, *3*, 31–35. [CrossRef]
37. Hackett, T.L.; Warner, S.M.; Stefanowicz, D.; Shaheen, F.; Pechkovsky, D.V.; Murray, L.A.; Argentieri, R.; Kicic, A.; Stick, S.M.; Bai, T.R.; et al. Induction of epithelial-mesenchymal transition in primary airway epithelial cells from patients with asthma by transforming growth factor-beta1. *Am. J. Respir. Crit. Care Med.* **2009**, *180*, 122–133. [CrossRef]
38. Omori, K.; Hattori, N.; Senoo, T.; Takayama, Y.; Masuda, T.; Nakashima, T.; Iwamoto, H.; Fujitaka, K.; Hamada, H.; Kohno, N. Inhibition of Plasminogen Activator Inhibitor-1 Attenuates Transforming Growth Factor-beta-Dependent Epithelial Mesenchymal Transition and Differentiation of Fibroblasts to Myofibroblasts. *PLoS ONE* **2016**, *11*, e0148969. [CrossRef]
39. Michael, S.; Montag, M.; Dott, W. Pro-inflammatory effects and oxidative stress in lung macrophages and epithelial cells induced by ambient particulate matter. *Environ. Pollut.* **2013**, *183*, 19–29. [CrossRef]
40. Aoshiba, K.; Nagai, A. Oxidative stress, cell death, and other damage to alveolar epithelial cells induced by cigarette smoke. *Tob. Induc. Dis.* **2003**, *1*, 219–226. [CrossRef]
41. Tsuji, T.; Aoshiba, K.; Nagai, A. Cigarette smoke induces senescence in alveolar epithelial cells. *Am. J. Respir. Cell Mol. Biol.* **2004**, *31*, 643–649. [CrossRef] [PubMed]
42. Parimon, T.; Chen, P.; Stripp, B.R.; Liang, J.; Jiang, D.; Noble, P.W.; Parks, W.C.; Yao, C. Senescence of alveolar epithelial progenitor cells: A critical driver of lung fibrosis. *Am. J. Physiol. Cell Physiol.* **2023**, *325*, C483–C495. [CrossRef] [PubMed]

43. Kim, S.J.; Cheresh, P.; Jablonski, R.P.; Williams, D.B.; Kamp, D.W. The Role of Mitochondrial DNA in Mediating Alveolar Epithelial Cell Apoptosis and Pulmonary Fibrosis. *Int. J. Mol. Sci.* **2015**, *16*, 21486–21519. [CrossRef] [PubMed]
44. Cheng, P.; Li, S.; Chen, H. Macrophages in Lung Injury, Repair, and Fibrosis. *Cells* **2021**, *10*, 436. [CrossRef] [PubMed]
45. Frangogiannis, N. Transforming growth factor-beta in tissue fibrosis. *J. Exp. Med.* **2020**, *217*, e20190103. [CrossRef]
46. Khalil, N.; Bereznay, O.; Sporn, M.; Greenberg, A.H. Macrophage production of transforming growth factor beta and fibroblast collagen synthesis in chronic pulmonary inflammation. *J. Exp. Med.* **1989**, *170*, 727–737. [CrossRef]
47. Assoian, R.K.; Fleurdelys, B.E.; Stevenson, H.C.; Miller, P.J.; Madtes, D.K.; Raines, E.W.; Ross, R.; Sporn, M.B. Expression and secretion of type beta transforming growth factor by activated human macrophages. *Proc. Natl. Acad. Sci. USA* **1987**, *84*, 6020–6024. [CrossRef]
48. Verrecchia, F.; Mauviel, A. Transforming growth factor-beta signaling through the Smad pathway: Role in extracellular matrix gene expression and regulation. *J. Investig. Dermatol.* **2002**, *118*, 211–215. [CrossRef]
49. Han, Y.Y.; Shen, P.; Chang, W.X. Involvement of epithelial-to-mesenchymal transition and associated transforming growth factor-beta/Smad signaling in paraquat-induced pulmonary fibrosis. *Mol. Med. Rep.* **2015**, *12*, 7979–7984. [CrossRef]
50. Xiao, L.; Du, Y.; Shen, Y.; He, Y.; Zhao, H.; Li, Z. TGF-beta 1 induced fibroblast proliferation is mediated by the FGF-2/ERK pathway. *Front. Biosci. (Landmark Ed.)* **2012**, *17*, 2667–2674. [CrossRef]
51. Kadota, T.; Yoshioka, Y.; Fujita, Y.; Araya, J.; Minagawa, S.; Hara, H.; Miyamoto, A.; Suzuki, S.; Fujimori, S.; Kohno, T.; et al. Extracellular Vesicles from Fibroblasts Induce Epithelial-Cell Senescence in Pulmonary Fibrosis. *Am. J. Respir. Cell Mol. Biol.* **2020**, *63*, 623–636. [CrossRef] [PubMed]
52. Brigstock, D.R. Extracellular Vesicles in Organ Fibrosis: Mechanisms, Therapies, and Diagnostics. *Cells* **2021**, *10*, 1596. [CrossRef] [PubMed]
53. Fujita, Y. Extracellular vesicles in idiopathic pulmonary fibrosis: Pathogenesis and therapeutics. *Inflamm. Regen.* **2022**, *42*, 23. [CrossRef] [PubMed]
54. Chanda, D.; Otoupalova, E.; Hough, K.P.; Locy, M.L.; Bernard, K.; Deshane, J.S.; Sanderson, R.D.; Mobley, J.A.; Thannickal, V.J. Fibronectin on the Surface of Extracellular Vesicles Mediates Fibroblast Invasion. *Am. J. Respir. Cell Mol. Biol.* **2019**, *60*, 279–288. [CrossRef] [PubMed]
55. Huang, X.; Yang, N.; Fiore, V.F.; Barker, T.H.; Sun, Y.; Morris, S.W.; Ding, Q.; Thannickal, V.J.; Zhou, Y. Matrix stiffness-induced myofibroblast differentiation is mediated by intrinsic mechanotransduction. *Am. J. Respir. Cell Mol. Biol.* **2012**, *47*, 340–348. [CrossRef]
56. Hinz, B. Mechanical aspects of lung fibrosis: A spotlight on the myofibroblast. *Proc. Am. Thorac. Soc.* **2012**, *9*, 137–147. [CrossRef]
57. Serezani, C.H.; Ballinger, M.N.; Aronoff, D.M.; Peters-Golden, M. Cyclic AMP: Master regulator of innate immune cell function. *Am. J. Respir. Cell Mol. Biol.* **2008**, *39*, 127–132. [CrossRef]
58. Della Latta, V.; Cabiati, M.; Rocchiccioli, S.; Del Ry, S.; Morales, M.A. The role of the adenosinergic system in lung fibrosis. *Pharmacol. Res.* **2013**, *76*, 182–189. [CrossRef]
59. Cash, E.; Goodwin, A.T.; Tatler, A.L. Adenosine receptor signalling as a driver of pulmonary fibrosis. *Pharmacol. Ther.* **2023**, *249*, 108504. [CrossRef]
60. Schiller, M.; Verrecchia, F.; Mauviel, A. Cyclic adenosine 3′,5′-monophosphate-elevating agents inhibit transforming growth factor-beta-induced SMAD3/4-dependent transcription via a protein kinase A-dependent mechanism. *Oncogene* **2003**, *22*, 8881–8890. [CrossRef]
61. Selige, J.; Hatzelmann, A.; Dunkern, T. The differential impact of PDE4 subtypes in human lung fibroblasts on cytokine-induced proliferation and myofibroblast conversion. *J. Cell. Physiol.* **2011**, *226*, 1970–1980. [CrossRef] [PubMed]
62. Koga, K.; Takaesu, G.; Yoshida, R.; Nakaya, M.; Kobayashi, T.; Kinjyo, I.; Yoshimura, A. Cyclic adenosine monophosphate suppresses the transcription of proinflammatory cytokines via the phosphorylated c-Fos protein. *Immunity* **2009**, *30*, 372–383. [CrossRef] [PubMed]
63. Kolb, M.; Crestani, B.; Maher, T.M. Phosphodiesterase 4B inhibition: A potential novel strategy for treating pulmonary fibrosis. *Eur. Respir. Rev.* **2023**, *32*, 220206. [CrossRef] [PubMed]
64. Lin, M.E.; Herr, D.R.; Chun, J. Lysophosphatidic acid (LPA) receptors: Signaling properties and disease relevance. *Prostaglandins Other Lipid Mediat.* **2010**, *91*, 130–138. [CrossRef]
65. Nakamura, Y.; Shimizu, Y. Cellular and Molecular Control of Lipid Metabolism in Idiopathic Pulmonary Fibrosis: Clinical Application of the Lysophosphatidic Acid Pathway. *Cells* **2023**, *12*, 548. [CrossRef]
66. Sakai, N.; Chun, J.; Duffield, J.S.; Wada, T.; Luster, A.D.; Tager, A.M. LPA1-induced cytoskeleton reorganization drives fibrosis through CTGF-dependent fibroblast proliferation. *FASEB J.* **2013**, *27*, 1830–1846. [CrossRef]
67. Tang, N.; Zhao, Y.; Feng, R.; Liu, Y.; Wang, S.; Wei, W.; Ding, Q.; An, M.S.; Wen, J.; Li, L. Lysophosphatidic acid accelerates lung fibrosis by inducing differentiation of mesenchymal stem cells into myofibroblasts. *J. Cell. Mol. Med.* **2014**, *18*, 156–169. [CrossRef]
68. Xu, M.Y.; Porte, J.; Knox, A.J.; Weinreb, P.H.; Maher, T.M.; Violette, S.M.; McAnulty, R.J.; Sheppard, D.; Jenkins, G. Lysophosphatidic acid induces alphavbeta6 integrin-mediated TGF-beta activation via the LPA2 receptor and the small G protein G alpha(q). *Am. J. Pathol.* **2009**, *174*, 1264–1279. [CrossRef]
69. Jiang, S.; Yang, H.; Li, M. Emerging Roles of Lysophosphatidic Acid in Macrophages and Inflammatory Diseases. *Int. J. Mol. Sci.* **2023**, *24*, 12524. [CrossRef]

70. Goodwin, A.; Jenkins, G. Role of integrin-mediated TGFbeta activation in the pathogenesis of pulmonary fibrosis. *Biochem. Soc. Trans.* **2009**, *37 Pt 4*, 849–854. [CrossRef]
71. Madala, S.K.; Korfhagen, T.R.; Schmidt, S.; Davidson, C.; Edukulla, R.; Ikegami, M.; Violette, S.M.; Weinreb, P.H.; Sheppard, D.; Hardie, W.D. Inhibition of the alphavbeta6 integrin leads to limited alteration of TGF-alpha-induced pulmonary fibrosis. *Am. J. Physiol. Lung Cell. Mol. Physiol.* **2014**, *306*, L726–L735. [CrossRef] [PubMed]
72. Kim, K.K.; Wei, Y.; Szekeres, C.; Kugler, M.C.; Wolters, P.J.; Hill, M.L.; Frank, J.A.; Brumwell, A.N.; Wheeler, S.E.; Kreidberg, J.A.; et al. Epithelial cell alpha3beta1 integrin links beta-catenin and Smad signaling to promote myofibroblast formation and pulmonary fibrosis. *J. Clin. Investig.* **2009**, *119*, 213–224. [CrossRef] [PubMed]
73. Sonbol, H.S. Extracellular Matrix Remodeling in Human Disease. *J. Microsc. Ultrastruct.* **2018**, *6*, 123–128. [CrossRef] [PubMed]
74. Upagupta, C.; Shimbori, C.; Alsilmi, R.; Kolb, M. Matrix abnormalities in pulmonary fibrosis. *Eur. Respir. Rev.* **2018**, *27*, 180033. [CrossRef]
75. Jessen, H.; Hoyer, N.; Prior, T.S.; Frederiksen, P.; Karsdal, M.A.; Leeming, D.J.; Bendstrup, E.; Sand, J.M.B.; Shaker, S.B. Turnover of type I and III collagen predicts progression of idiopathic pulmonary fibrosis. *Respir. Res.* **2021**, *22*, 205. [CrossRef]
76. Snijder, J.; Peraza, J.; Padilla, M.; Capaccione, K.; Salvatore, M.M. Pulmonary fibrosis: A disease of alveolar collapse and collagen deposition. *Expert. Rev. Respir. Med.* **2019**, *13*, 615–619. [CrossRef]
77. Leask, A.; Holmes, A.; Black, C.M.; Abraham, D.J. Connective tissue growth factor gene regulation. Requirements for its induction by transforming growth factor-beta 2 in fibroblasts. *J. Biol. Chem.* **2003**, *278*, 13008–13015. [CrossRef]
78. Deng, Z.; Fear, M.W.; Suk Choi, Y.; Wood, F.M.; Allahham, A.; Mutsaers, S.E.; Prele, C.M. The extracellular matrix and mechanotransduction in pulmonary fibrosis. *Int. J. Biochem. Cell Biol.* **2020**, *126*, 105802. [CrossRef]
79. Blokland, K.E.C.; Pouwels, S.D.; Schuliga, M.; Knight, D.A.; Burgess, J.K. Regulation of cellular senescence by extracellular matrix during chronic fibrotic diseases. *Clin. Sci.* **2020**, *134*, 2681–2706. [CrossRef]
80. Mahalanobish, S.; Saha, S.; Dutta, S.; Sil, P.C. Matrix metalloproteinase: An upcoming therapeutic approach for idiopathic pulmonary fibrosis. *Pharmacol. Res.* **2020**, *152*, 104591. [CrossRef]
81. Pardo, A.; Cabrera, S.; Maldonado, M.; Selman, M. Role of matrix metalloproteinases in the pathogenesis of idiopathic pulmonary fibrosis. *Respir. Res.* **2016**, *17*, 23. [CrossRef] [PubMed]
82. Sokai, A.; Handa, T.; Tanizawa, K.; Oga, T.; Uno, K.; Tsuruyama, T.; Kubo, T.; Ikezoe, K.; Nakatsuka, Y.; Tanimura, K.; et al. Matrix metalloproteinase-10: A novel biomarker for idiopathic pulmonary fibrosis. *Respir. Res.* **2015**, *16*, 120. [CrossRef] [PubMed]
83. Fujishima, S.; Shiomi, T.; Yamashita, S.; Yogo, Y.; Nakano, Y.; Inoue, T.; Nakamura, M.; Tasaka, S.; Hasegawa, N.; Aikawa, N.; et al. Production and activation of matrix metalloproteinase 7 (matrilysin 1) in the lungs of patients with idiopathic pulmonary fibrosis. *Arch. Pathol. Lab. Med.* **2010**, *134*, 1136–1142. [CrossRef] [PubMed]
84. Vuorinen, K.; Myllarniemi, M.; Lammi, L.; Piirila, P.; Rytila, P.; Salmenkivi, K.; Kinnula, V.L. Elevated matrilysin levels in bronchoalveolar lavage fluid do not distinguish idiopathic pulmonary fibrosis from other interstitial lung diseases. *APMIS* **2007**, *115*, 969–975. [CrossRef] [PubMed]
85. Inoue, R.; Yasuma, T.; Fridman D'Alessandro, V.; Toda, M.; Ito, T.; Tomaru, A.; D'Alessandro-Gabazza, C.N.; Tsuruga, T.; Okano, T.; Takeshita, A.; et al. Amelioration of Pulmonary Fibrosis by Matrix Metalloproteinase-2 Overexpression. *Int. J. Mol. Sci.* **2023**, *24*, 6695. [CrossRef]
86. Bormann, T.; Maus, R.; Stolper, J.; Tort Tarres, M.; Brandenberger, C.; Wedekind, D.; Jonigk, D.; Welte, T.; Gauldie, J.; Kolb, M.; et al. Role of matrix metalloprotease-2 and MMP-9 in experimental lung fibrosis in mice. *Respir. Res.* **2022**, *23*, 180. [CrossRef]
87. Perng, D.W.; Chang, K.T.; Su, K.C.; Wu, Y.C.; Chen, C.S.; Hsu, W.H.; Tsai, C.M.; Lee, Y.C. Matrix metalloprotease-9 induces transforming growth factor-beta(1) production in airway epithelium via activation of epidermal growth factor receptors. *Life Sci.* **2011**, *89*, 204–212. [CrossRef]
88. Lagente, V.; Le Quement, C.; Boichot, E. Macrophage metalloelastase (MMP-12) as a target for inflammatory respiratory diseases. *Expert. Opin. Ther. Targets* **2009**, *13*, 287–295. [CrossRef]
89. Kang, H.R.; Cho, S.J.; Lee, C.G.; Homer, R.J.; Elias, J.A. Transforming growth factor (TGF)-beta1 stimulates pulmonary fibrosis and inflammation via a Bax-dependent, bid-activated pathway that involves matrix metalloproteinase-12. *J. Biol. Chem.* **2007**, *282*, 7723–7732. [CrossRef]
90. Manoury, B.; Nenan, S.; Guenon, I.; Boichot, E.; Planquois, J.M.; Bertrand, C.P.; Lagente, V. Macrophage metalloelastase (MMP-12) deficiency does not alter bleomycin-induced pulmonary fibrosis in mice. *J. Inflamm.* **2006**, *3*, 2. [CrossRef]
91. Lauer, M.E.; Dweik, R.A.; Garantziotis, S.; Aronica, M.A. The Rise and Fall of Hyaluronan in Respiratory Diseases. *Int. J. Cell Biol.* **2015**, *2015*, 712507. [CrossRef] [PubMed]
92. Bjermer, L.; Lundgren, R.; Hallgren, R. Hyaluronan and type III procollagen peptide concentrations in bronchoalveolar lavage fluid in idiopathic pulmonary fibrosis. *Thorax* **1989**, *44*, 126–131. [CrossRef] [PubMed]
93. Milman, N.; Kristensen, M.S.; Bentsen, K. Hyaluronan and procollagen type III aminoterminal peptide in serum and bronchoalveolar lavage fluid from patients with pulmonary fibrosis. *APMIS* **1995**, *103*, 749–754. [CrossRef] [PubMed]
94. Li, Y.; Jiang, D.; Liang, J.; Meltzer, E.B.; Gray, A.; Miura, R.; Wogensen, L.; Yamaguchi, Y.; Noble, P.W. Severe lung fibrosis requires an invasive fibroblast phenotype regulated by hyaluronan and CD44. *J. Exp. Med.* **2011**, *208*, 1459–1471. [CrossRef] [PubMed]
95. Xia, H.; Herrera, J.; Smith, K.; Yang, L.; Gilbertsen, A.; Benyumov, A.; Racila, E.; Bitterman, P.B.; Henke, C.A. Hyaluronan/CD44 axis regulates S100A4-mediated mesenchymal progenitor cell fibrogenicity in idiopathic pulmonary fibrosis. *Am. J. Physiol. Lung Cell. Mol. Physiol.* **2021**, *320*, L926–L941. [CrossRef]

96. Li, Y.; Liang, J.; Yang, T.; Monterrosa Mena, J.; Huan, C.; Xie, T.; Kurkciyan, A.; Liu, N.; Jiang, D.; Noble, P.W. Hyaluronan synthase 2 regulates fibroblast senescence in pulmonary fibrosis. *Matrix Biol.* **2016**, *55*, 35–48. [CrossRef]
97. Kliment, C.R.; Oury, T.D. Oxidative stress, extracellular matrix targets, and idiopathic pulmonary fibrosis. *Free Radic. Biol. Med.* **2010**, *49*, 707–717. [CrossRef]
98. Chapman, K.E.; Sinclair, S.E.; Zhuang, D.; Hassid, A.; Desai, L.P.; Waters, C.M. Cyclic mechanical strain increases reactive oxygen species production in pulmonary epithelial cells. *Am. J. Physiol. Lung Cell. Mol. Physiol.* **2005**, *289*, L834–L841. [CrossRef]
99. Bueno, M.; Calyeca, J.; Rojas, M.; Mora, A.L. Mitochondria dysfunction and metabolic reprogramming as drivers of idiopathic pulmonary fibrosis. *Redox Biol.* **2020**, *33*, 101509. [CrossRef]
100. Liu, X.; Chen, Z. The pathophysiological role of mitochondrial oxidative stress in lung diseases. *J. Transl. Med.* **2017**, *15*, 207. [CrossRef]
101. Ge, Z.; Chen, Y.; Ma, L.; Hu, F.; Xie, L. Macrophage polarization and its impact on idiopathic pulmonary fibrosis. *Front. Immunol.* **2024**, *15*, 1444964. [CrossRef]
102. Kishore, A.; Petrek, M. Roles of Macrophage Polarization and Macrophage-Derived miRNAs in Pulmonary Fibrosis. *Front. Immunol.* **2021**, *12*, 678457. [CrossRef] [PubMed]
103. Canton, M.; Sanchez-Rodriguez, R.; Spera, I.; Venegas, F.C.; Favia, M.; Viola, A.; Castegna, A. Reactive Oxygen Species in Macrophages: Sources and Targets. *Front. Immunol.* **2021**, *12*, 734229. [CrossRef] [PubMed]
104. Cho, S.J.; Hong, K.S.; Jeong, J.H.; Lee, M.; Choi, A.M.K.; Stout-Delgado, H.W.; Moon, J.S. DROSHA-Dependent AIM2 Inflammasome Activation Contributes to Lung Inflammation during Idiopathic Pulmonary Fibrosis. *Cells* **2019**, *8*, 938. [CrossRef]
105. Lopes-Paciencia, S.; Saint-Germain, E.; Rowell, M.C.; Ruiz, A.F.; Kalegari, P.; Ferbeyre, G. The senescence-associated secretory phenotype and its regulation. *Cytokine* **2019**, *117*, 15–22. [CrossRef]
106. Mebratu, Y.A.; Soni, S.; Rosas, L.; Rojas, M.; Horowitz, J.C.; Nho, R. The aged extracellular matrix and the profibrotic role of senescence-associated secretory phenotype. *Am. J. Physiol. Cell Physiol.* **2023**, *325*, C565–C579. [CrossRef]
107. Tu, M.; Wei, T.; Jia, Y.; Wang, Y.; Wu, J. Molecular mechanisms of alveolar epithelial cell senescence and idiopathic pulmonary fibrosis: A narrative review. *J. Thorac. Dis.* **2023**, *15*, 186–203. [CrossRef]
108. Campbell, R.A.; Docherty, M.H.; Ferenbach, D.A.; Mylonas, K.J. The Role of Ageing and Parenchymal Senescence on Macrophage Function and Fibrosis. *Front. Immunol.* **2021**, *12*, 700790. [CrossRef]
109. Okuda, R.; Aoshiba, K.; Matsushima, H.; Ogura, T.; Okudela, K.; Ohashi, K. Cellular senescence and senescence-associated secretory phenotype: Comparison of idiopathic pulmonary fibrosis, connective tissue disease-associated interstitial lung disease, and chronic obstructive pulmonary disease. *J. Thorac. Dis.* **2019**, *11*, 857–864. [CrossRef]
110. Han, D.; Xu, Y.; Peng, W.P.; Feng, F.; Wang, Z.; Gu, C.; Zhou, X. Citrus Alkaline Extracts Inhibit Senescence of A549 Cells to Alleviate Pulmonary Fibrosis via the beta-Catenin/P53 Pathway. *Med. Sci. Monit.* **2021**, *27*, e928547. [CrossRef]
111. Yamada, Z.; Nishio, J.; Motomura, K.; Mizutani, S.; Yamada, S.; Mikami, T.; Nanki, T. Senescence of alveolar epithelial cells impacts initiation and chronic phases of murine fibrosing interstitial lung disease. *Front. Immunol.* **2022**, *13*, 935114. [CrossRef] [PubMed]
112. Rana, T.; Jiang, C.; Liu, G.; Miyata, T.; Antony, V.; Thannickal, V.J.; Liu, R.M. PAI-1 Regulation of TGF-beta1-induced Alveolar Type II Cell Senescence, SASP Secretion, and SASP-mediated Activation of Alveolar Macrophages. *Am. J. Respir. Cell Mol. Biol.* **2020**, *62*, 319–330. [CrossRef] [PubMed]
113. Minagawa, S.; Araya, J.; Numata, T.; Nojiri, S.; Hara, H.; Yumino, Y.; Kawaishi, M.; Odaka, M.; Morikawa, T.; Nishimura, S.L.; et al. Accelerated epithelial cell senescence in IPF and the inhibitory role of SIRT6 in TGF-beta-induced senescence of human bronchial epithelial cells. *Am. J. Physiol. Lung Cell. Mol. Physiol.* **2011**, *300*, L391–L401. [CrossRef] [PubMed]
114. Sisson, T.H.; Christensen, P.J.; Muraki, Y.; Dils, A.J.; Chibucos, L.; Subbotina, N.; Tohyama, K.; Horowitz, J.C.; Matsuo, T.; Bailie, M.; et al. Phosphodiesterase 4 inhibition reduces lung fibrosis following targeted type II alveolar epithelial cell injury. *Physiol. Rep.* **2018**, *6*, e13753. [CrossRef]
115. Richeldi, L.; Azuma, A.; Cottin, V.; Hesslinger, C.; Stowasser, S.; Valenzuela, C.; Wijsenbeek, M.S.; Zoz, D.F.; Voss, F.; Maher, T.M.; et al. Trial of a Preferential Phosphodiesterase 4B Inhibitor for Idiopathic Pulmonary Fibrosis. *N. Engl. J. Med.* **2022**, *386*, 2178–2187. [CrossRef]
116. Sakkas, L.I.; Mavropoulos, A.; Bogdanos, D.P. Phosphodiesterase 4 Inhibitors in Immune-mediated Diseases: Mode of Action, Clinical Applications, Current and Future Perspectives. *Curr. Med. Chem.* **2017**, *24*, 3054–3067. [CrossRef]
117. Spina, D. Phosphodiesterase-4 inhibitors in the treatment of inflammatory lung disease. *Drugs* **2003**, *63*, 2575–2594. [CrossRef]
118. Crilly, A.; Robertson, S.E.; Reilly, J.H.; Gracie, J.A.; Lai, W.Q.; Leung, B.P.; Life, P.F.; McInnes, I.B. Phosphodiesterase 4 (PDE4) regulation of proinflammatory cytokine and chemokine release from rheumatoid synovial membrane. *Ann. Rheum. Dis.* **2011**, *70*, 1130–1137. [CrossRef]
119. Griswold, D.E.; Webb, E.F.; Badger, A.M.; Gorycki, P.D.; Levandoski, P.A.; Barnette, M.A.; Grous, M.; Christensen, S.; Torphy, T.J. SB 207499 (Ariflo), a second generation phosphodiesterase 4 inhibitor, reduces tumor necrosis factor alpha and interleukin-4 production in vivo. *J. Pharmacol. Exp. Ther.* **1998**, *287*, 705–711.
120. Maher, T.M.; Schlecker, C.; Luedtke, D.; Bossert, S.; Zoz, D.F.; Schultz, A. Phase I studies of BI 1015550, a preferential phosphodiesterase 4B inhibitor, in healthy males and patients with idiopathic pulmonary fibrosis. *ERJ Open Res.* **2022**, *8*, 00240-2022. [CrossRef]

121. Nikitopoulou, I.; Manitsopoulos, N.; Kotanidou, A.; Tian, X.; Petrovic, A.; Magkou, C.; Ninou, I.; Aidinis, V.; Schermuly, R.T.; Kosanovic, D.; et al. Orotracheal treprostinil administration attenuates bleomycin-induced lung injury, vascular remodeling, and fibrosis in mice. *Pulm. Circ.* **2019**, *9*, 2045894019881954. [CrossRef] [PubMed]
122. Corboz, M.R.; Zhang, J.; LaSala, D.; DiPetrillo, K.; Li, Z.; Malinin, V.; Brower, J.; Kuehl, P.J.; Barrett, T.E.; Perkins, W.R.; et al. Therapeutic administration of inhaled INS1009, a treprostinil prodrug formulation, inhibits bleomycin-induced pulmonary fibrosis in rats. *Pulm. Pharmacol. Ther.* **2018**, *49*, 95–103. [CrossRef] [PubMed]
123. Fang, L.; Chen, W.C.; Jaksch, P.; Molino, A.; Saglia, A.; Roth, M.; Lambers, C. Treprostinil Reconstitutes Mitochondrial Organisation and Structure in Idiopathic Pulmonary Fibrosis Cells. *Int. J. Mol. Sci.* **2023**, *24*, 12148. [CrossRef] [PubMed]
124. Waxman, A.; Restrepo-Jaramillo, R.; Thenappan, T.; Ravichandran, A.; Engel, P.; Bajwa, A.; Allen, R.; Feldman, J.; Argula, R.; Smith, P.; et al. Inhaled Treprostinil in Pulmonary Hypertension Due to Interstitial Lung Disease. *N. Engl. J. Med.* **2021**, *384*, 325–334. [CrossRef]
125. Nathan, S.D.; Waxman, A.; Rajagopal, S.; Case, A.; Johri, S.; DuBrock, H.; De La Zerda, D.J.; Sahay, S.; King, C.; Melendres-Groves, L.; et al. Inhaled treprostinil and forced vital capacity in patients with interstitial lung disease and associated pulmonary hypertension: A post-hoc analysis of the INCREASE study. *Lancet Respir. Med.* **2021**, *9*, 1266–1274. [CrossRef]
126. Nathan, S.D.; Tapson, V.F.; Elwing, J.; Rischard, F.; Mehta, J.; Shapiro, S.; Shen, E.; Deng, C.; Smith, P.; Waxman, A. Efficacy of Inhaled Treprostinil on Multiple Disease Progression Events in Patients with Pulmonary Hypertension due to Parenchymal Lung Disease in the INCREASE Trial. *Am. J. Respir. Crit. Care Med.* **2022**, *205*, 198–207. [CrossRef]
127. Nathan, S.D.; Behr, J.; Cottin, V.; Lancaster, L.; Smith, P.; Deng, C.Q.; Pearce, N.; Bell, H.; Peterson, L.; Flaherty, K.R. Study design and rationale for the TETON phase 3, randomised, controlled clinical trials of inhaled treprostinil in the treatment of idiopathic pulmonary fibrosis. *BMJ Open Respir. Res.* **2022**, *9*, e001310. [CrossRef]
128. Chen, S.; Gao, D.; Sun, R.; Bao, J.; Lu, C.; Zhang, Z.; Xiao, T.; Gu, X.; Zhou, H. Anlotinib prove to be a potential therapy for the treatment of pulmonary fibrosis complicated with lung adenocarcinoma. *Pulm. Pharmacol. Ther.* **2023**, *80*, 102202. [CrossRef]
129. Wu, Y.T.; Li, Q.Z.; Zhao, X.K.; Mu, M.; Zou, G.L.; Zhao, W.F. Anlotinib Attenuates Liver Fibrosis by Regulating the Transforming Growth Factor beta1/Smad3 Signaling Pathway. *Dig. Dis. Sci.* **2023**, *68*, 4186–4195. [CrossRef]
130. Ruan, H.; Lv, Z.; Liu, S.; Zhang, L.; Huang, K.; Gao, S.; Gan, W.; Liu, X.; Zhang, S.; Helian, K.; et al. Anlotinib attenuated bleomycin-induced pulmonary fibrosis via the TGF-beta1 signalling pathway. *J. Pharm. Pharmacol.* **2020**, *72*, 44–55. [CrossRef]
131. Chen, W.; Zhang, J.; Zhong, W.; Liu, Y.; Lu, Y.; Zeng, Z.; Huang, H.; Wan, X.; Meng, X.; Zou, F.; et al. Anlotinib Inhibits PFKFB3-Driven Glycolysis in Myofibroblasts to Reverse Pulmonary Fibrosis. *Front. Pharmacol.* **2021**, *12*, 744826. [CrossRef] [PubMed]
132. Li, Y.; Sun, Z.; Sun, W.; Wang, H.; Zu, J. Effectiveness and Safety of Anlotinib Monotherapy for Patients with Extensive-stage Small-Cell Lung Cancer Who Progressed to Chemotherapy: A Real-world Exploratory Study. *Clin. Med. Insights Oncol.* **2022**, *16*, 11795549211067184. [CrossRef] [PubMed]
133. Ramos, R.; Vale, N. Dual Drug Repurposing: The Example of Saracatinib. *Int. J. Mol. Sci.* **2024**, *25*, 4565. [CrossRef] [PubMed]
134. Du, G.; Wang, J.; Zhang, T.; Ding, Q.; Jia, X.; Zhao, X.; Dong, J.; Yang, X.; Lu, S.; Zhang, C.; et al. Targeting Src family kinase member Fyn by Saracatinib attenuated liver fibrosis in vitro and in vivo. *Cell Death Dis.* **2020**, *11*, 118. [CrossRef] [PubMed]
135. Hu, M.; Che, P.; Han, X.; Cai, G.Q.; Liu, G.; Antony, V.; Luckhardt, T.; Siegal, G.P.; Zhou, Y.; Liu, R.M.; et al. Therapeutic targeting of SRC kinase in myofibroblast differentiation and pulmonary fibrosis. *J. Pharmacol. Exp. Ther.* **2014**, *351*, 87–95. [CrossRef]
136. Ahangari, F.; Becker, C.; Foster, D.G.; Chioccioli, M.; Nelson, M.; Beke, K.; Wang, X.; Justet, A.; Adams, T.; Readhead, B.; et al. Saracatinib, a Selective Src Kinase Inhibitor, Blocks Fibrotic Responses in Preclinical Models of Pulmonary Fibrosis. *Am. J. Respir. Crit. Care Med.* **2022**, *206*, 1463–1479. [CrossRef]
137. Baselga, J.; Cervantes, A.; Martinelli, E.; Chirivella, I.; Hoekman, K.; Hurwitz, H.I.; Jodrell, D.I.; Hamberg, P.; Casado, E.; Elvin, P.; et al. Phase I safety, pharmacokinetics, and inhibition of SRC activity study of saracatinib in patients with solid tumors. *Clin. Cancer Res.* **2010**, *16*, 4876–4883. [CrossRef]
138. Yanagihara, T.; Tsubouchi, K.; Gholiof, M.; Chong, S.G.; Lipson, K.E.; Zhou, Q.; Scallan, C.; Upagupta, C.; Tikkanen, J.; Keshavjee, S.; et al. Connective-Tissue Growth Factor Contributes to TGF-beta1-induced Lung Fibrosis. *Am. J. Respir. Cell Mol. Biol.* **2022**, *66*, 260–270. [CrossRef]
139. Kono, M.; Nakamura, Y.; Suda, T.; Kato, M.; Kaida, Y.; Hashimoto, D.; Inui, N.; Hamada, E.; Miyazaki, O.; Kurashita, S.; et al. Plasma CCN2 (connective tissue growth factor; CTGF) is a potential biomarker in idiopathic pulmonary fibrosis (IPF). *Clin. Chim. Acta* **2011**, *412*, 2211–2215. [CrossRef]
140. Richeldi, L.; Fernandez Perez, E.R.; Costabel, U.; Albera, C.; Lederer, D.J.; Flaherty, K.R.; Ettinger, N.; Perez, R.; Scholand, M.B.; Goldin, J.; et al. Pamrevlumab, an anti-connective tissue growth factor therapy, for idiopathic pulmonary fibrosis (PRAISE): A phase 2, randomised, double-blind, placebo-controlled trial. *Lancet Respir. Med.* **2020**, *8*, 25–33. [CrossRef]
141. Song, L.L.; Zhou, H.Y.; Ye, P.P.; Li, Q.; Chen, K.G.; Zhang, Y.H.; Zhao, F.R.; Shi, J.Y.; Luo, Y.; Zhu, M.; et al. A first-in-human phase I study of SHR-1906, a humanized monoclonal antibody against connective tissue growth factor, in healthy participants. *Clin. Transl. Sci.* **2023**, *16*, 2604–2613. [CrossRef] [PubMed]
142. Murphy, B.; Sum, C.-S.; Wang, T.; Heiry, R.; Kalinowski, S.; Hung, C.-P.; Chu, C.-H.; Azzara, A.; Milinda, Z.; Burns, L. LPA1 antagonist BMS-986278 for idiopathic pulmonary fibrosis: Preclinical pharmacological in vitro and in vivo evaluation. *Eur. Respir. J.* **2019**, *54*, PA5383.

143. Cheng, P.T.; Kaltenbach III, R.F.; Zhang, H.; Shi, J.; Tao, S.; Li, J.; Kennedy, L.J.; Walker, S.J.; Shi, Y.; Wang, Y. Discovery of an oxycyclohexyl acid lysophosphatidic acid receptor 1 (LPA1) antagonist BMS-986278 for the treatment of pulmonary fibrotic diseases. *J. Med. Chem.* **2021**, *64*, 15549–15581. [CrossRef] [PubMed]
144. Gill, M.W.; Murphy, B.J.; Cheng, P.T.; Sivaraman, L.; Davis, M.; Lehman-McKeeman, L. Mechanism of hepatobiliary toxicity of the LPA1 antagonist BMS-986020 developed to treat idiopathic pulmonary fibrosis: Contrasts with BMS-986234 and BMS-986278. *Toxicol. Appl. Pharmacol.* **2022**, *438*, 115885. [CrossRef] [PubMed]
145. Corte, T.J.; Lancaster, L.; Swigris, J.J.; Maher, T.M.; Goldin, J.G.; Palmer, S.M.; Suda, T.; Ogura, T.; Minnich, A.; Zhan, X.; et al. Phase 2 trial design of BMS-986278, a lysophosphatidic acid receptor 1 (LPA(1)) antagonist, in patients with idiopathic pulmonary fibrosis (IPF) or progressive fibrotic interstitial lung disease (PF-ILD). *BMJ Open Respir. Res.* **2021**, *8*, e001026. [CrossRef]
146. Corte, T.; Cottin, V.; Glassberg, M.; Kreuter, M.; Ogura, T.; Suda, T.; Goldin, J.; Berkowitz, E.; Elpers, B.; Kim, S. BMS-986278, an oral lysophosphatidic acid receptor 1 (LPA1) antagonist, for patients with idiopathic pulmonary fibrosis: Results from a phase 2 randomized trial. In *B17. Emerging Data on Disease and Symptom Based Therapeutics for Patients with IPF*; American Thoracic Society: New York, NY, USA, 2023; p. A2785.
147. Song, Y.; Ali, F.N.; Ye, Z.; Zarzoso, J.; Rogowski, J.; Sun, Y.; Xin, Y. Pharmacokinetics of Fipaxalparant, a Small-Molecule Selective Negative Allosteric Modulator of Lysophosphatidic Acid Receptor 1, and the Effect of Food in Healthy Volunteers. *Clin. Pharmacol. Drug Dev.* **2024**, *13*, 819–827. [CrossRef]
148. Allanore, Y.; Distler, O.; Jagerschmidt, A.; Illiano, S.; Ledein, L.; Boitier, E.; Agueusop, I.; Denton, C.P.; Khanna, D. Lysophosphatidic Acid Receptor 1 Antagonist SAR100842 for Patients With Diffuse Cutaneous Systemic Sclerosis: A Double-Blind, Randomized, Eight-Week Placebo-Controlled Study Followed by a Sixteen-Week Open-Label Extension Study. *Arthritis Rheumatol.* **2018**, *70*, 1634–1643. [CrossRef]
149. Kim, J.S.; Shin, M.J.; Lee, S.Y.; Choi, S.M.; Choi, K.U.; Suh, D.S.; Kim, D.K.; Kim, J.H. BBT-877, a Novel Autotaxin Inhibitor, Abrogates Drug Resistance in Epithelial Ovarian Cancer Stem Cells. *Anticancer. Res.* **2024**, *44*, 1131–1142. [CrossRef]
150. Lee, J.H.; Khin, P.P.; Lee, G.; Lim, O.K.; Jun, H.S. Effect of BBT-877, a novel inhibitor of ATX, on a mouse model of type 1 diabetic nephropathy. *Aging* **2022**, *14*, 6467–6480. [CrossRef]
151. Lee, G.; Kang, S.U.; Ryou, J.-H.; Lim, J.-J.; Lee, D.-Y.; Kwon, H.-J.; Ha, G.-H.; Lee, Y.-H. BBT-877, a potent autotaxin inhibitor in clinical development to treat idiopathic pulmonary fibrosis. *PAT* **2019**, *505*, 100.
152. Bellani, S.; Molyneaux, P.L.; Maher, T.M.; Spagnolo, P. Potential of alphavbeta6 and alphavbeta1 integrin inhibition for treatment of idiopathic pulmonary fibrosis. *Expert. Opin. Ther. Targets* **2024**, *28*, 575–585. [CrossRef] [PubMed]
153. An, M.; Ho, S.; Rao, V.; Ho, B.; Ahn, R.; Yuzon, J.; Budi, E.; Lau, J.; Her, C.; Wolters, P. Bexotegrast Targets TGF-β Inhibition to Specific Cell Types in the Fibrotic Human Lung. *Artery* **2024**, *51*, 41.
154. Raghu, G.; Mouded, M.; Chambers, D.C.; Martinez, F.J.; Richeldi, L.; Lancaster, L.H.; Hamblin, M.J.; Gibson, K.F.; Rosas, I.O.; Prasse, A.; et al. A Phase IIb Randomized Clinical Study of an Anti-alpha(v)beta(6) Monoclonal Antibody in Idiopathic Pulmonary Fibrosis. *Am. J. Respir. Crit. Care Med.* **2022**, *206*, 1128–1139. [CrossRef] [PubMed]
155. Peyraud, F.; Cousin, S.; Italiano, A. CSF-1R Inhibitor Development: Current Clinical Status. *Curr. Oncol. Rep.* **2017**, *19*, 70. [CrossRef] [PubMed]
156. Meziani, L.; Mondini, M.; Petit, B.; Boissonnas, A.; Thomas de Montpreville, V.; Mercier, O.; Vozenin, M.C.; Deutsch, E. CSF1R inhibition prevents radiation pulmonary fibrosis by depletion of interstitial macrophages. *Eur. Respir. J.* **2018**, *51*, 1702120. [CrossRef]
157. Watson, C.K.; Schloesser, D.; Fundel-Clemens, K.; Lerner, C.; Gabler, S.; Baskaran, P.; Wohnhaas, C.T.; Dichtl, S.; Huber, H.J.; Ask, K.; et al. Antifibrotic Drug Nintedanib Inhibits CSF1R to Promote IL-4-associated Tissue Repair Macrophages. *Am. J. Respir. Cell Mol. Biol.* **2023**, *68*, 366–380. [CrossRef]
158. Kitko, C.L.; Arora, M.; DeFilipp, Z.; Zaid, M.A.; Di Stasi, A.; Radojcic, V.; Betts, C.B.; Coussens, L.M.; Meyers, M.L.; Qamoos, H.; et al. Axatilimab for Chronic Graft-Versus-Host Disease After Failure of at Least Two Prior Systemic Therapies: Results of a Phase I/II Study. *J. Clin. Oncol.* **2023**, *41*, 1864–1875. [CrossRef]
159. Wolff, D.; Cutler, C.; Lee, S.J.; Pusic, I.; Bittencourt, H.; White, J.; Hamadani, M.; Arai, S.; Salhotra, A.; Perez-Simon, J.A.; et al. Axatilimab in Recurrent or Refractory Chronic Graft-versus-Host Disease. *N. Engl. J. Med.* **2024**, *391*, 1002–1014. [CrossRef]
160. Milara, J.; Hernandez, G.; Ballester, B.; Morell, A.; Roger, I.; Montero, P.; Escriva, J.; Lloris, J.M.; Molina-Molina, M.; Morcillo, E.; et al. The JAK2 pathway is activated in idiopathic pulmonary fibrosis. *Respir. Res.* **2018**, *19*, 24. [CrossRef]
161. Zhang, Y.; Zhang, Q.; Liu, Q.; Dang, H.; Gao, S.; Wang, W.; Zhou, H.; Chen, Y.; Ma, L.; Wang, J.; et al. Safety and efficacy of jaktinib (a novel JAK inhibitor) in patients with myelofibrosis who are relapsed or refractory to ruxolitinib: A single-arm, open-label, phase 2, multicenter study. *Am. J. Hematol.* **2023**, *98*, 1579–1587. [CrossRef]
162. Park, E.; Park, S.; Lee, S.J.; Jeong, D.; Jin, H.; Moon, H.; Cha, B.; Kim, D.; Ma, S.; Seo, W.; et al. Identification and Biological Evaluation of a Potent and Selective JAK1 Inhibitor for the Treatment of Pulmonary Fibrosis. *J. Med. Chem.* **2023**, *66*, 16342–16363. [CrossRef] [PubMed]
163. Silva-Carmona, M.; Vogel, T.P.; Marchal, S.; Guesmi, M.; Dubus, J.C.; Leroy, S.; Fabre, A.; Barlogis, V.; Forbes, L.R.; Giovannini-Chami, L. Successful Treatment of Interstitial Lung Disease in STAT3 Gain-of-Function Using JAK Inhibitors. *Am. J. Respir. Crit. Care Med.* **2020**, *202*, 893–897. [CrossRef] [PubMed]
164. Montero, P.; Milara, J.; Roger, I.; Cortijo, J. Role of JAK/STAT in Interstitial Lung Diseases; Molecular and Cellular Mechanisms. *Int. J. Mol. Sci.* **2021**, *22*, 6211. [CrossRef]

165. Zhao, M.; Zhang, H.; Ma, S.; Gong, S.; Wei, C.; Miao, L.; Zhao, W. Clinical pharmacokinetic characteristics of Jaktinib in subjects with hepatic impairment in a phase I trial. *Drug Metab. Pharmacokinet.* **2024**, 101030. [CrossRef]
166. Thannickal, V.J.; Jandeleit-Dahm, K.; Szyndralewiez, C.; Torok, N.J. Pre-clinical evidence of a dual NADPH oxidase 1/4 inhibitor (setanaxib) in liver, kidney and lung fibrosis. *J. Cell. Mol. Med.* **2023**, *27*, 471–481. [CrossRef] [PubMed]
167. Invernizzi, P.; Carbone, M.; Jones, D.; Levy, C.; Little, N.; Wiesel, P.; Nevens, F.; the study investigators. Setanaxib, a first-in-class selective NADPH oxidase 1/4 inhibitor for primary biliary cholangitis: A randomized, placebo-controlled, phase 2 trial. *Liver Int.* **2023**, *43*, 1507–1522. [CrossRef] [PubMed]
168. Hecker, L.; Vittal, R.; Jones, T.; Jagirdar, R.; Luckhardt, T.R.; Horowitz, J.C.; Pennathur, S.; Martinez, F.J.; Thannickal, V.J. NADPH oxidase-4 mediates myofibroblast activation and fibrogenic responses to lung injury. *Nat. Med.* **2009**, *15*, 1077–1081. [CrossRef] [PubMed]
169. Louzada, R.A.; Corre, R.; Ameziane El Hassani, R.; Meziani, L.; Jaillet, M.; Cazes, A.; Crestani, B.; Deutsch, E.; Dupuy, C. NADPH oxidase DUOX1 sustains TGF-beta1 signalling and promotes lung fibrosis. *Eur. Respir. J.* **2021**, *57*, 1901949. [CrossRef]
170. Jiang, F.; Liu, G.S.; Dusting, G.J.; Chan, E.C. NADPH oxidase-dependent redox signaling in TGF-beta-mediated fibrotic responses. *Redox Biol.* **2014**, *2*, 267–272. [CrossRef]
171. Duvic, M. Tazarotene: A review of its pharmacological profile and potential for clinical use in psoriasis. *Expert. Opin. Investig. Drugs* **1997**, *6*, 1537–1551. [CrossRef]
172. Zhou, T.B.; Drummen, G.P.; Qin, Y.H. The controversial role of retinoic acid in fibrotic diseases: Analysis of involved signaling pathways. *Int. J. Mol. Sci.* **2012**, *14*, 226–243. [CrossRef] [PubMed]
173. Tabata, C.; Kadokawa, Y.; Tabata, R.; Takahashi, M.; Okoshi, K.; Sakai, Y.; Mishima, M.; Kubo, H. All-trans-retinoic acid prevents radiation- or bleomycin-induced pulmonary fibrosis. *Am. J. Respir. Crit. Care Med.* **2006**, *174*, 1352–1360. [CrossRef] [PubMed]
174. So, P.L.; Fujimoto, M.A.; Epstein, E.H., Jr. Pharmacologic retinoid signaling and physiologic retinoic acid receptor signaling inhibit basal cell carcinoma tumorigenesis. *Mol. Cancer Ther.* **2008**, *7*, 1275–1284. [CrossRef] [PubMed]
175. Al Haj Zen, A.; Nawrot, D.A.; Howarth, A.; Caporali, A.; Ebner, D.; Vernet, A.; Schneider, J.E.; Bhattacharya, S. The Retinoid Agonist Tazarotene Promotes Angiogenesis and Wound Healing. *Mol. Ther.* **2016**, *24*, 1745–1759. [CrossRef] [PubMed]
176. Calamita, E.; Liu, W.H.; Ogger, P.P.; Griffin, L.; Michalaki, C.; Murphy, F.; Worrell, J.; McCarthy, C.; Agro, A.; Hertz, M.; et al. Type 1 Invariant Natural Killer T Cells Drive Lung Fibrosis. *Am. J. Respir. Crit. Care Med.* **2024**, *210*, 521–523. [CrossRef]
177. Kumar, V.; Hertz, M.; Agro, A.; Byrne, A.J. Type 1 invariant natural killer T cells in chronic inflammation and tissue fibrosis. *Front. Immunol.* **2023**, *14*, 1260503. [CrossRef]
178. Jandl, K.; Marsh, L.M.; Mutgan, A.C.; Crnkovic, S.; Valzano, F.; Zabini, D.; Hoffmann, J.; Foris, V.; Gschwandtner, E.; Klepetko, W.; et al. Impairment of the NKT-STAT1-CXCL9 Axis Contributes to Vessel Fibrosis in Pulmonary Hypertension Caused by Lung Fibrosis. *Am. J. Respir. Crit. Care Med.* **2022**, *206*, 981–998. [CrossRef]
179. Kim, J.H.; Kim, H.Y.; Kim, S.; Chung, J.H.; Park, W.S.; Chung, D.H. Natural killer T (NKT) cells attenuate bleomycin-induced pulmonary fibrosis by producing interferon-gamma. *Am. J. Pathol.* **2005**, *167*, 1231–1241. [CrossRef]
180. Grabarz, F.; Aguiar, C.F.; Correa-Costa, M.; Braga, T.T.; Hyane, M.I.; Andrade-Oliveira, V.; Landgraf, M.A.; Camara, N.O.S. Protective role of NKT cells and macrophage M2-driven phenotype in bleomycin-induced pulmonary fibrosis. *Inflammopharmacology* **2018**, *26*, 491–504. [CrossRef]
181. Zhang, F.; Qi, X.; Wang, X.; Wei, D.; Wu, J.; Feng, L.; Cai, H.; Wang, Y.; Zeng, N.; Xu, T.; et al. Structural basis of the therapeutic anti-PD-L1 antibody atezolizumab. *Oncotarget* **2017**, *8*, 90215–90224. [CrossRef]
182. Jiang, A.; Liu, N.; Wang, J.; Zheng, X.; Ren, M.; Zhang, W.; Yao, Y. The role of PD-1/PD-L1 axis in idiopathic pulmonary fibrosis: Friend or foe? *Front. Immunol.* **2022**, *13*, 1022228. [CrossRef] [PubMed]
183. Kronborg-White, S.; Madsen, L.B.; Bendstrup, E.; Poletti, V. PD-L1 Expression in Patients with Idiopathic Pulmonary Fibrosis. *J. Clin. Med.* **2021**, *10*, 5562. [CrossRef] [PubMed]
184. Fukasawa, T.; Yoshizaki, A.; Ebata, S.; Nakamura, K.; Saigusa, R.; Miura, S.; Yamashita, T.; Hirabayashi, M.; Ichimura, Y.; Taniguchi, T.; et al. Contribution of Soluble Forms of Programmed Death 1 and Programmed Death Ligand 2 to Disease Severity and Progression in Systemic Sclerosis. *Arthritis Rheumatol.* **2017**, *69*, 1879–1890. [CrossRef] [PubMed]
185. Geng, Y.; Liu, X.; Liang, J.; Habiel, D.M.; Kulur, V.; Coelho, A.L.; Deng, N.; Xie, T.; Wang, Y.; Liu, N.; et al. PD-L1 on invasive fibroblasts drives fibrosis in a humanized model of idiopathic pulmonary fibrosis. *JCI Insight* **2019**, *4*, 125326. [CrossRef] [PubMed]
186. Ahmadvand, N.; Carraro, G.; Jones, M.R.; Shalashova, I.; Noori, A.; Wilhelm, J.; Baal, N.; Khosravi, F.; Chen, C.; Zhang, J.S.; et al. Cell-Surface Programmed Death Ligand-1 Expression Identifies a Sub-Population of Distal Epithelial Cells Enriched in Idiopathic Pulmonary Fibrosis. *Cells* **2022**, *11*, 1593. [CrossRef]
187. Ni, K.; Liu, M.; Zheng, J.; Wen, L.; Chen, Q.; Xiang, Z.; Lam, K.T.; Liu, Y.; Chan, G.C.; Lau, Y.L.; et al. PD-1/PD-L1 Pathway Mediates the Alleviation of Pulmonary Fibrosis by Human Mesenchymal Stem Cells in Humanized Mice. *Am. J. Respir. Cell Mol. Biol.* **2018**, *58*, 684–695. [CrossRef]
188. Zhao, Y.; Hao, C.; Li, M.; Qu, Y.; Guo, Y.; Deng, X.; Si, H.; Yao, W. PD-1/PD-L1 inhibitor ameliorates silica-induced pulmonary fibrosis by maintaining systemic immune homeostasis. *Biomed. Pharmacother.* **2022**, *148*, 112768. [CrossRef]
189. Lu, Y.; Zhong, W.; Liu, Y.; Chen, W.; Zhang, J.; Zeng, Z.; Huang, H.; Qiao, Y.; Wan, X.; Meng, X.; et al. Anti-PD-L1 antibody alleviates pulmonary fibrosis by inducing autophagy via inhibition of the PI3K/Akt/mTOR pathway. *Int. Immunopharmacol.* **2022**, *104*, 108504. [CrossRef]

190. Zhou, P.; Zhao, X.; Wang, G. Risk Factors for Immune Checkpoint Inhibitor-Related Pneumonitis in Cancer Patients: A Systemic Review and Meta-Analysis. *Respiration* **2022**, *101*, 1035–1050. [CrossRef]
191. Atchley, W.T.; Alvarez, C.; Saxena-Beem, S.; Schwartz, T.A.; Ishizawar, R.C.; Patel, K.P.; Rivera, M.P. Immune Checkpoint Inhibitor-Related Pneumonitis in Lung Cancer: Real-World Incidence, Risk Factors, and Management Practices Across Six Health Care Centers in North Carolina. *Chest* **2021**, *160*, 731–742. [CrossRef]
192. Su, Q.; Zhu, E.C.; Wu, J.B.; Li, T.; Hou, Y.L.; Wang, D.Y.; Gao, Z.H. Risk of Pneumonitis and Pneumonia Associated With Immune Checkpoint Inhibitors for Solid Tumors: A Systematic Review and Meta-Analysis. *Front. Immunol.* **2019**, *10*, 108. [CrossRef] [PubMed]
193. Ikeda, S.; Kato, T.; Kenmotsu, H.; Ogura, T.; Iwasawa, S.; Sato, Y.; Harada, T.; Kubota, K.; Tokito, T.; Okamoto, I.; et al. A Phase 2 Study of Atezolizumab for Pretreated NSCLC With Idiopathic Interstitial Pneumonitis. *J. Thorac. Oncol.* **2020**, *15*, 1935–1942. [CrossRef] [PubMed]

Journal of
Clinical Medicine

MDPI

Review

The Management of Interstitial Lung Disease in the ICU: A Comprehensive Review

Zehra Dhanani [1] and Rohit Gupta [2,]*

1 Thoracic Medicine and Surgery, Temple University Hospital, Philadelphia, PA 19140, USA; zehra.dhanani@tuhs.temple.edu
2 Thoracic Medicine and Surgery, Lewis Katz School of Medicine at Temple University, Philadelphia, PA 19140, USA
* Correspondence: rohit.gupta@tuhs.temple.edu; Tel.: +1-267-563-2151

Abstract: Interstitial lung disease (ILD) encompasses a diverse group of parenchymal lung diseases characterized by varying degrees of inflammation and/or fibrosis. Patients with ILD frequently require hospitalization, with many needing intensive care unit (ICU) admission, most often due to respiratory failure. The diagnosis and management of ILD in the ICU present unique challenges. Diagnosis primarily relies on chest CT imaging to identify fibrosis and inflammation. Acute exacerbations, whether in idiopathic pulmonary fibrosis (IPF) or non-IPF ILD, require careful evaluation of potential triggers and differential diagnoses. Bronchoalveolar lavage may provide valuable information, such as the identification of infections, but carries risks of complications. Biopsies, whether transbronchial or surgical, can also be informative but pose significant procedural risks. Corticosteroids are the cornerstone of treatment for acute exacerbations of IPF, with higher doses potentially benefiting non-IPF ILD. Additional immunosuppressive agents may be used in cases with evidence of inflammation. Oxygen supplementation, particularly with high-flow nasal cannula, is often employed to manage severe hypoxemia, while noninvasive ventilation can be useful for worsening hypoxemia and/or hypercapnia. When mechanical ventilation is used, it is recommended to target low tidal volumes to minimize lung injury; high PEEP may be less effective and even associated with increased mortality. Prone positioning can improve oxygenation in severely hypoxemic patients. In addition to ventilatory strategies, careful fluid management and addressing concomitant pulmonary hypertension are essential components of care. Extracorporeal membrane oxygenation is a high-risk intervention reserved for the most severe cases. Lung transplantation may be considered for end-stage ILD patients in the ICU, with outcomes dependent on the urgency of transplantation and the patient's overall condition. Managing ILD in the ICU requires a multidisciplinary approach, and despite recent advances, mortality remains high, emphasizing the need for continued research and individualized treatment strategies.

Keywords: interstitial lung disease; pulmonary fibrosis; acute exacerbation; mechanical ventilation; lung transplantation

1. Introduction

Interstitial lung disease (ILD) comprises a heterogeneous group of parenchymal lung diseases characterized by varying degrees of inflammation and/or fibrosis. Based on radiographic features, ILD can be broadly classified into two main groups: the fibrosis-predominant group and the inflammation- or cellular-predominant group [1,2]. Idiopathic pulmonary fibrosis (IPF), a classic example of fibrosis-predominant ILD, is characterized by the usual interstitial pneumonia pattern on imaging [3]. IPF is associated with a poor prognosis, with an estimated 5-year survival rate of approximately 50% [4]. In a large IPF registry study by Kim et al. involving over 1000 patients, 56.7% experienced at least one hospitalization during a two-year follow-up period, and 21.1% required ventilatory support [5].

Among ILD patients, admission to the intensive care unit (ICU) is most often necessitated by acute hypoxemic respiratory failure, frequently in the setting of an acute exacerbation. However, other etiologies, such as extra-parenchymal causes including pneumothorax, pleural effusion, and pulmonary embolism, must be ruled out [6,7] (Table 1). Exacerbations are particularly well documented in patients with IPF, where the incidence rate of exacerbations ranges from 4% to 20%, with those requiring ICU care generally exhibiting shorter survival compared to non-exacerbating patients [4,7]. By contrast, patients with non-IPF ILD typically experience fewer exacerbations and have lower mortality rates [8]. Factors such as poor baseline lung function, as indicated by reduced forced vital capacity (FVC) and diffusion capacity of the lung for carbon monoxide (DLCO), older age, and radiographic patterns of honeycombing are associated with an increased risk of exacerbations and poor prognosis [9–11].

Table 1. Common causes of acute respiratory decompensation in patients with ILD [2,12].

Causes of Acute Decompensation in Patients with ILD
1. Extra-parenchymal causes:
a. Pneumothorax
b. Pulmonary embolism
c. Pleural effusion
2. Pulmonary edema
3. Acute exacerbation of ILD (triggers: infection, occupational/environmental exposure, aspiration)

Given the scarcity of comprehensive research addressing the care of ILD patients in the ICU and the high morbidity and mortality associated with ICU admission in this population, consolidating current evidence is crucial for guiding clinicians in optimizing management strategies. Furthermore, a thorough understanding of these management strategies is essential, particularly as more end-stage ILD patients undergo rapid evaluation for lung transplantation while in the ICU. This knowledge can increase the likelihood of successful transplantation and improve survival outcomes. Despite the importance of these clinical issues, much of the available data stem from observational studies or are extrapolated from general ICU management principles. This review aims to address these gaps by providing a comprehensive overview of ILD management in the ICU, focusing on diagnostic and therapeutic considerations critical for improving outcomes, and highlighting potential avenues for future research.

1.1. The Diagnosis and Evaluation of Patients with ILD in the ICU

Diagnosing ILD in the ICU presents unique challenges, as this patient population may include both those who are newly diagnosed with ILD during their ICU stay and those with a pre-existing diagnosis of ILD. The diagnosis of ILD primarily relies on imaging findings, particularly high-resolution CT (HRCT) scans. HRCT features indicative of fibrosis include reticulations, interstitial thickening, traction bronchiectasis, and honeycombing [3] (Figure 1). In contrast, inflammation may be characterized by ground-glass opacities (GGOs) [13] (Figure 2). However, it is important to note that GGOs are nonspecific and can represent the intra-alveolar filling process of any etiology such as infection, fluid accumulation, and cellular infiltration [14]. Some imaging features might point toward a diagnosis of a specific ILD, but distinguishing between different ILDs involves combining these imaging characteristics and distribution, along with a thorough history and laboratory investigations, including but not limited to an autoimmune panel, drug use, and exposure history [1]. A multidisciplinary approach can be particularly valuable in managing complex cases and refining the diagnostic process [15].

In the context of a pre-existing ILD diagnosis, an acute exacerbation of ILD (AE-ILD) should be considered a possible cause of acute decompensation [6]. Comparing baseline HRCT findings taken during the stable disease state with those obtained during acute decompensation can provide crucial insights into disease progression, superimposed inflammation, or other potential causes of decline (Figure 3). An acute exacerbation of IPF (AE-IPF) is defined as acute respiratory decompensation occurring within 30 days, with parenchymal findings of ground-glass opacities (GGOs) or consolidation on CT scans that cannot be fully explained by pulmonary edema [7,16]. Acute exacerbation of non-IPF ILD (AE-non-IPF) is less well defined but follows a similar approach, where extra-parenchymal causes of acute respiratory decompensation, such as pneumothorax and pulmonary embolism, must be ruled out [6]. The overall annual incidence of AE-non-IPF, which is 1–3% for connective tissue disease-related ILD with a nonspecific interstitial pneumonia pattern, tends to be lower compared to that of AE-IPF, which ranges from 4 to 20% [7,8].

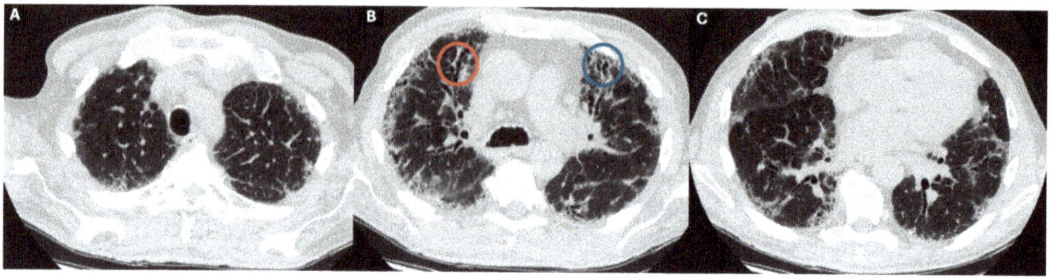

Figure 1. Chest CT images of a patient with fibrosis-predominant ILD showing honeycombing (image (**B**)), traction bronchiectasis (image (**B**)), and interstitial thickening. Image (**A–C**) show cross-sectional views of chest CT images of a patient with fibrosis-predominant ILD. Red circle shows traction bronchiectasis and blue circle shows honeycombing.

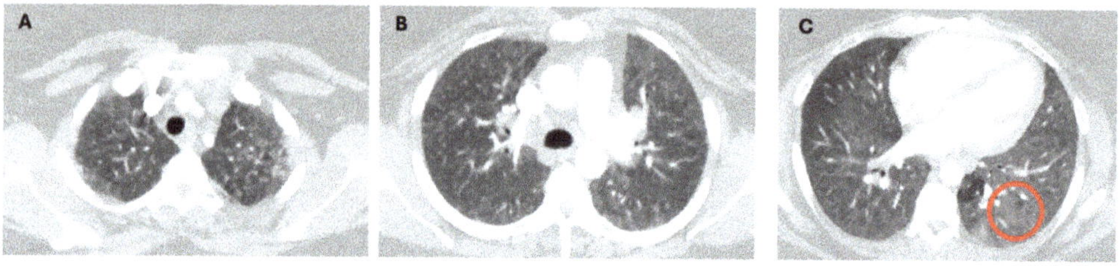

Figure 2. Chest CT images of a patient with inflammation-predominant ILD showing ground-glass opacities (image (**C**)). Image (**A–C**) show cross-sectional views of chest CT images of a patient with inflammation-predominant ILD. Red circle shows an area of ground-glass opacities.

These acute exacerbations can be triggered by various factors, such as infections, procedures, and exposure to drugs or toxins [6,7]. Patients with an identified trigger generally have better outcomes compared to those with idiopathic exacerbations, likely because the underlying cause(s) can potentially be treated [17]. Since infections are the most common trigger of AE-ILD, obtaining a sputum sample is crucial. When sputum collection is not feasible, bronchoalveolar lavage (BAL) can be considered an alternative. BAL not only allows for the evaluation of infections but also provides important insights into cellular patterns and cytology, which help narrow down the diagnosis. While BAL is commonly obtained in the outpatient setting, its role in the ICU for diagnosing infections and/or ILD is less well understood [18]. Chang et al. demonstrated that a significant number of ICU patients received a new or alternative ILD diagnosis based on BAL results [19]. Conversely, Arcadu et al. found that only a small proportion of BAL procedures yielded positive results and that the procedure was associated with a high rate of patients requiring mechanical ventilation and reintubation [20]. BAL holds significant value in diagnosing opportunistic infections, such as Pneumocystis jirovecii pneumonia (PJP), where it serves as the gold standard for diagnosis [21]. BAL can also assist in diagnosing noninfectious conditions, such as diffuse alveolar hemorrhage, which is identified by a progressively bloody return on serial aliquot administration. However, BAL is not without risks. In a study of 167 critically ill, mechanically ventilated patients who underwent bronchoscopy with BAL, post-procedural hypoxia and bronchospasm occurred in 29% and 9% of cases, respectively. Notably, only 38% had a respiratory diagnosis, and complications may be higher among ILD patients due to limited respiratory reserve [22]. The decision to perform BAL may hinge on intubation status, as it is more feasible in already intubated patients. Therefore, BAL should be used selectively, with clear diagnostic aims.

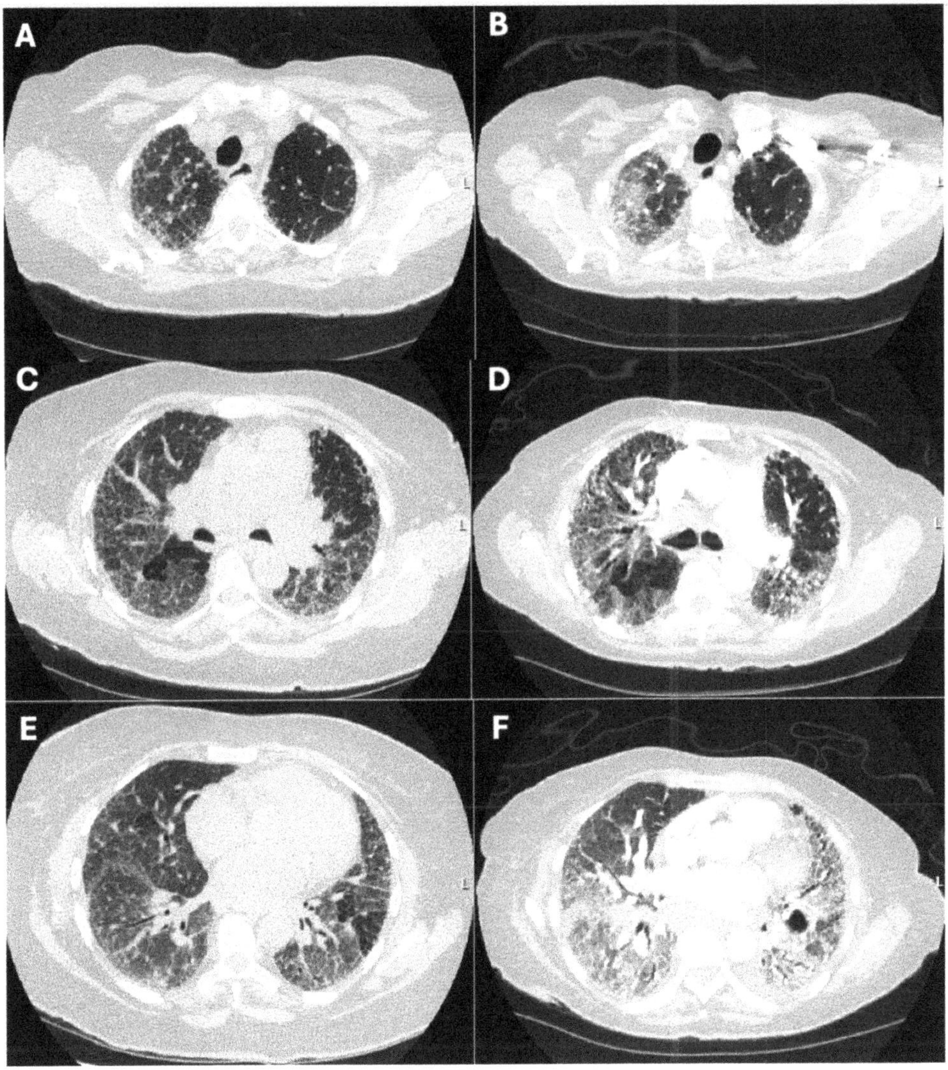

Figure 3. Chest CT images of a patient with ILD at baseline and with an acute exacerbation (a few months after). The images (**A**,**C**,**E**) show the baseline disease involving interstitial thickening, reticulations, and mosaicism, while the images (**B**,**D**,**F**) show pronounced ground-glass opacities and increased interstitial infiltrates, indicative of an exacerbation when the patient was in the ICU.

Obtaining transbronchial or surgical biopsies may be tempting but carries significant risks for patients with ILD in the ICU. Studies suggest that transbronchial biopsy has variable yield and a high complication rate. A review of 42 patients with unexplained respiratory failure (18% with ILD) who underwent transbronchial lung biopsies reported a 12.5% incidence of pneumothorax and 7.1% of significant bleeding [23,24]. Similarly, while surgical lung biopsy is associated with high mortality, it can provide significant diagnostic yield and lead to changes in management [25,26]. Additionally, as many ILDs progress to fibrosis, biopsy may not always yield meaningful information. Therefore, while biopsy has a role, it should be performed with great caution.

1.2. The Treatment of Patients with ILD in the ICU

The management of ILD in the ICU is complex, requiring careful consideration of coexisting morbidities. The backbone of treatment includes identifying and addressing the trigger for acute decompensation, assessing the need for immunosuppression, and ensuring appropriate oxygen supplementation. Special attention should be given to the patient's volume status and right heart function. When applicable, timely initiation of lung transplant evaluation and the potential use of extracorporeal membrane oxygenation (ECMO) should be considered. A multidisciplinary approach is essential to provide comprehensive care for these critically ill patients. A simplified overview of these management strategies is shown in Figure 4.

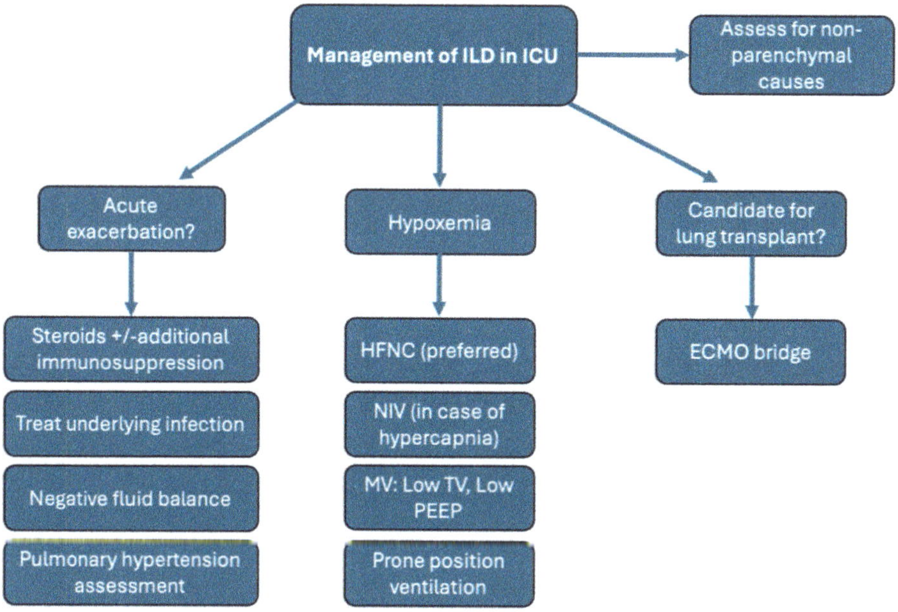

Figure 4. The management of patients with ILD in the ICU. ILD (interstitial lung disease), ICU (intensive care unit), HFNC (high-flow nasal cannula), NIV (noninvasive ventilation), MV (mechanical ventilation), TV (tidal volume), and PEEP (positive end-expiratory pressure). The flowchart outlines a comprehensive approach to managing interstitial lung disease (ILD) in the ICU. Non-parenchymal causes must be ruled out. Acute exacerbations may be managed by using corticosteroids or other immunosuppressives, and careful fluid management, along with pulmonary hypertension assessment/management. For hypoxemia, various oxygenation strategies like HFNC and mechanical ventilation are utilized, tailored to patient needs. In severe cases, candidacy for lung transplantation is considered, potentially utilizing ECMO as a bridge to transplant.

2. Immunosuppression

Corticosteroids remain the mainstay of therapy for AE-IPF. This approach is primarily based on expert opinion, as there are no large randomized controlled trials supporting its use in IPF exacerbations. Guidelines emphasize the anecdotal utility of corticosteroids and the poor prognosis associated with AE-IPF. The usual prescribed dose of corticosteroids is 0.5–1.0 mg/kg per day [3]. However, extra caution is necessary in patients with concomitant infections. Naccache et al. investigated the addition of cyclophosphamide to corticosteroids for treating AE-IPF and found that it increased 3-month all-cause mortality, although not to a statistically significant degree [27]. Observational cohort studies have explored other immunosuppressive agents, such as azathioprine, tacrolimus, rituximab with plasma exchange, and intravenous immunoglobulin (IVIG), which show mixed outcomes [28–30]. However, their true efficacy is yet to be determined, and they are not widely used in clinical practice.

There is somewhat stronger evidence for using corticosteroids in the management of acute exacerbations of non-IPF ILD. Jang et al. demonstrated that higher doses of corticosteroids (1–2 mg/kg in divided doses) improved survival in patients with non-IPF ILD compared to those with IPF [31]. Pulse-dose corticosteroids may be employed in patients with severe, rapidly progressive ILD; however, caution should be exercised.

For patients with systemic sclerosis, the Scleroderma Lung Study 1 (SLS 1) showed that cyclophosphamide was effective in improving lung function, dyspnea, and health-related quality of life among patients with systemic sclerosis who had active alveolitis [32]. Similarly, the Scleroderma Lung Study 2 (SLS 2) found that both cyclophosphamide and mycophenolate significantly improved lung function, dyspnea, and other disease parameters, with mycophenolate being better tolerated than cyclophosphamide [33]. Notably, these studies did not include acutely ill patients admitted to the ICU; however, their findings may still be relevant for patients with acute exacerbations, as the patients included in both studies exhibited signs of active ongoing lung inflammation, as evidenced by imaging. Cyclophosphamide was significantly associated with side effects, such as leukopenia, and had a shorter time to withdrawal, which may be particularly concerning for ICU patients predisposed to these adverse effects. However, there are limited data examining these immunosuppressive drugs in the intensive care setting. A small cohort study of patients with severe respiratory failure due to systemic sclerosis and ANCA-associated ILD demonstrated positive outcomes with cyclophosphamide in the ICU [34].

Among other immunosuppressive therapies, azathioprine, once commonly used, has fallen out of favor in systemic sclerosis after its inferiority to cyclophosphamide (and, by extension, mycophenolate) was shown in terms of patient outcomes, including pulmonary function [35]. Rituximab has emerged as a valuable treatment option in systemic sclerosis. The DESIRES study showed that rituximab improved lung function (FVC) in patients with systemic sclerosis, and the EVER-ILD trial found that rituximab combined with mycophenolate delayed lung function decline in patients with ILD with an inflammatory pattern [36,37]. Extrapolating these findings to critically ill patients, Keir et al. reported favorable outcomes with rituximab in a series of eight patients with ILDs associated with various connective tissue diseases [38].

Biologics, such as tocilizumab, have gained popularity over the last decade. Trials in 2016 and 2020 assessed the use of tocilizumab in systemic sclerosis and showed delayed lung function decline (secondary outcome) compared to placebo [39,40]. However, its role in the ICU during acute exacerbations remains unclear, and data in this setting are limited.

In cases of rapidly progressive non-IPF ILD, such as MDA-5 dermatomyositis-associated ILD, there are recommendations for initiating treatment with multiple immunosuppressive agents rather than using a step-up approach [41]. A case series by Matsushita et al. demonstrated remission in all patients treated with a combination of corticosteroids, tacrolimus, and cyclophosphamide [42]. Similarly, rituximab has shown favorable outcomes in patients with rapidly progressive ILD, particularly in those with anti-melanoma differentiation-associated protein 5 (MDA-5) dermatomyositis-associated ILD [43]. The use of IVIG and plasmapheresis may be considered in resistant disease states, depending on the underlying condition; for example, both IVIG and plasmaphereses have been associated with improved survival among patients with anti-MDA-5 dermatomyositis-related ILD [44,45], while plasmapheresis has also been linked to increased mortality among patients with SLE-associated DAH [46]. We agree with the approach suggested by Hallowell et al., where the authors recommend starting with a combination of corticosteroids and another immunosuppressive agent, such as mycophenolate, azathioprine, or tacrolimus, along with IVIG upfront, with the consideration of plasmapheresis in cases where the disease remains refractory, for rapidly progressive ILD with severe symptoms [47].

Another important setting where immunosuppression plays a crucial role is in managing DAH, a significant and often severe complication of inflammatory ILD. High-dose steroids are commonly employed to target the inflammatory component, although their effectiveness in critically ill patients remains uncertain [48,49]. Other immunosuppressive agents, such as rituximab, offer an alternative for refractory cases, with studies showing effectiveness in reducing autoantibody production and controlling disease activity [50]. Plasmapheresis may also be used as adjunctive therapy, particularly in autoimmune conditions, though evidence on its long-term benefit remains limited [51].

3. Oxygenation and Ventilation Strategies

Patients with ILD are often hospitalized with respiratory complaints, with hypoxemia being the most common presenting sign [5]. These patients often require increasing amounts of supplemental oxygen to maintain oxygenation, including high-flow nasal cannula (HFNC), noninvasive ventilation (NIV), or mechanical ventilation (MV), necessitating ICU stay.

3.1. High-Flow Nasal Cannula (HFNC)

High-flow nasal oxygen provides high flows of noninvasive oxygenation, with FiO_2 potentially reaching 100%. It also offers the added advantages of a small amount of PEEP and a more comfortable interface [2]. Koyauchi et al. demonstrated that HFNC is effective in improving oxygenation in patients with ILD [52].

3.2. Noninvasive Ventilation (NIV)

Noninvasive ventilation is associated with reduced mortality and shorter hospital stays among patients with COPD [53]. However, limited data are available on its utility in ILD patients. Positive end-expiratory pressure (PEEP) in NIV is expected to improve oxygenation, while bilevel pressure assists with ventilation, which could be beneficial for ILD patients experiencing hypoxia and hypercapnia [54]. A meta-analysis by Sanguanwong et al. showed that NIV significantly improved oxygenation, as evidenced by higher P/F ratios compared to conventional oxygenation therapy [55]. It is important to note that there was no difference in survival between patients receiving NIV and those receiving invasive ventilation [56].

A few studies directly comparing NIV to HFNC have shown that NIV improves the P/F ratio more effectively [52,57,58]. However, there was no difference in mortality or the need for invasive ventilation between the two methods [52,57–59].

3.3. Mechanical Ventilation (MV)

Patients with ILD are at high risk of respiratory decompensation, which often necessitates MV [60]. While mechanical ventilation is frequently used as a rescue strategy in severe respiratory failure, it is associated with high mortality rates among ILD patients. Mollica et al. demonstrated that all patients with IPF who required MV died within the same hospitalization [56]. The high mortality was shown again by Martin et al., who reported a 75% mortality rate among fibrosis-predominant ILD patients requiring MV [60]. MV-related predictors of in-hospital mortality include the inability to achieve early targeted plateau pressure ($\geq$30 cm H_2O), severe hypoxemia as suggested by a reduced P/F ratio and high initial FiO_2, and high initial mean airway pressures [60]. However, a recent study by Matsunashi et al. demonstrated a 54% survival rate among patients with fibrosis-predominant ILD who required invasive mechanical ventilation. Although this study had a small sample size, the results suggest that improved ventilatory techniques may help mitigate complications such as barotrauma and volutrauma, potentially enhancing survival outcomes [61].

To avoid ventilator-induced lung injury, various aspects of respiratory physiology must be carefully considered. In patients with pulmonary fibrosis, an imbalance between collagen and elastin deposition in the extracellular matrix leads to increased collagen accumulation, making the lungs stiffer and less compliant in areas affected by fibroblastic foci [62]. Although low tidal volume ventilation (6 mL/kg) has been a cornerstone in managing acute respiratory distress syndrome (ARDS) due to its association with decreased mortality, less is known about the optimal ventilatory strategy for patients with ILD [63]. Nonetheless, experts recommend using low tidal volumes to prevent barotrauma and minimize the proinflammatory effects of lung overstretching, which can lead to the accumulation of inflammatory cells and the release of cytokines and chemokines that exacerbate lung injury [62,64,65].

In contrast to the approach for ARDS, where high positive end-expiratory pressure (PEEP) is used to improve oxygenation and keep alveoli open, high PEEP may not be suitable for ILD patients. Unlike ARDS, ILD patients may not have recruitable alveolar units [64]. In fact, some retrospective studies have linked high PEEP with increased mortality in patients with ILD [66]. There is a theoretical risk of pneumothorax in ILD patients due to high PEEP, resulting from reduced elastance in the non-recruitable lung units and overdistension of the normal lung units, though data supporting this risk are limited.

3.4. Prone Position Ventilation

Prone position ventilation is a well-established tool in the management of ARDS, with robust evidence demonstrating improvement in oxygenation and 30-day mortality [67]. However, its utility in ILD patients remains less clear. Lung mechanics in ILD differ from those in ARDS, with reduced compliance due to fibrosis, which limits the recruiting ability of the alveolar units in the prone position. Despite this, limited studies have explored prone positioning in ILD populations. Xu et al. demonstrated that prone position ventilation improved oxygenation and hemodynamics in ILD patients, suggesting potential benefits even in this distinct group [68].

3.5. Suggested Approach to Respiratory Support

In our opinion, when managing a patient with ILD and acute hypoxic respiratory failure, the best initial step is to employ HFNC. This method offers high FiO_2 and flow rates (resulting in a small amount of PEEP), while being generally well tolerated and presenting a lower risk of complications like pneumothorax. For patients who remain hypoxemic or exhibit significant hypercapnia despite HFNC, we believe a trial of NIV is reasonable.

The decision to proceed with intubation is complex and should be individualized based on the specific ILD subtype. Given the particularly poor outcomes associated with mechanical ventilation in IPF, we agree with guidelines recommending against intubation in these patients when clinical judgment indicates minimal chances of recovery and the patient is not a candidate for transplantation. This further highlights the importance of early discussions around goals of care, ideally while the patient can still participate in decision-making.

That being said, in cases where a reversible cause of exacerbation is identified, intubation and mechanical ventilation may serve as supportive measures while targeted therapies are given time to take effect. In such instances, we suggest using low tidal volumes and low PEEP, recognizing the non-recruitable nature of ILD lungs. However, in select cases with evidence of recruitable lung units, a higher PEEP may be cautiously considered, though careful monitoring is essential to avoid complications such as barotrauma.

4. Other Interventions and Supportive Care

Managing ILD in the ICU requires comprehensive supportive measures tailored to their complex needs. Key interventions include antibiotic and antifibrotic therapies, fluid management, and strategies for managing pulmonary hypertension. Additionally, the role of ECMO and urgent consideration for lung transplantation are essential, highlighting the importance of a multidisciplinary approach in optimizing patient outcomes.

4.1. Antibiotic Therapy

Empiric antibiotics are routinely initiated in critically ill ILD patients while awaiting culture results. This is particularly important for patients who are starting high-dose corticosteroids or other immunosuppressive therapies, as these treatments increase the risk of superimposed infections. The choice of antibiotics may be informed by prior culture and sensitivity data, as well as pre-existing comorbid conditions. Careful selection of antibiotics is particularly crucial in non-IPF ILD patients who may be on chronic immunosuppressives, as they are at an increased risk of opportunistic infections [9,16]. In particular, PJP pneumonia must be considered. A review of patients with rheumatoid arthritis-associated ILD on biologic therapies revealed a high incidence of PJP, affecting 50% of the 26 patients examined [69]. Notably, PJP can present with imaging findings that mimic ILD exacerbations, making it essential to include PJP in the differential diagnosis for all ILD patients, especially those on chronic immunosuppressives. Obtaining a BAL sample, or sputum if BAL is not feasible, is critical for diagnosis. In cases where there is a delay in testing and clinical suspicion is high, empirical treatment for PJP should be initiated without waiting for confirmatory results [19,21].

Clinicians should also be aware of potential chronic or atypical infections, such as Aspergillus and non-tuberculous mycobacteria, which may require empirical treatment, especially when heavy immunosuppression is used, as these infections can lead to fulminant disease [70].

4.2. Antifibrotic Therapy

Antifibrotics have been shown to reduce the rate of lung function decline in both IPF and non-IPF ILD [71–73]. Data also demonstrate their effectiveness in reducing the rates of acute exacerbations [74]. However, these medications primarily serve a preventive function, and there are currently little to no recommendations for initiating antifibrotic therapy in patients experiencing an acute exacerbation in the ICU [75].

4.3. Fluid Management

The importance of maintaining a net negative or neutral fluid balance in patients with AE-ILD is being increasingly recognized [12]. Overall fluid status has also been identified as a predictor of mortality in ventilated patients with AE-ILD [6,60]. Aggressive fluid management is also essential in the management of concomitant pulmonary hypertension as right ventricular (RV) offloading may be necessary in cases of RV failure [76].

4.4. Management of Concomitant Pulmonary Hypertension

Patients with severe ILD often have concomitant pulmonary hypertension. These patients may present with signs of RV failure as their initial presentation or develop RV failure during their ICU stay [77]. The signs of RV failure are often nonspecific, such as severe hypoxemia and hypotension, and can be confused with other potential etiologies, leading to delays in diagnosis and management. Frequent echocardiographic assessments and a high index of suspicion are required, as these patients can deteriorate rapidly [76] (Figure 5). Pulmonary hypertension is associated with a poor prognosis among patients with ILD and can be particularly detrimental when coupled with RV failure in the ICU [78–81].

Managing acute RV failure in these patients is challenging due to the pressure-sensitive nature of RV failure. Treatment may include inhaled vasodilators such as nitric oxide or epoprostenol to induce vasodilation in the ventilated units of the lungs [82,83]. Intravenous vasodilators should be used cautiously, as they can worsen ventilation/perfusion mismatch, potentially leading to worsening hypoxemia [84,85]. In terms of ventilatory strategies, high PEEP should be avoided, as it can increase intrathoracic pressure and reduce RV preload. For patients who do not respond to less invasive supportive interventions, mechanical circulatory support devices, such as veno-arterial ECMO and RV Impella, may be considered in severe cases [76].

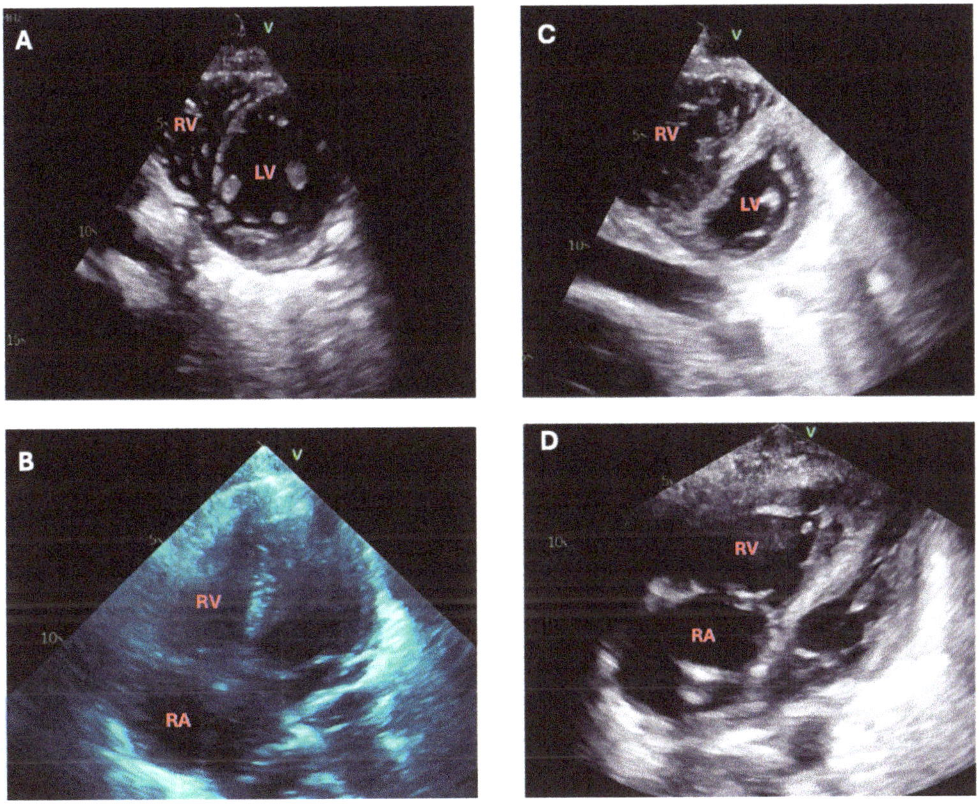

Figure 5. Echocardiographic images from a patient with rapidly progressive interstitial lung disease admitted to the ICU. Images (**A**,**B**), taken at initial presentation, show a normal right ventricle (RV), left ventricle (LV), and right atrium (RA). Five days later, repeat imaging reveals acute right ventricular dilation in both the parasternal short-axis (image (**C**)) and apical 4-chamber (image (**D**)) views, consistent with rapid development of right ventricular failure in the setting of ILD exacerbation.

4.5. Extracorporeal Membrane Oxygenation (ECMO)

In recent years, the emergence and increasing use of ECMO has revolutionized the management of respiratory failure in the ICU. In the context of ILD, ECMO offers a potential modality to support oxygenation and gas exchange while allowing for 'lung rest' and offering a bridge for patients awaiting lung transplantation or undergoing urgent transplant evaluation when outpatient assessment is not possible [86]. Studies have shown that ECMO is associated with high mortality in patients who are not eligible for lung transplantation compared to those eligible for transplantation. For patients on ECMO as a bridge to transplantation, survival rates are comparable to critically ill pre-transplant patients not requiring ECMO. Additionally, patients who underwent urgent transplant evaluation and listing while on ECMO had similar long-term survival and allograft function to those listed as outpatients [86–88]. Although ECMO has opened new avenues for managing patients with end-stage ILD, it carries serious complications; therefore, its use should be individualized and based on thorough, patient-centric multidisciplinary discussions.

4.6. Lung Transplantation

ILD is the leading indication for lung transplantation, which may be the only salvage option for advanced ILD patients. Typically, lung transplantation evaluation and workup are completed in the outpatient setting. However, in some cases, patients admitted to the ICU with advanced fibrosis may need urgent evaluation for transplantation. Several relative and absolute contraindications to lung transplantation are particularly relevant for ICU patients, including multiorgan failure, sepsis, and a glomerular filtration rate (GFR) <60 mL/min/1.73 m^2 [89].

A single-center study by Dotan et al. showed that patients with *an acute exacerbation of IPF (already listed)* who underwent transplantation had worse short- and long-term survival compared to patients with stable IPF (1-year and 3-year survival rates of 94% and 90% for stable IPF vs. 71% and 60% for patients who were transplanted during AE-IPF) [90]. In contrast, a large study by Tang et al. found that patients who were *urgently listed* for lung transplantation—75% of whom had *restrictive lung disease*—had similar outcomes to those listed electively (1-year survival of 75% in the elective group vs. 78% in the urgent group) [91]. These findings suggest a hopeful outlook for patients who may otherwise have no salvageable treatment options. It also reflects improvements in our ability to provide advanced life support through mechanical ventilation, pulmonary vasodilators, and ECMO, enabling us to sustain critically ill patients longer and facilitate their eligibility for transplantation.

Despite these advancements, contraindications such as multiorgan failure, poor functional status, and the inability to participate in rehabilitation remain crucial factors when considering lung transplantation in ICU patients [92]. Aggressive efforts are being made to improve the nutrition and functional status of patients who are being considered for or are listed for lung transplantation; however, these interventions lack specific evidence supporting their effectiveness.

4.7. Multidisciplinary Approach

The management of patients with ILD requires the involvement of multiple specialists and services. Rheumatologists play a crucial role in diagnosing new cases of connective tissue disease-related ILD and in navigating the complex decisions regarding the administration and choice of immunosuppressive agents. Castelino et al. demonstrated that, with rheumatology input, one-third of patients in the ICU received a CTD diagnosis different from their initial referral diagnosis [93].

Similarly, palliative care is vital for patients with advanced ILD who often suffer from debilitating symptoms such as severe dyspnea, fatigue, and cough, as well as psychosocial distress due to their progressive and life-limiting condition. These patients also face high ICU-related mortality, particularly during acute exacerbations. Palliative care in ILD goes beyond end-of-life care; it involves the early management of symptoms, discussions about goals of care, and psychosocial support for both patients and their families. This is particularly important for those newly diagnosed with ILD in the ICU who may face overwhelming emotional and physical challenges. Studies have shown that early integration of palliative care into the treatment plan of patients with ILD in an outpatient setting improves symptom control, enhances quality of life, and facilitates advanced care planning, leading to better alignment between patient wishes and the care they receive [94].

Early palliative care involvement can also help in navigating challenging decisions if patients become critically ill, such as the appropriateness of invasive therapies like mechanical ventilation or ECMO in patients with advanced ILD. For example, in patients with progressive ILD, timely conversations around the goals of care can prevent unwanted interventions and focus on comfort-oriented measures if they need hospitalization or ICU stay.

5. Prognosis

Several studies have shown that patients with ILD requiring ICU admission face high mortality rates [2,87,95]. A systematic review by Huapaya et al. found that IPF is associated with higher mortality in the ICU setting compared to other forms of ILD [96]. Specifically, in-hospital mortality for IPF was 79% between 1993 and 2004, which decreased to 65% in 2005–2017. In contrast, non-IPF ILD patients had lower, yet still high, mortality rates of 62% in 2001–2009, which dropped to 48% in 2010–2017. This decline is attributed to the development of antifibrotic therapies, improved understanding and application of immunosuppressives, increased use of CT imaging for better diagnosis and characterization of ILD subtypes, advances in ICU management strategies, and the availability of ECMO and lung transplantation. Despite this decline in mortality, the prognosis remains poor and overall mortality remains high, along with high morbidity. Additionally, evidence suggests that patients with IPF who survive ICU admission often die within a few months after hospital discharge, indicating a high out-of-hospital mortality rate [97]. Mechanical ventilation and hypoxia during hospitalization were identified as risk factors regardless of the type of ILD [96,97].

6. Future Directions

A significant gap remains in our understanding of the management of ILD, particularly in the ICU setting, highlighting the need for further investigation and an individualized, evidence-based medical approach. Looking ahead, ongoing prospective randomized controlled trials, such as STRIVE-IPF [NCT03286556] and EXCHANGE_IPF (NCT03584802), are exploring the efficacy and safety of combination therapy involving plasma exchange, IVIG, and rituximab for managing AE-IPF. Another trial, EXAFIP2 (NCT05674994), is comparing the use of glucocorticoids with placebo in AE-IPF, while NCT05842681 is examining the use of azithromycin in this context. In addition to the ongoing work on management strategies, the REACT (NCT06445686) and IERATIC (NCT05313672) trials are investigating patient hemodynamics before and after an exacerbation and respiratory mechanics in patients with AE-IPF.

Furthermore, there is a growing interest in identifying biomarkers to more reliably characterize acute exacerbations across various ILDs. Biomarkers related to alveolar epithelial cells, fibroproliferation, and immune molecules are being investigated to improve our understanding of these acute events and potentially refine treatment strategies [98].

These future studies are crucial for expanding our knowledge of ILD management in the ICU, and they hold the potential to significantly improve patient outcomes.

7. Conclusions

Managing patients with ILD in the ICU setting requires a nuanced and multifaceted approach due to the complexity of the disease and its associated complications. Accurate diagnosis relies heavily on imaging and thorough investigations. Treatment often involves a combination of corticosteroids, cautious use of other immunosuppressive agents, and careful application of oxygenation and ventilation strategies, as well supportive ICU care. The role of multidisciplinary care, including rheumatologists and palliative care teams, is crucial in optimizing patient outcomes. For patients with advanced disease, urgent evaluation for lung transplantation, possibly with ECMO support, may be considered a lifesaving intervention. Despite advancements in life support and management strategies, the high mortality rates among patients with ILD in the ICU underscore the need for ongoing research and tailored interventions.

Funding: This research received no external funding.

Conflicts of Interest: This research received no external funding. R.G. has had research grants, been a consultant/speaker for Kinevant, Mallinckrodt, ANI, and United Therapeutics.

References

1. Adegunsoye, A.; Ryerson, C.J. Diagnostic Classification of Interstitial Lung Disease in Clinical Practice. *Clin. Chest Med.* **2021**, *42*, 251–261. [CrossRef] [PubMed]
2. Krishnan, A.; Janz, D.R.; Lammi, M.R. ICU Management of the Patient with Fibrotic Interstitial Lung Disease. *CHEST Crit. Care* **2023**, *1*, 100020. [CrossRef]
3. Raghu, G.; Remy-Jardin, M.; Richeldi, L.; Thomson, C.C.; Inoue, Y.; Johkoh, T.; Kreuter, M.; Lynch, D.A.; Maher, T.M.; Martinez, F.J.; et al. Idiopathic Pulmonary Fibrosis (an Update) and Progressive Pulmonary Fibrosis in Adults: An Official ATS/ERS/JRS/ALAT Clinical Practice Guideline. *Am. J. Respir. Crit. Care Med.* **2022**, *205*, e18–e47. [CrossRef] [PubMed]
4. Tsubouchi, K.; Hamada, N.; Tokunaga, S.; Ichiki, K.; Takata, S.; Ishii, H.; Kitasato, Y.; Okamoto, M.; Kawakami, S.; Yatera, K.; et al. Survival and acute exacerbation for patients with idiopathic pulmonary fibrosis (IPF) or non-IPF idiopathic interstitial pneumonias: 5-year follow-up analysis of a prospective multi-institutional patient registry. *BMJ Open Respir. Res.* **2023**, *10*, e001864. [CrossRef] [PubMed]
5. Kim, H.J.; Snyder, L.D.; Adegunsoye, A.; Neely, M.L.; Bender, S.; White, E.S.; Conoscenti, C.S.; Strek, M.E. IPF-PRO Registry Investigators Hospitalizations in patients with idiopathic pulmonary fibrosis. *Respir. Res.* **2021**, *22*, 257. [CrossRef]
6. Charokopos, A.; Moua, T.; Ryu, J.H.; Smischney, N.J. Acute exacerbation of interstitial lung disease in the intensive care unit. *World J. Crit. Care Med.* **2022**, *11*, 22–32. [CrossRef]
7. Collard, H.R.; Ryerson, C.J.; Corte, T.J.; Jenkins, G.; Kondoh, Y.; Lederer, D.J.; Lee, J.S.; Maher, T.M.; Wells, A.U.; Antoniou, K.M.; et al. Acute Exacerbation of Idiopathic Pulmonary Fibrosis. An International Working Group Report. *Am. J. Respir. Crit. Care Med.* **2016**, *194*, 265–275. [CrossRef]
8. Leuschner, G.; Behr, J. Acute Exacerbation in Interstitial Lung Disease. *Front. Med.* **2017**, *4*, 176. [CrossRef]
9. Suzuki, A.; Kondoh, Y.; Brown, K.K.; Johkoh, T.; Kataoka, K.; Fukuoka, J.; Kimura, T.; Matsuda, T.; Yokoyama, T.; Fukihara, J.; et al. Acute exacerbations of fibrotic interstitial lung diseases. *Respirology* **2020**, *25*, 525–534. [CrossRef]
10. Alhamad, E.H.; Cal, J.G.; Alrajhi, N.N.; AlBoukai, A.A. Acute exacerbation in interstitial lung disease. *Ann. Thorac. Med.* **2021**, *16*, 178–187. [CrossRef]
11. Xie, M.; Zhu, C.; Ye, Y. Incidence, risk factors, and prognosis of acute exacerbation of rheumatoid arthritis-associated interstitial lung disease: A systematic review and meta-analysis. *BMC Pulm. Med.* **2023**, *23*, 255. [CrossRef] [PubMed]
12. Azadeh, N.; Moua, T.; Baqir, M.; Ryu, J.H. Treatment of acute exacerbations of interstitial lung disease. *Expert Rev. Respir. Med.* **2018**, *12*, 309–313. [CrossRef] [PubMed]
13. Solomon, J.J.; Fischer, A. Connective Tissue Disease-Associated Interstitial Lung Disease: A Focused Review. *J. Intensive Care Med.* **2015**, *30*, 392–400. [CrossRef] [PubMed]
14. Miller, W.T.; Shah, R.M. Isolated Diffuse Ground-Glass Opacity in Thoracic CT: Causes and Clinical Presentations. *Am. J. Roentgenol.* **2005**, *184*, 613–622. [CrossRef] [PubMed]
15. Furini, F.; Carnevale, A.; Casoni, G.L.; Guerrini, G.; Cavagna, L.; Govoni, M.; Sciré, C.A. The Role of the Multidisciplinary Evaluation of Interstitial Lung Diseases: Systematic Literature Review of the Current Evidence and Future Perspectives. *Front. Med.* **2019**, *6*, 246. [CrossRef] [PubMed]
16. Collard, H.R.; Moore, B.B.; Flaherty, K.R.; Brown, K.K.; Kaner, R.J.; King, T.E.; Lasky, J.A.; Loyd, J.E.; Noth, I.; Olman, M.A.; et al. Acute Exacerbations of Idiopathic Pulmonary Fibrosis. *Am. J. Respir. Crit. Care Med.* **2007**, *176*, 636–643. [CrossRef] [PubMed]
17. Moua, T.; Westerly, B.D.; Dulohery, M.M.; Daniels, C.E.; Ryu, J.H.; Lim, K.G. Patients with Fibrotic Interstitial Lung Disease Hospitalized for Acute Respiratory Worsening. *Chest* **2016**, *149*, 1205–1214. [CrossRef]
18. Molyneaux, P.L.; Smith, J.J.; Saunders, P.; Chua, F.; Wells, A.U.; Renzoni, E.A.; Nicholson, A.G.; Fahy, W.A.; Jenkins, R.G.; Maher, T.M. BAL Is Safe and Well Tolerated in Individuals with Idiopathic Pulmonary Fibrosis: An Analysis of the PROFILE Study. *Am. J. Respir. Crit. Care Med.* **2021**, *203*, 136–139. [CrossRef] [PubMed]
19. Chang, S.-L.; Tsai, H.-C.; Lin, F.-C.; Chao, H.-S.; Chou, C.-W.; Chang, S.-C. Clinical usefulness of bronchoalveolar lavage in patients with interstitial lung diseases: A pilot study. *J. Thorac. Dis.* **2020**, *12*, 3125–3134. [CrossRef]
20. Arcadu, A.; Moua, T. Bronchoscopy assessment of acute respiratory failure in interstitial lung disease. *Respirology* **2017**, *22*, 352–359. [CrossRef]
21. Ibrahim, A.; Chattaraj, A.; Iqbal, Q.; Anjum, A.; Rehman, M.E.U.; Aijaz, Z.; Nasir, F.; Ansar, S.; Zangeneh, T.T.; Iftikhar, A. Pneumocystis jiroveci Pneumonia: A Review of Management in Human Immunodeficiency Virus (HIV) and Non-HIV Immunocompromised Patients. *Avicenna J. Med.* **2023**, *13*, 23–34. [CrossRef] [PubMed]
22. Schnabel, R.M.; van der Velden, K.; Osinski, A.; Rohde, G.; Roekaerts, P.M.H.J.; Bergmans, D.C.J.J. Clinical course and complications following diagnostic bronchoalveolar lavage in critically ill mechanically ventilated patients. *BMC Pulm. Med.* **2015**, *15*, 107. [CrossRef]
23. Ghiani, A.; Neurohr, C. Diagnostic yield, safety, and impact of transbronchial lung biopsy in mechanically ventilated, critically ill patients: A retrospective study. *BMC Pulm. Med.* **2021**, *21*, 15. [CrossRef] [PubMed]
24. Helgeson, S.A.; Imam, J.S.; Burnside, R.C.; Fernandez-Bussy, S.; Brigham, T.J.; Patel, N.M. Transbronchial Forceps Biopsy in the Intensive Care Unit: A Systematic Review and Meta-analysis. *J. Bronchol. Interv. Pulmonol.* **2021**, *28*, 281–289. [CrossRef] [PubMed]

25. Donaldson, L.H.; Gill, A.J.; Hibbert, M. Utility of surgical lung biopsy in critically ill patients with diffuse pulmonary infiltrates: A retrospective review. *Intern. Med. J.* **2016**, *46*, 1306–1310. [CrossRef] [PubMed]
26. Almotairi, A.; Biswas, S.; Shahin, J. The Role of Open Lung Biopsy in Critically Ill Patients with Hypoxic Respiratory Failure: A Retrospective Cohort Study. *Can. Respir. J.* **2016**, *2016*, 1–8. [CrossRef]
27. Naccache, J.-M.; Jouneau, S.; Didier, M.; Borie, R.; Cachanado, M.; Bourdin, A.; Reynaud-Gaubert, M.; Bonniaud, P.; Israël-Biet, D.; Prévot, G.; et al. Cyclophosphamide added to glucocorticoids in acute exacerbation of idiopathic pulmonary fibrosis (EXAFIP): A randomised, double-blind, placebo-controlled, phase 3 trial. *Lancet Respir. Med.* **2022**, *10*, 26–34. [CrossRef]
28. Horita, N.; Akahane, M.; Okada, Y.; Kobayashi, Y.; Arai, T.; Amano, I.; Takezawa, T.; To, M.; To, Y. Tacrolimus and Steroid Treatment for Acute Exacerbation of Idiopathic Pulmonary Fibrosis. *Intern. Med.* **2011**, *50*, 189–195. [CrossRef]
29. Sakamoto, S.; Homma, S.; Miyamoto, A.; Kurosaki, A.; Fujii, T.; Yoshimura, K. Cyclosporin A in the Treatment of Acute Exacerbation of Idiopathic Pulmonary Fibrosis. *Intern. Med.* **2010**, *49*, 109–115. [CrossRef]
30. Donahoe, M.; Valentine, V.G.; Chien, N.; Gibson, K.F.; Raval, J.S.; Saul, M.; Xue, J.; Zhang, Y.; Duncan, S.R. Correction: Autoantibody-Targeted Treatments for Acute Exacerbations of Idiopathic Pulmonary Fibrosis. *PLoS ONE* **2015**, *10*, e0133684. [CrossRef]
31. Jang, H.J.; Yong, S.H.; Leem, A.Y.; Lee, S.H.; Kim, S.Y.; Lee, S.H.; Kim, E.Y.; Chung, K.S.; Jung, J.Y.; Kang, Y.A.; et al. Corticosteroid responsiveness in patients with acute exacerbation of interstitial lung disease admitted to the emergency department. *Sci. Rep.* **2021**, *11*, 5762. [CrossRef] [PubMed]
32. Tashkin, D.P.; Elashoff, R.; Clements, P.J.; Goldin, J.; Roth, M.D.; Furst, D.E.; Arriola, E.; Silver, R.; Strange, C.; Bolster, M.; et al. Cyclophosphamide versus Placebo in Scleroderma Lung Disease. *N. Engl. J. Med.* **2006**, *354*, 2655–2666. [CrossRef] [PubMed]
33. Tashkin, D.P.; Roth, M.D.; Clements, P.J.; Furst, D.E.; Khanna, D.; Kleerup, E.C.; Goldin, J.; Arriola, E.; Volkmann, E.R.; Kafaja, S.; et al. Mycophenolate mofetil versus oral cyclophosphamide in scleroderma-related interstitial lung disease (SLS II): A randomised controlled, double-blind, parallel group trial. *Lancet Respir. Med.* **2016**, *4*, 708–719. [CrossRef] [PubMed]
34. Schulze, A.B.; Evers, G.; Kümmel, A.; Rosenow, F.; Sackarnd, J.; Hering, J.P.; Schülke, C.; Engelbertz, J.A.; Görlich, D.; Barth, P.J.; et al. Cyclophosphamide pulse therapy as treatment for severe interstitial lung diseases. *Sarcoidosis Vasc. Diffuse Lung Dis.* **2019**, *36*, 157–166. [CrossRef]
35. Nadashkevich, O.; Davis, P.; Fritzler, M.; Kovalenko, W. A randomized unblinded trial of cyclophosphamide versus azathioprine in the treatment of systemic sclerosis. *Clin. Rheumatol.* **2006**, *25*, 205–212. [CrossRef]
36. Mankikian, J.; Caille, A.; Reynaud-Gaubert, M.; Agier, M.-S.; Bermudez, J.; Bonniaud, P.; Borie, R.; Brillet, P.-Y.; Cadranel, J.; Court-Fortune, I.; et al. Rituximab and mycophenolate mofetil combination in patients with interstitial lung disease (EVER-ILD): A double-blind, randomised, placebo-controlled trial. *Eur. Respir. J.* **2023**, *61*, 2202071. [CrossRef]
37. Ebata, S.; Yoshizaki, A.; Oba, K.; Kashiwabara, K.; Ueda, K.; Uemura, Y.; Watadani, T.; Fukasawa, T.; Miura, S.; Yoshizaki-Ogawa, A.; et al. Safety and efficacy of rituximab in systemic sclerosis (DESIRES): A double-blind, investigator-initiated, randomised, placebo-controlled trial. *Lancet Rheumatol.* **2021**, *3*, e489–e497. [CrossRef]
38. Keir, G.J.; Maher, T.M.; Hansell, D.M.; Denton, C.P.; Ong, V.H.; Singh, S.; Wells, A.U.; Renzoni, E.A. Severe interstitial lung disease in connective tissue disease: Rituximab as rescue therapy. *Eur. Respir. J.* **2012**, *40*, 641–648. [CrossRef]
39. Khanna, D.; Lin, C.J.F.; Furst, D.E.; Goldin, J.; Kim, G.; Kuwana, M.; Allanore, Y.; Matucci-Cerinic, M.; Distler, O.; Shima, Y.; et al. Tocilizumab in systemic sclerosis: A randomised, double-blind, placebo-controlled, phase 3 trial. *Lancet Respir. Med.* **2020**, *8*, 963–974. [CrossRef]
40. Khanna, D.; Denton, C.P.; Jahreis, A.; Van Laar, J.M.; Frech, T.M.; Anderson, M.E.; Baron, M.; Chung, L.; Fierlbeck, G.; Lakshminarayanan, S.; et al. Safety and efficacy of subcutaneous tocilizumab in adults with systemic sclerosis (faSScinate): A phase 2, randomised, controlled trial. *Lancet* **2016**, *387*, 2630–2640. [CrossRef]
41. Romero-Bueno, F.; Diaz Del Campo, P.; Trallero-Araguás, E.; Ruiz-Rodríguez, J.C.; Castellvi, I.; Rodriguez-Nieto, M.J.; Martínez-Becerra, M.J.; Sanchez-Pernaute, O.; Pinal-Fernandez, I.; Solanich, X.; et al. Recommendations for the treatment of anti-melanoma differentiation-associated gene 5-positive dermatomyositis-associated rapidly progressive interstitial lung disease. *Semin. Arthritis Rheum.* **2020**, *50*, 776–790. [CrossRef] [PubMed]
42. Matsushita, T.; Mizumaki, K.; Kano, M.; Yagi, N.; Tennichi, M.; Takeuchi, A.; Okamoto, Y.; Hamaguchi, Y.; Murakami, A.; Hasegawa, M.; et al. Antimelanoma differentiation-associated protein 5 antibody level is a novel tool for monitoring disease activity in rapidly progressive interstitial lung disease with dermatomyositis. *Br. J. Dermatol.* **2017**, *176*, 395–402. [CrossRef] [PubMed]
43. Ge, Y.; Li, S.; Tian, X.; He, L.; Lu, X.; Wang, G. Anti-melanoma differentiation-associated gene 5 (MDA5) antibody-positive dermatomyositis responds to rituximab therapy. *Clin. Rheumatol.* **2021**, *40*, 2311–2317. [CrossRef] [PubMed]
44. Shirakashi, M.; Nakashima, R.; Tsuji, H.; Tanizawa, K.; Handa, T.; Hosono, Y.; Akizuki, S.; Murakami, K.; Hashimoto, M.; Yoshifuji, H.; et al. Efficacy of plasma exchange in anti-MDA5-positive dermatomyositis with interstitial lung disease under combined immunosuppressive treatment. *Rheumatology* **2020**, *59*, 3284–3292. [CrossRef] [PubMed]
45. Wang, L.-M.; Yang, Q.-H.; Zhang, L.; Liu, S.-Y.; Zhang, P.-P.; Zhang, X.; Liu, X.-J.; Han, L.-S.; Li, T.-F. Intravenous immunoglobulin for interstitial lung diseases of anti-melanoma differentiation-associated gene 5-positive dermatomyositis. *Rheumatology* **2022**, *61*, 3704–3710. [CrossRef] [PubMed]

46. Jiang, M.; Chen, R.; Zhao, L.; Zhang, X. Risk factors for mortality of diffuse alveolar hemorrhage in systemic lupus erythematosus: A systematic review and meta-analysis. *Arthritis Res. Ther.* **2021**, *23*, 57. [CrossRef]
47. Hallowell, R.W.; Danoff, S.K. Diagnosis and Management of Myositis-Associated Lung Disease. *Chest* **2023**, *163*, 1476–1491. [CrossRef]
48. Park, J.A. Treatment of Diffuse Alveolar Hemorrhage: Controlling Inflammation and Obtaining Rapid and Effective Hemostasis. *Int. J. Mol. Sci.* **2021**, *22*, 793. [CrossRef]
49. Newsome, B.R.; Morales, J.E. Diffuse Alveolar Hemorrhage. *South. Med. J.* **2011**, *104*, 269–274. [CrossRef]
50. Stone, J.H.; Merkel, P.A.; Spiera, R.; Seo, P.; Langford, C.A.; Hoffman, G.S.; Kallenberg, C.G.M.; St. Clair, E.W.; Turkiewicz, A.; Tchao, N.K.; et al. Rituximab versus Cyclophosphamide for ANCA-Associated Vasculitis. *N. Engl. J. Med.* **2010**, *363*, 221–232. [CrossRef] [PubMed]
51. Klemmer, P.J.; Chalermskulrat, W.; Reif, M.S.; Hogan, S.L.; Henke, D.C.; Falk, R.J. Plasmapheresis therapy for diffuse alveolar hemorrhage in patients with small-vessel vasculitis. *Am. J. Kidney Dis.* **2003**, *42*, 1149–1153. [CrossRef] [PubMed]
52. Koyauchi, T.; Hasegawa, H.; Kanata, K.; Kakutani, T.; Amano, Y.; Ozawa, Y.; Matsui, T.; Yokomura, K.; Suda, T. Efficacy and Tolerability of High-Flow Nasal Cannula Oxygen Therapy for Hypoxemic Respiratory Failure in Patients with Interstitial Lung Disease with Do-Not-Intubate Orders: A Retrospective Single-Center Study. *Respiration* **2018**, *96*, 323–329. [CrossRef] [PubMed]
53. Lindenauer, P.K.; Stefan, M.S.; Shieh, M.-S.; Pekow, P.S.; Rothberg, M.B.; Hill, N.S. Outcomes Associated with Invasive and Noninvasive Ventilation Among Patients Hospitalized With Exacerbations of Chronic Obstructive Pulmonary Disease. *JAMA Intern. Med.* **2014**, *174*, 1982. [CrossRef] [PubMed]
54. Plantier, L.; Cazes, A.; Dinh-Xuan, A.-T.; Bancal, C.; Marchand-Adam, S.; Crestani, B. Physiology of the lung in idiopathic pulmonary fibrosis. *Eur. Respir. Rev.* **2018**, *27*, 170062. [CrossRef] [PubMed]
55. Sanguanwong, N.; Jantarangsi, N.; Ngeyvijit, J.; Owattanapanich, N.; Phoophiboon, V. Effect of Noninvasive Respiratory Support on Interstitial Lung Disease with Acute Respiratory Failure: A Systematic Review and Meta-Analysis. *Can. J. Respir. Ther.* **2023**, *59*, 232–244. [CrossRef]
56. Mollica, C.; Paone, G.; Conti, V.; Ceccarelli, D.; Schmid, G.; Mattia, P.; Perrone, N.; Petroianni, A.; Sebastiani, A.; Cecchini, L.; et al. Mechanical Ventilation in Patients with End-Stage Idiopathic Pulmonary Fibrosis. *Respiration* **2010**, *79*, 209–215. [CrossRef]
57. Imai, R.; Tsugitomi, R.; Nakaoka, H.; Jinta, T.; Tamura, T. Noninvasive Oxygenation Strategies for Acute Exacerbation of Interstitial Lung Disease: A Retrospective Single-center Study and a Review of the Literature. *Clin. Pulm. Med.* **2019**, *26*, 87–91. [CrossRef]
58. Omote, N.; Matsuda, N.; Hashimoto, N.; Nishida, K.; Sakamoto, K.; Ando, A.; Nakahara, Y.; Nishikimi, M.; Higashi, M.; Matsui, S.; et al. High-flow nasal cannula therapy for acute respiratory failure in patients with interstitial pneumonia: A retrospective observational study. *Nagoya J. Med. Sci.* **2020**, *82*, 301–313. [CrossRef]
59. Shebl, E.; Embarak, S. High-flow nasal oxygen therapy versus noninvasive ventilation in chronic interstitial lung disease patients with acute respiratory failure. *Egypt. J. Chest Dis. Tuberc.* **2018**, *67*, 270. [CrossRef]
60. Martin, M.J.; Moua, T. Mechanical Ventilation and Predictors of In-Hospital Mortality in Fibrotic Interstitial Lung Disease with Acute Respiratory Failure: A Cohort Analysis Through the Paradigm of Acute Respiratory Distress Syndrome. *Crit. Care Med.* **2020**, *48*, 993–1000. [CrossRef]
61. Matsunashi, A.; Nagata, K.; Morimoto, T.; Tomii, K. Mechanical ventilation for acute exacerbation of fibrosing interstitial lung diseases. *Respir. Investig.* **2023**, *61*, 306–313. [CrossRef] [PubMed]
62. Marchioni, A.; Tonelli, R.; Rossi, G.; Spagnolo, P.; Luppi, F.; Cerri, S.; Cocconcelli, E.; Pellegrino, M.R.; Fantini, R.; Tabbì, L.; et al. Ventilatory support and mechanical properties of the fibrotic lung acting as a "squishy ball". *Ann. Intensive Care* **2020**, *10*, 13. [CrossRef] [PubMed]
63. The Acute Respiratory Distress Syndrome Network. Ventilation with Lower Tidal Volumes as Compared with Traditional Tidal Volumes for Acute Lung Injury and the Acute Respiratory Distress Syndrome. *N. Engl. J. Med.* **2000**, *342*, 1301–1308. [CrossRef] [PubMed]
64. Baydur, A. Mechanical Ventilation in Interstitial Lung Disease. *Chest* **2008**, *133*, 1062–1063. [CrossRef]
65. Luo, Z.; Yang, L.; Liu, S.; Hu, Y.; Cao, Z.; Zhu, J.; Wang, J.; Ma, Y. Mechanical ventilation for acute respiratory failure due to idiopathic pulmonary fibrosis versus connective tissue disease-associated interstitial lung disease: Effectiveness and risk factors for death. *Clin. Respir. J.* **2020**, *14*, 918–932. [CrossRef]
66. Fernández-Pérez, E.R.; Yilmaz, M.; Jenad, H.; Daniels, C.E.; Ryu, J.H.; Hubmayr, R.D.; Gajic, O. Ventilator Settings and Outcome of Respiratory Failure in Chronic Interstitial Lung Disease. *Chest* **2008**, *133*, 1113–1119. [CrossRef]
67. Guérin, C.; Reignier, J.; Richard, J.-C.; Beuret, P.; Gacouin, A.; Boulain, T.; Mercier, E.; Badet, M.; Mercat, A.; Baudin, O.; et al. Prone Positioning in Severe Acute Respiratory Distress Syndrome. *N. Engl. J. Med.* **2013**, *368*, 2159–2168. [CrossRef]
68. Xu, Y.; Sun, Q.; Yu, Y.; Liang, W.; Liu, X.; Yang, C.; Xu, Y.; Nong, L.; Chen, S.; He, W.; et al. Prone position ventilation support for acute exacerbation of interstitial lung disease? *Clin. Respir. J.* **2018**, *12*, 1372–1380. [CrossRef]
69. Kameda, H.; Tokuda, H.; Sakai, F.; Johkoh, T.; Mori, S.; Yoshida, Y.; Takayanagi, N.; Taki, H.; Hasegawa, Y.; Hatta, K.; et al. Clinical and Radiological Features of Acute-Onset Diffuse Interstitial Lung Diseases in Patients with Rheumatoid Arthritis Receiving Treatment with Biological Agents: Importance of *Pneumocystis* Pneumonia in Japan Revealed by a Multicenter Study. *Intern. Med.* **2011**, *50*, 305–313. [CrossRef]
70. Kousha, M.; Tadi, R.; Soubani, A.O. Pulmonary aspergillosis: A clinical review. *Eur. Respir. Rev.* **2011**, *20*, 156–174. [CrossRef]

71. Distler, O.; Highland, K.B.; Gahlemann, M.; Azuma, A.; Fischer, A.; Mayes, M.D.; Raghu, G.; Sauter, W.; Girard, M.; Alves, M.; et al. Nintedanib for Systemic Sclerosis–Associated Interstitial Lung Disease. *N. Engl. J. Med.* **2019**, *380*, 2518–2528. [CrossRef]
72. Flaherty, K.R.; Wells, A.U.; Cottin, V.; Devaraj, A.; Walsh, S.L.F.; Inoue, Y.; Richeldi, L.; Kolb, M.; Tetzlaff, K.; Stowasser, S.; et al. Nintedanib in Progressive Fibrosing Interstitial Lung Diseases. *N. Engl. J. Med.* **2019**, *381*, 1718–1727. [CrossRef]
73. Maher, T.M.; Strek, M.E. Antifibrotic therapy for idiopathic pulmonary fibrosis: Time to treat. *Respir. Res.* **2019**, *20*, 205. [CrossRef]
74. Petnak, T.; Lertjitbanjong, P.; Thongprayoon, C.; Moua, T. Impact of Antifibrotic Therapy on Mortality and Acute Exacerbation in Idiopathic Pulmonary Fibrosis. *Chest* **2021**, *160*, 1751–1763. [CrossRef]
75. Kreuter, M.; Polke, M.; Walsh, S.L.F.; Krisam, J.; Collard, H.R.; Chaudhuri, N.; Avdeev, S.; Behr, J.; Calligaro, G.; Corte, T.; et al. Acute exacerbation of idiopathic pulmonary fibrosis: International survey and call for harmonisation. *Eur. Respir. J.* **2020**, *55*, 1901760. [CrossRef]
76. Arrigo, M.; Price, S.; Harjola, V.-P.; Huber, L.C.; Schaubroeck, H.A.I.; Vieillard-Baron, A.; Mebazaa, A.; Masip, J. Diagnosis and treatment of right ventricular failure secondary to acutely increased right ventricular afterload (acute *cor pulmonale*): A clinical consensus statement of the Association for Acute CardioVascular Care of the European Society of Cardiology. *Eur. Heart J. Acute Cardiovasc. Care* **2024**, *13*, 304–312. [CrossRef]
77. Behr, J.; Ryu, J.H. Pulmonary hypertension in interstitial lung disease. *Eur. Respir. J.* **2008**, *31*, 1357–1367. [CrossRef]
78. Nathan, S.D.; Hassoun, P.M. Pulmonary Hypertension due to Lung Disease and/or Hypoxia. *Clin. Chest Med.* **2013**, *34*, 695–705. [CrossRef]
79. Lettieri, C.J.; Nathan, S.D.; Browning, R.F.; Barnett, S.D.; Ahmad, S.; Shorr, A.F. The distance-saturation product predicts mortality in idiopathic pulmonary fibrosis. *Respir. Med.* **2006**, *100*, 1734–1741. [CrossRef]
80. Caminati, A.; Cassandro, R.; Harari, S. Pulmonary hypertension in chronic interstitial lung diseases. *Eur. Respir. Rev.* **2013**, *22*, 292–301. [CrossRef]
81. Baughman, R.P.; Shlobin, O.A.; Wells, A.U.; Alhamad, E.H.; Culver, D.A.; Barney, J.; Cordova, F.C.; Carmona, E.M.; Scholand, M.B.; Wijsenbeek, M.; et al. Clinical features of sarcoidosis associated pulmonary hypertension: Results of a multi-national registry. *Respir. Med.* **2018**, *139*, 72–78. [CrossRef] [PubMed]
82. Strange, C.; Bolster, M.; Mazur, J.; Taylor, M.; Gossage, J.R.; Silver, R. Hemodynamic Effects of Epoprostenol in Patients with Systemic Sclerosis and Pulmonary Hypertension. *Chest* **2000**, *118*, 1077–1082. [CrossRef] [PubMed]
83. Olschewski, H.; Ardeschir Ghofrani, H.; Walmrath, D.; Schermuly, R.; Temmesfeld-Wollbrück, B.; Grimminger, F.; Seeger, W. Inhaled Prostacyclin and Iloprost in Severe Pulmonary Hypertension Secondary to Lung Fibrosis. *Am. J. Respir. Crit. Care Med.* **1999**, *160*, 600–607. [CrossRef]
84. Nathan, S.D. Progress in the Treatment of Pulmonary Hypertension Associated with Interstitial Lung Disease. *Am. J. Respir. Crit. Care Med.* **2023**, *208*, 238–246. [CrossRef]
85. Hinkamp, C.A.; Shah, T.; Bartolome, S.; Torres, F.; Chin, K.M. Parenteral prostanoids for severe Group 3 pulmonary hypertension with right ventricular dysfunction. *J. Thorac. Dis.* **2021**, *13*, 1466–1475. [CrossRef]
86. Hoopes, C.W.; Kukreja, J.; Golden, J.; Davenport, D.L.; Diaz-Guzman, E.; Zwischenberger, J.B. Extracorporeal membrane oxygenation as a bridge to pulmonary transplantation. *J. Thorac. Cardiovasc. Surg.* **2013**, *145*, 862–868. [CrossRef]
87. Trudzinski, F.C.; Kaestner, F.; Schäfers, H.-J.; Fähndrich, S.; Seiler, F.; Böhmer, P.; Linn, O.; Kaiser, R.; Haake, H.; Langer, F.; et al. Outcome of Patients with Interstitial Lung Disease Treated with Extracorporeal Membrane Oxygenation for Acute Respiratory Failure. *Am. J. Respir. Crit. Care Med.* **2016**, *193*, 527–533. [CrossRef] [PubMed]
88. Daar, J.A.; Toyoda, Y.; Shigemura, N.; Baskin, S.M.; Desai, P.; Gordon, M. Extracorporeal membrane oxygenation as a bridge to lung transplantation: 5-year outcomes and bridge to decision in a large, older cohort. *Respir. Res.* **2024**, *25*, 350. [CrossRef]
89. Leard, L.E.; Holm, A.M.; Valapour, M.; Glanville, A.R.; Attawar, S.; Aversa, M.; Campos, S.V.; Christon, L.M.; Cypel, M.; Dellgren, G.; et al. Consensus document for the selection of lung transplant candidates: An update from the International Society for Heart and Lung Transplantation. *J. Heart Lung Transplant.* **2021**, *40*, 1349–1379. [CrossRef]
90. Dotan, Y.; Vaidy, A.; Shapiro, W.B.; Zhao, H.; Dass, C.; Toyoda, Y.; Marchetti, N.; Shenoy, K.; Cordova, F.C.; Criner, G.J.; et al. Effect of Acute Exacerbation of Idiopathic Pulmonary Fibrosis on Lung Transplantation Outcome. *Chest* **2018**, *154*, 818–826. [CrossRef]
91. Tang, A.; Thuita, L.; Siddiqui, H.U.; Rappaport, J.; Blackstone, E.H.; McCurry, K.R.; Ahmad, U.; Tong, M.Z.; Bribriesco, A.; Johnston, D.R.; et al. Urgently listed lung transplant patients have outcomes similar to those of electively listed patients. *J. Thorac. Cardiovasc. Surg.* **2021**, *161*, 306–317.e8. [CrossRef] [PubMed]
92. Weill, D. Lung transplantation: Indications and contraindications. *J. Thorac. Dis.* **2018**, *10*, 4574–4587. [CrossRef] [PubMed]
93. Castelino, F.V.; Goldberg, H.; Dellaripa, P.F. The impact of rheumatological evaluation in the management of patients with interstitial lung disease. *Rheumatology* **2011**, *50*, 489–493. [CrossRef] [PubMed]
94. Wijsenbeek, M.S.; Moor, C.C. Palliative Care in Interstitial Lung Disease. In *Palliative Care in Lung Disease*; Lindell, K.O., Danoff, S.K., Eds.; Respiratory Medicine; Springer International Publishing: Cham, Switzerland, 2021; pp. 189–207. ISBN 978-3-030-81787-9.
95. Güngör, G.; Tatar, D.; Saltürk, C.; Çimen, P.; Karakurt, Z.; Kirakli, C.; Adıgüzel, N.; Ediboğlu, Ö.; Yılmaz, H.; Moçin, Ö.Y.; et al. Why Do Patients with Interstitial Lung Diseases Fail in the ICU? A 2-Center Cohort Study. *Respir. Care* **2013**, *58*, 525–531. [CrossRef]
96. Huapaya, J.A.; Wilfong, E.M.; Harden, C.T.; Brower, R.G.; Danoff, S.K. Risk factors for mortality and mortality rates in interstitial lung disease patients in the intensive care unit. *Eur. Respir. Rev.* **2018**, *27*, 180061. [CrossRef]

97. Lain, W.-L.; Chang, S.-C.; Chen, W.-C. Outcome and prognostic factors of interstitial lung disease patients with acute respiratory failure in the intensive care unit. *Ther. Adv. Respir. Dis.* **2020**, *14*, 175346662092695. [CrossRef]
98. Drakopanagiotakis, F.; Markart, P.; Steiropoulos, P. Acute Exacerbations of Interstitial Lung Diseases: Focus on Biomarkers. *Int. J. Mol. Sci.* **2023**, *24*, 10196. [CrossRef] [PubMed]

Journal of
Clinical Medicine

MDPI

Article

Exercise-Induced Oxygen Desaturation and Outcomes After Nintedanib Therapy for Fibrosing Interstitial Lung Disease in Patients Without Dyspnea

Masaki Okamoto [1,2,*], Toyoshi Yanagihara [3], Kiminori Fujimoto [4], Tomonori Chikasue [4], Kazuhiro Tabata [5], Yoshiaki Zaizen [2], Masaki Tominaga [2], Akiko Sumi [4], Yuuya Nishii [1,2], Norikazu Matsuo [1,2], Takashi Nouno [1,2], Shuji Matsuura [6], Atsushi Kawaguchi [7] and Tomoaki Hoshino [2]

1 Department of Respirology, NHO Kyushu Medical Center, Jigyohama 1-8-1, Chuo-ku, Fukuoka 810-0065, Japan
2 Division of Respirology, Neurology and Rheumatology, Department of Internal Medicine, Kurume University School of Medicine, Asahi-Machi 67, Kurume 830-0011, Japan
3 Department of Respiratory Medicine, Fukuoka University Hospital, 7-45-1 Nanakuma, Jonan-ku, Fukuoka 814-0180, Japan
4 Department of Radiology, Kurume University School of Medicine, Asahi-Machi 67, Kurume 830-0011, Japan
5 Department of Pathology, Kagoshima University Graduate School of Medical and Dental Sciences, 8-35-1 Sakuragaoka, Kagoshima 890-8544, Japan
6 Department of Radiology, NHO Kyushu Medical Center, Jigyohama 1-8-1, Chuo-ku, Fukuoka 810-0065, Japan
7 Education and Research Center for Community Medicine, Faculty of Medicine, Saga Medical School, 5-1-1 Nabeshima, Saga 849-8501, Japan
* Correspondence: okamoto_masaki@med.kurume-u.ac.jp; Tel.: +81-92-852-0700

Abstract: Background: The degree of exercise-induced oxygen desaturation and outcomes following antifibrotic drug therapy in asymptomatic patients with fibrosing interstitial lung disease (FILD) remain unclear. **Methods:** We compared clinical data, incidence of annual FILD progression, overall survival, and tolerability after initiating nintedanib between 58 patients with dyspnea and 18 patients without. Annual FILD progression was defined as >10% decrease in forced vital capacity (FVC), >15% decrease in diffusing capacity of the lungs for carbon monoxide (D_{LCO}), developing acute exacerbations, or FILD-related death within 1 year of starting nintedanib. Outcomes between the two groups were adjusted for covariates, including age, gender, FVC, D_{LCO}, and diagnosis of idiopathic pulmonary fibrosis, all known prognostic factors for FILD. **Results:** In 6-min walk test, incidence of decrease to <90% of SpO_2 was significantly lower in non-dyspnea group than in dyspnea group (24% vs. 55%, $p = 0.028$), but incidence of >4% decreases showed no significant difference (71% vs. 89%, $p = 0.11$) The incidence of annual progression was significantly lower in non-dyspnea than in dyspnea group (17% vs. 53%, adjusted $p = 0.026$). The relative change in D_{LCO} was significantly slower in non-dyspnea group (adjusted $p = 0.036$), but FVC was not (adjusted $p = 0.067$). Overall survival was longer in non-dyspnea group (adjusted $p = 0.0089$). The discontinuation rate and therapeutic period of nintedanib were not significantly different between the groups. **Conclusions:** Asymptomatic patients with FILD have severe exercise-induced oxygen desaturation and better outcomes after nintedanib therapy than symptomatic patients. Antifibrotic drug therapy should not be avoided solely because of a lack of symptoms.

Keywords: fibrosing interstitial lung disease; nintedanib; dyspnea

1. Introduction

Fibrosing interstitial lung disease (FILD) encompasses various subtypes characterized by specific patterns of lung parenchymal fibrosis with or without inflammation [1–4]. Idiopathic pulmonary fibrosis (IPF), which pathologically manifests as usual interstitial pneumonia (UIP), is the most common type of idiopathic interstitial pneumonia [1–4]. Patients with IPF have a grave prognosis with a median survival of approximately 3 years [5]. A proportion of patients with non-IPF FILD exhibit progressive characteristics, defined as progressive pulmonary fibrosis by global guidelines and various studies, and have similarly poor survival rates as patients with IPF [1,6]. Two randomized controlled trials and one meta-analysis have shown that the antifibrotic agents nintedanib and pirfenidone slow the decline in forced vital capacity (FVC), reduce the incidence of acute exacerbation (AE) and/or lower all-cause mortality in patients with IPF [7–9]. The recent phase 3 INBUILD trial revealed that nintedanib reduced the decline in FVC in patients with progressive non-IPF FILD [10]. Consequently, both the global guidelines and the Japanese guidelines moderately recommend antifibrotic drug therapy for these patients [1,11].

Recently, some studies have suggested the effectiveness of antifibrotic drugs in patients with early FILD [12,13]. In the INMARK, a phase 3 trial involving patients with early IPF who had an FVC of >80%, nintedanib reduced the decrease in FVC for 12 weeks [12]. In the subgroup analysis of the INBUILD trial, nintedanib suppressed the decrease in FVC over 52 weeks regardless of severity markers, such as the gender–age–pulmonary physiology (GAP) score and baseline FVC [10,13]. However, antifibrotic drug therapy for patients without dyspnea is often avoided because patients and respiratory physicians often consider such therapy to be unnecessary before the disease becomes severe. In fact, a lower score on the modified Medical Research Council (mMRC) scale evaluating the severity of dyspnea in daily life was associated with better survival in patients with IPF [14]. By contrast, in the subgroup analysis of the SENSCIS, a phase 3 trial involving patients with systemic sclerosis (SSc)-associated ILD, the nintedanib group showed a numerically greater reduction in the FVC decline compared with placebo in patients without than with dyspnea, although the difference was not statistically significant [15]. The high effectiveness of antifibrotic drugs in asymptomatic patients with FILD may be associated with the presence of potential exercise-induced oxygen desaturation. Desaturation during the 6 min walk test (6MWT) has been reported as a predictor of survival and/or disease progression in patients with IPF [16,17], especially in those with early-stage disease classified as stage I in the Japanese Respiratory Society disease severity system [18,19]. Nishiyama et al. [20] suggested that dyspnea may not present in patients with FILD despite high disease severity, because patients with IPF may experience more severe desaturation but milder dyspnea than those with chronic obstructive pulmonary disease (COPD).

In the present study, we attempted to clarify the degree of exercise-induced oxygen desaturation and the outcomes following nintedanib therapy in patients with FILD without dyspnea.

2. Materials and Methods

2.1. Patient Selection

We retrospectively analyzed consecutive patients with FILD who received nintedanib therapy in our hospital from 2015 to 2022. The inclusion criteria were as follows: patients diagnosed with FILD according to a multidisciplinary discussion based on global guidelines on IPF, idiopathic interstitial pneumonia, SSc, polymyositis, rheumatoid arthritis, and Sjögren's syndrome [1,4,21–24]. The exclusion criteria were patients who could not regularly visit our hospital at least 1 year after starting nintedanib and patients who could not undergo pulmonary function testing at least every 6 months, because the annual progression of FILD could not be accurately analyzed in such patients. AE of FILD was diagnosed in accordance with the criteria detailed in a previous report [25]. Disease severity was staged in accordance with the GAP model, classifying patients into three stages based on clinical variables, e.g., sex or age, FVC, and the diffusing capacity of the lung for carbon monoxide (D_{LCO})] [26]. The GAP score and chronic pulmonary emphysema assessment test (CAT) result, as patient-reported outcomes [27,28], were collected upon starting nintedanib. According to a previous report, the patients were classified into four groups based on their GAP scores: 0 or 1, 2 or 3, 4 or 5, and 6 to 8, with increasing severity [26].

2.2. Study Protocol

The patients' clinical data upon starting nintedanib were collected to determine factors predicting the progression of FILD. The mMRC scale includes five grades (0–4) and is used to evaluate dyspnea in daily life [14]. Patients with an mMRC scale score of 0 were classified into the non-dyspnea group, and the remaining patients were classified into the dyspnea group. In the present study, a single physical therapist used the mMRC scale to evaluate the patients.

Annual progression of FILD was defined as a >10% decrease in FVC or a >15% decrease in D_{LCO}, the development of AE, or death of FILD at 1 year after starting nintedanib. Overall survival (OS) was measured from the day of starting nintedanib to the final observation day (24 February 2024). When measuring OS, events were defined in two ways: death from any cause and FILD.

The treatment protocol with nintedanib was based on recommendations provided in the INPULSIS trials [7]. The recommended starting dose was 150 mg twice a day. Dose reductions of up to 100 mg twice a day and treatment interruptions were recommended to manage adverse events. After the improvement of adverse events, nintedanib could be reintroduced at the discretion of the physician.

2.3. Pulmonary Function Tests

Pulmonary function tests and measurement of FVC and forced expiratory volume in 1 s were performed using a spirometer (CHESTAC-8900, Chest, Tokyo, Japan). The D_{LCO} was measured using the single-breath technique. These techniques were performed according to the guidelines of the American Thoracic Society/European Respiratory Society [29].

2.4. 6MWT

The 6MWT was performed according to the American Thoracic Society statement [30]. The patients were instructed to walk as fast as possible and were allowed to slow down or stop if necessary during examination. The SpO_2 and 6MWT distance were monitored and recorded.

2.5. Statistical Analysis

The data are expressed as the median (25th–75th percentiles of the interquartile range) or least squares (LS) mean $\pm$ standard error (SE) as appropriate. We analyzed the differences in clinical data between the non-dyspnea and dyspnea groups using the Wilcoxon rank-sum test, Fisher's exact test, and multiple regression analysis as appropriate. The cut-off levels of the lowest and decreased SpO_2 and the CAT score for comparison between the two groups were set at 90%, 4%, and 10, respectively. These levels were based on previous reports, indicating that they were prognostic factors of FILD or COPD [17,18,28]. In the logistic regression analysis using backward elimination and multiple regression analysis, we adjusted for covariates including age, gender, FVC, D_{LCO}, and diagnosis with IPF as prognostic factors based on previous reports [1–3,26]. In the Kaplan–Meier analysis of OS using the log-rank test, we adjusted for the above covariates by Cox hazard proportional analysis with or without backward elimination. In the logistic regression analysis, a p value of <0.05 in the univariate analysis was set as the criterion for variable selection in the multivariate analysis. A p value of <0.05 was considered statistically significant. All statistical analyses were performed using JMP 14.0 (SAS Institute Japan, Tokyo, Japan).

3. Results

3.1. Patient Selection and Characteristics

The patient selection process based on the inclusion and exclusion criteria is shown in Figure 1. Among 83 identified patients with FILD, 7 patients did not meet the study criteria because of failure to undergo observation for more than 1 year. In total, 76 patients were selected for the study, including 56 (74%) male patients and 60 (79%) smokers, with a median age of 72.2 (65.9–76.2) years. Eighteen (24%) of seventy-three patients were assigned to the non-dyspnea group. The patients' characteristics and comparison of clinical data upon starting nintedanib between the non-dyspnea and dyspnea groups are shown in Table 1 and Figure 2. The patients' FILD subtypes included IPF in 53 (70%) patients, unclassifiable ILD in 11 (15%), fibrotic hypersensitivity pneumonia in 7 (9%), connective tissue disease-associated ILD (CTD-ILD) in 4 (5%), and smoking-related ILD in 1 (1%). Among the four patients with CTD-ILD, the disease subtypes of CTD were SSc, polymyositis, rheumatoid arthritis, and SSc with secondary Sjögren's syndrome, in one patient each. According to the GAP models, the patients' disease severity was classified as 0 or 1 in 9 (12%) patients, 2 or 3 in 38 (50%), 4 or 5 in 28 (37%), and 6 to 8 in 1 (1%). The radiological ILD patterns based on the global IPF guidelines [1] were definite UIP in 25 (33%) patients, probable UIP in 17 (22%), indeterminate for UIP in 21 (28%), and an alternative diagnosis in 13 (17%). Among the 73 patients, none had pulmonary hypertension. In the comparison of clinical data between the two groups, the non-dyspnea group included significantly more male patients; more patients with a lower mMRC scale score (median, 0 vs. 1), GAP score (median, 3 vs. 3), decrease in SpO_2 (median, 5.0% vs. 7.0%) during the 6MWT, C-reactive protein level (median, 0.11 vs. 0.25 mg/dL), Krebs von den Lungen-6 (KL-6) level (median, 584.5 vs. 875.0 IU/mL), monocyte count, and CAT score (median, 6.0 vs. 17.0); and more patients with a higher FVC (median, 84.2% vs. 78.8%), D_{LCO} (median, 72.2% vs. 58.2%) and the lowest SpO_2 (median, 92.0% vs. 88.0%) during the 6MWT compared to the dyspnea group ($p < 0.05$). Among the 76 patients, the incidence of a decrease of up to <90% in the SpO_2 during the 6MWT was significantly lower in the non-dyspnea group than in the dyspnea group, but not significantly (24% vs. 55%, $p = 0.028$) (Table 1 and Figure 2A). The incidence of a >4% decrease in SpO_2 during the 6MWT was not significantly different between the non-dyspnea and dyspnea groups (71% vs. 89%, $p = 0.11$) (Table 1 and Figure 2B). The rate of patients with a CAT score of >10 was significantly lower in the non-dyspnea group than in the dyspnea group (40% vs. 82%, $p = 0.0025$) (Table 1 and Figure 2C). There was no difference in the percentage of patients with a reduced starting dose of nintedanib between the non-dyspnea and dyspnea groups (6% vs. 10%, $p = 1.0$). The present study suggests that a certain proportion of patients who have FILD without dyspnea and require nintedanib therapy have severe exercise-induced oxygen desaturation.

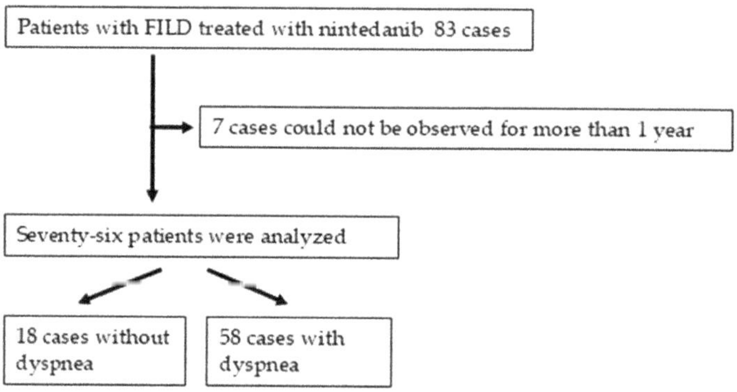

Figure 1. Inclusion and exclusion criteria for study patients. FILD, fibrosing interstitial pneumonia.

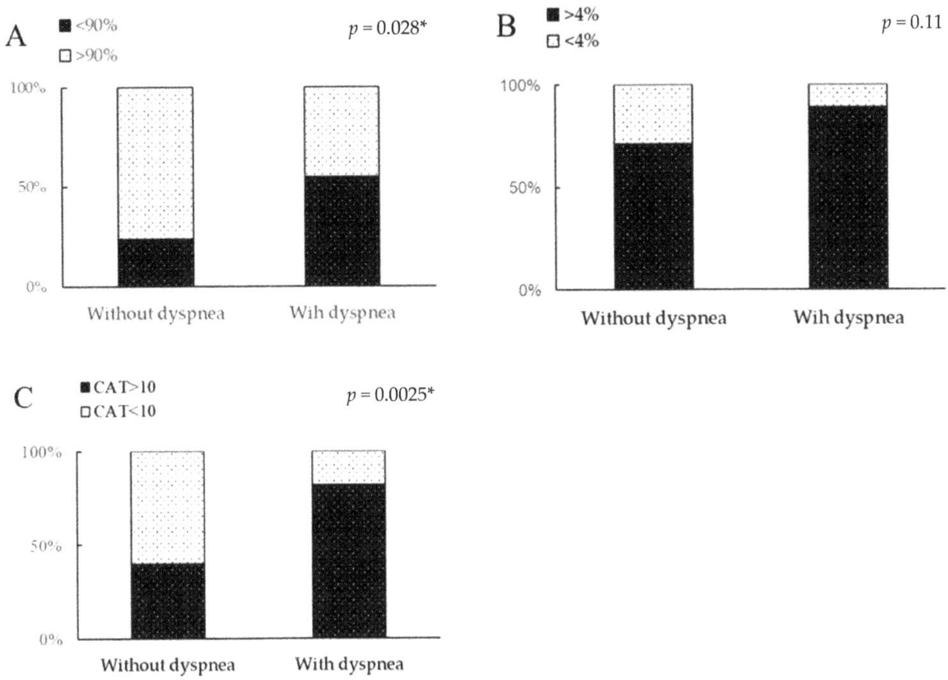

Figure 2. Comparison of desaturation and patient-reported outcomes among patients with FILD with versus without dyspnea. Comparison of (**A**) lowest and (**B**) highest decrease in SpO_2 in the 6MWT and (**C**) CAT score between non-dyspnea and dyspnea groups. Cut-off levels were set at 90% of the lowest SpO_2 in the 6MWT, 4% for the decrease in SpO_2 in the 6MWT, and 10 for the CAT score as prognostic factors of FILD or chronic obstructive pulmonary disease based on previous reports. 6MWT, 6-min walk test; CAT, chronic obstructive pulmonary disease assessment test. * $p < 0.05$ is regarded as statistically significant.

Table 1. Patients' characteristics.

	Overall	Non-Dyspnea Group	Dyspnea Group	*p* Value
Number	76	18 (24%)	58 (74%)	
Age (years)	72.2 (65.9–76.2)	70.8 (65.2–74.4)	72.5 (66.2–76.6)	0.17
Male gender	56 (74%)	17 (94%)	39 (69%)	0.030 *
FILD subtype (FILD/UC-ILD/ HP/CTD/SR-ILD)	53 (70%)/11 (15%)/ 7 (9%)/4 (5%)/1 (1%)	14 (77%)/1(6%)/ 2 (11%)/1(6%)/0	39 (67%)/10 (17%)/ 5 (9%)/3(5%)/1 (2%)	
Smoker	60 (79%)	17 (94%)	43 (74%)	0.097
Body mass index (kg/m^2)	24.3 (22.0–26.7)	24.5 (22.0–26.3)	24.0 (21.8–27.0)	0.67
mMRC scale	1 (1–2)	0 (0–0)	1 (1–2)	<0.00010 *
GAP score (0 or 1/2 or 3/4 or 5/6 to 8)	9 (12%)/38 (50%) /28 (37%)/1 (1%)	3 (17%)/13 (72%) /2 (11%)/0	6 (10%)/25 (43%) /26 (45%)/1 (2%)	0.030 *
HRCT pattern				
Definite UIP	25 (33%)	7 (39%)	18 (31%)	0.57
Probable UIP	17 (22%)	5 (28%)	12 (21%)	
Indeterminate for UIP	21 (28%)	3 (17%)	18 (31%)	
Alternative diagnosis	13 (17%)	3 (17%)	10 (17%)	
Pulmonary function				
FVC (%)	81.5 (66.3–92.8)	84.2 (79.1–99.4)	78.8 (64.6–91.3)	0.025 *
D_{LCO} (%)	61.3 (48.4–72.6)	72.2 (63.4–84.8)	58.2 (43.5–67.8)	0.00070 *

Table 1. *Cont.*

	Overall	Non-Dyspnea Group	Dyspnea Group	*p* Value
Six-minutes walk test				
Lowest SpO_2 (%)	90.0 (85.0–92.5)	92.0 (89.5–94.0)	88.0 (84.3–92.0)	0.0015 *
Less than 90%	35 (48%)	4 (24%)	31 (55%)	0.028 *
Decrease in SpO_2 (%)	6.0 (4.0–10.5)	5.0 (2.5–6.5)	7.0 (5.0–11.5)	0.0068 *
More than 4%	62 (82%)	12 (71%)	50 (89%)	0.11
Walk distance (m)	375.0 (307.5–463.0)	420.0 (399.5–508.5)	359.0 (293.0–435.0)	0.0068 *
Serum biomarker				
CRP (mg/dL)	0.14 (0.070–0.43)	0.11 (0.050–0.16)	0.25 (0.073–0.48)	0.030 *
KL-6 (IU/mL)	782.0 (565.0–1233.0)	584.5 (437.3–869.0)	875.0 (601.5–1310.5)	0.014 *
LDH (IU/L)	210.0 (183.0–243.3)	200.0 (172.0–227.5)	218.5 (185.0–252.8)	0.13
Monocyte count (/uL)	414.5 (330.7–530.2)	370.9 (325.3–414.8)	457.3 (329.8–556.2)	0.054
CAT	14.0 (8.0–23.0)	6.0 (3.0–13.0)	17.0 (11.0–25.0)	0.00020 *
More than 10	48 (63%)	6 (40%)	42 (82%)	0.0025 *
Starting dose of nintedanib (mg/day) 200/300	7 (9%)/69 (91%)	1 (6%)/17 (94%)	6 (10%)/52 (90%)	1

Data are expressed as medians (25th to 75th percentiles of interquartile range) unless otherwise stated. FILD, fibrosing interstitial lung disease; IPF, idiopathic pulmonary fibrosis; UC-ILD, unclassifiable interstitial lung disease; HP, hypersensitivity pneumonia; CTD, connective tissue disease; SR-ILD, smoking-related interstitial pneumonia; mMRC, modified Medical Research Council; GAP, gender–age–physiology; UIP, usual interstitial pneumonia; CT, computed tomography; FVC, forced vital capacity; D_{LCO}, diffusing capacity of the lung for carbon monoxide; 6MWT, 6 min walk test; CRP, C-reactive protein; KL-6, Krebs von den Lungen-6; LDH, lactate dehydrogenase; CAT, chronic obstructive pulmonary disease assessment test. * $p < 0.05$ is regarded as statistically significant.

3.2. Patient Outcomes

A comparison of the patients' outcomes between the non-dyspnea and dyspnea groups is shown in Table 2. The median observation period was 861.0 (671.5–1488.5) days after starting nintedanib. Among the 76 patients, 24 (32%) and 17 (22%) patients died from any cause and from FILD, respectively. Compared with the dyspnea group, the non-dyspnea group showed significantly longer OS and significantly lower mortality from any cause and FILD ($p < 0.05$). In total, 34 (45%) of 76 patients exhibited annual progression (Table 2). Among the 76 patients, annual progression of FILD occurred in 3 (17%) of 18 patients in the non-dyspnea group and 31 (53%) of 58 patients in the dyspnea group, with a significant difference according to Fisher's exact test ($p = 0.0070$). In a similar comparison of the components of annual progression of FILD, only the incidence of a >15% decrease in D_{LCO} was significantly lower in the non-dyspnea group than in the dyspnea group ($p = 0.026$); the other components showed no significant differences between the two groups. Moreover, the incidence of annual progression of FILD was also significantly lower in the non-dyspnea group than in the dyspnea group after adjusting for covariates (adjusted $p = 0.026$) (Figure 3A). Comparisons of the relative decrease in FVC and D_{LCO} over 6 months are shown in Figure 3B–E. The relative decrease in FVC (median ± SE, 1.5% ± 2.7% vs. −0.39% ± 1.4%; $p = 0.011$) and D_{LCO} (median ± SE, −0.57% ± 3.7% vs. −11.2% ± 2.1%; $p = 0.017$) were significantly slower in the non-dyspnea group than in the dyspnea group. After adjusting for covariates, the relative change in D_{LCO} was also significantly slower in the non-dyspnea group than in the dyspnea group (LS mean ± SE, −0.80% ± 3.5% vs. −11.0% ± 2.9%; $p = 0.036$). Similarly, the relative change in FVC tended to be slower in the non-dyspnea group than in the dyspnea group (LS mean ± SE, 7.4% ± 3.0% vs. 1.3% ± 1.5%; $p = 0.067$), but not significantly. Comparisons of the relative decrease in pulmonary function over 12 months are shown in Figure 3F–I. The relative decrease in D_{LCO} was significantly slower in the non-dyspnea group than in the dyspnea group (median ± SE, −1.5% ± 4.0% vs. −16.7% ± 2.1%; $p = 0.0040$), but the relative change in FVC showed no difference between the two groups (median ± SE, 0.85% ± 3.2% vs. −2.0% ± 1.8%; $p = 0.17$). After adjusting for covariates, the relative change in D_{LCO} tended to be slower in the non-dyspnea group than in the dyspnea group (LS mean ± SE,

−7.0% ± 4.7% vs. −16.7% ± 2.4%; $p = 0.059$), but not significantly. Similarly, there was no significant difference in the relative change in FVC between the non-dyspnea and dyspnea group (LS mean ± SE, 0.76% ± 4.0% vs. −2.0% ± 2.2%; $p = 0.54$).

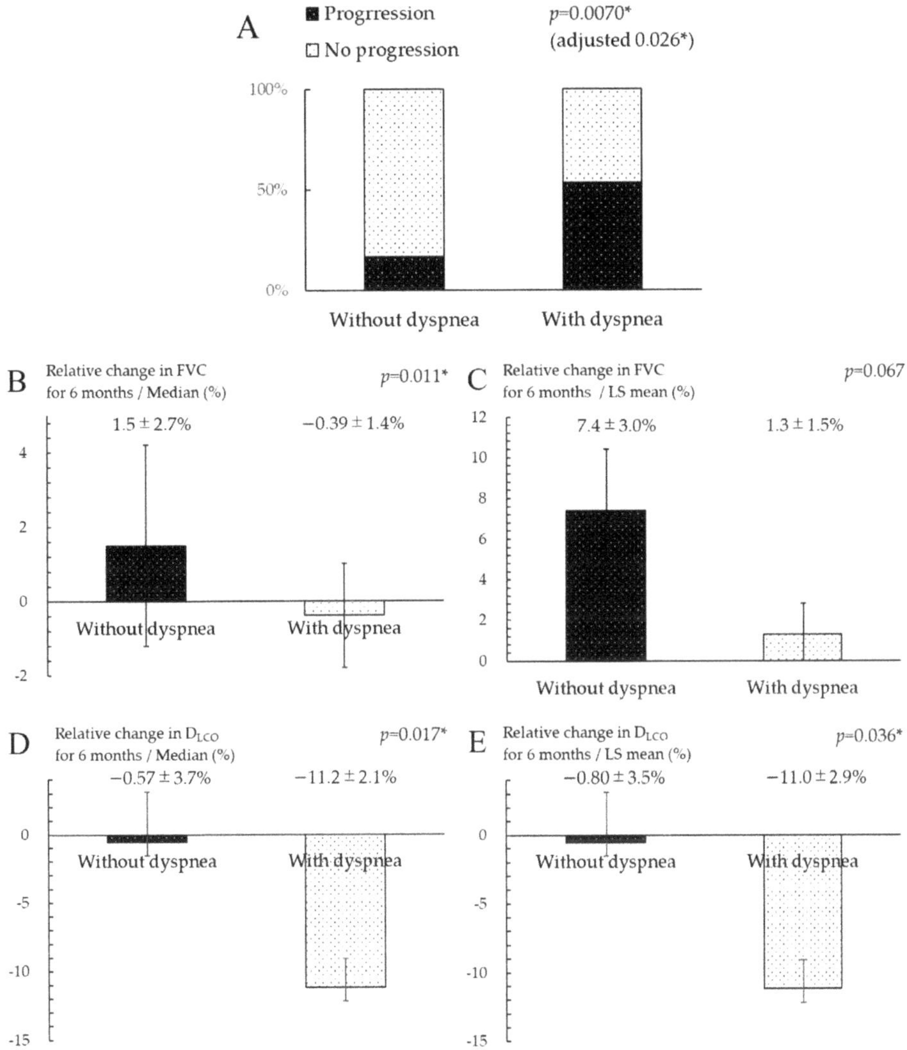

Figure 3. *Cont.*

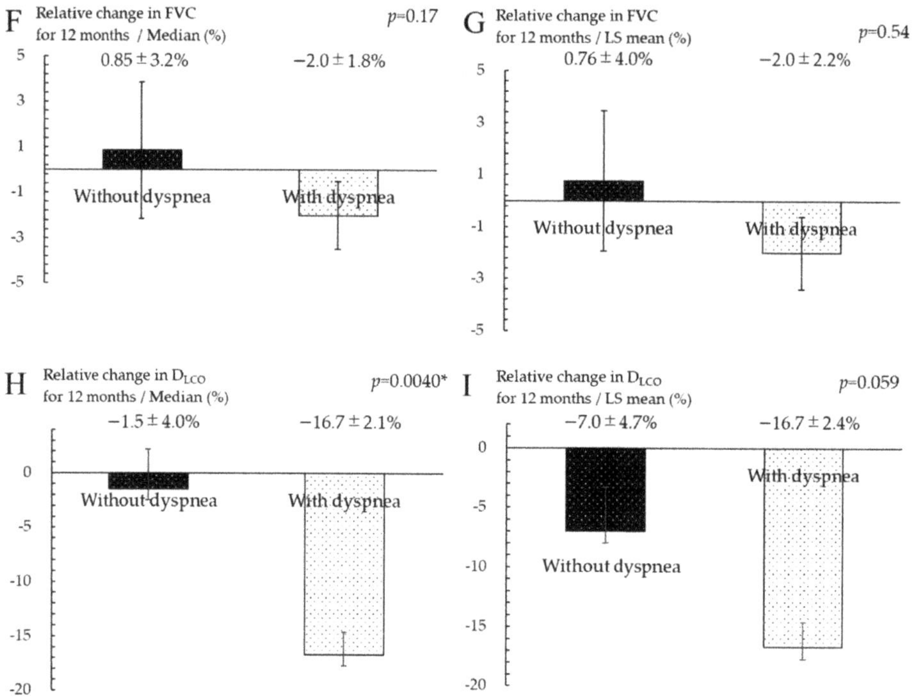

Figure 3. Comparison of progression among patients with FILD with versus without dyspnea. (**A**) Incidence of annual progression (defined as >10% relative decrease in FVC or 15% decrease in D_{LCO}, development of acute exacerbation, or death) was compared among patients with FILD with versus without dyspnea using Fisher's exact test. Adjustment for covariates including age, gender, FVC, D_{LCO}, and diagnosis with IPF as prognostic factors based on previous reports was performed using logistic regression analysis. We compared the relative decrease in (**B**,**C**) FVC and (**D**,**E**) D_{LCO} over 6 months using the (**B**,**D**) Wilcoxon rank-sum test or (**C**,**E**) multiple regression analysis. Similarly, we compared the relative decrease in (**F**,**G**) FVC and (**H**,**I**) D_{LCO} over 12 months using the (**F**,**H**) Wilcoxon rank-sum test or (**G**,**I**) multiple regression analysis. Decreases in FVC and D_{LCO} are shown as (**B**,**D**,**F**,**H**) median ± SE or (**C**,**E**,**G**,**I**) LS mean ± SE. Adjustment for covariates including age, sex, FVC, D_{LCO}, and diagnosis with IPF was performed using multiple regression analysis. FILD, fibrosing interstitial lung disease; FVC, forced vital capacity; D_{LCO}, diffusing capacity of the lung for carbon monoxide; IPF, idiopathic pulmonary fibrosis; SE, standard error; LS, least squares. * $p < 0.05$ is regarded as statistically significant.

The Kaplan–Meier curve is shown in Figure 4A,B. OS is defined by death from any cause (Figure 4A), and FILD (Figure 4B) was significantly longer in the non-dyspnea group than in the dyspnea group according to the log-rank test ($p = 0.014$ and $p = 0.0052$). After adjustment for covariates, the non-dyspnea group showed significantly longer OS defined by death due to FILD (adjusted $p = 0.0089$) than the dyspnea group. However, no significant difference in OS defined by death from any cause was observed between the two groups (adjusted $p = 0.11$).

Table 2. Patients' outcomes.

	Overall	Non-Dyspnea Group	Dyspnea Group	p Value
Number	76	18 (24%)	58 (74%)	
Overall survival (days)	861.0 (671.5–1488.5)	1382.5 (822.8–1540.3)	780.0 (604.0–1341.5)	0.017 *
Mortality from any cause	24 (32%)	2 (11%)	22 (38%)	0.042 *
Mortality due to FILD	17 (22%)	0	17 (29%)	0.0080 *
Annual disease progression	34 (45%)	3 (17%)	31 (53%)	0.0070 *
More than 10% decrease in FVC	12 (16%)	2 (11%)	10 (17%)	0.72
More than 15% decrease in D_{LCO}	30 (41%)	3 (17%)	27 (48%)	0.026 *
Developing acute exacerbation	2 (3%)	0	2 (3%)	1
ILD-specific mortality	2 (3%)	0	2 (3%)	1
Immunosuppressive therapy over 180 days	12 (16%)	1 (6%)	11 (19%)	0.27

Data are expressed as median (25th to 75th percentiles of interquartile range) unless otherwise stated. FILD, fibrosing interstitial lung disease; FVC, forced vital capacity; D_{LCO}, diffusing capacity of the lung for carbon monoxide; AE, acute exacerbation; ILD, interstitial lung disease. * $p < 0.05$ is regarded as statistically significant.

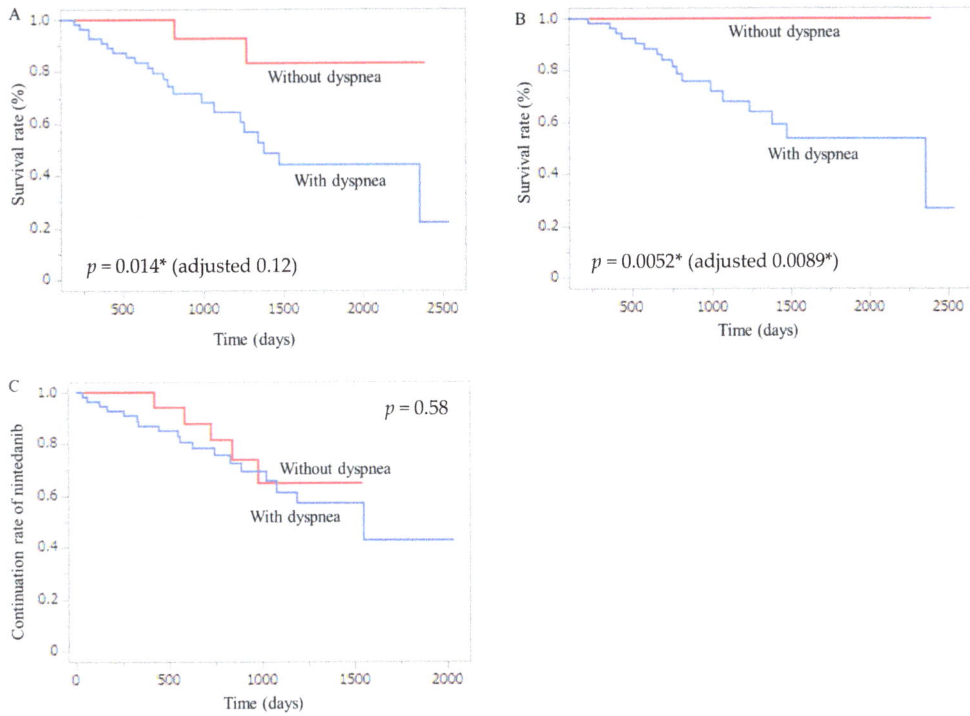

Figure 4. Comparison of survival between patients with FILD with versus without dyspnea. Kaplan Meier curves for mortality from (**A**) any cause and (**B**) FILD after start of nintedanib between patients who had FILD with versus without dyspnea using the log-rank test. Adjustment for covariates including age, sex, FVC, D_{LCO}, and diagnosis with IPF was performed using a Cox proportional hazard model. (**C**) Kaplan–Meier curves comparing the therapeutic period of nintedanib between patients with FILD with versus without dyspnea using the log-rank test. FILD, fibrosing interstitial lung disease; FVC, forced vital capacity; D_{LCO}, diffusing capacity of the lung for carbon monoxide; IPF, idiopathic pulmonary fibrosis. * $p < 0.05$ is regarded as statistically significant.

In summary, patients with FILD without dyspnea had a significantly lower incidence of annual progression and mortality and a slower short-term decrease in pulmonary function after starting nintedanib than patients with dyspnea, even after adjustment for covariates.

3.3. Analysis of Risk Factors for Annual Progression of FILD

The results of the analysis of risk factors for the annual progression of FILD are shown in Table 3. The univariate analysis showed that the absence of dyspnea (odds ratio (OR), 0.17; 95% confidence interval (CI), 0.037–0.60; $p = 0.011$), higher lowest SpO_2 during the 6MWT (OR, 0.90; 95% CI, 0.82–0.98; $p = 0.021$), lower decrease in SpO_2 (OR, 1.1; 95% CI, 1.0–1.3; $p = 0.029$), and longer 6MWT distance (OR, 0.95; 95% CI, 0.90–0.99; $p = 0.032$) were significantly associated with a lower incidence of annual progression of FILD (Table 3A). We next assessed the results of the multivariate analysis with or without backward elimination including variables with a p-value of <0.05 in the univariate analysis and covariates. In the multivariate analysis with backward elimination, only the absence of dyspnea was independently associated with a lower incidence of annual progression (OR, 0.17; 95% CI, 0.045–0.67; $p = 0.011$) (Table 3B). In the multivariate analysis without backward elimination, the absence of dyspnea (OR, 0.14; 95% CI, 0.022–0.83; $p = 0.031$) and no diagnosis of IPF (OR, 4.4; 95% CI, 1.1–16.6; $p = 0.031$) were independently associated with a lower incidence of annual progression (Table 3C).

Table 3. (**A**) Univariate analysis of factors associated with annual progression of FILD. (**B**) Multivariate analysis of factors associated with annual progression of FILD with backward elimination. (**C**) Multivariate analysis of factors associated with annual progression of FILD without backward elimination.

	Change in Variables	OR	95% CI	S.E.	p Value
		(A)			
Age (years)	5.0	1.07	0.79–1.5	0.0308	0.68
Male gender		0.43	0.15–1.2	0.266	0.11
ILD subtype					
IPF		1.8	0.36–9.4	0.258	0.25
Fibrotic HP		1.7	0.36–9.4	0.401	0.49
UC-ILD		0.41	0.084–1.6	0.361	0.22
CT-definite UIP pattern		1.5	0.59–4.1	0.246	0.37
Smoker		0.56	0.18–1.7	0.284	0.30
Body mass index (kg/m^2)	10.0	0.84	0.25–2.8	0.0616	0.78
mMRC scale (0/1/2/3/4)					
0 (without dyspnea)		0.17	0.037–0.60	0.343	0.011 *
<2		0.37	0.12–1.1	0.027	0.067
<3		0.36	0.071–1.5	0.375	0.17
GAP score	1.0	1.1	0.82–1.6	0.175	0.43
Pulmonary function					
FVC (%)	10.0	0.82	0.62–1.1	0.0137	0.16
D_{LCO} (%)	10.0	0.88	0.68–1.1	0.0127	0.32
Six-minutes walk test					
Lowest SpO_2 (%)	1.0	0.90	0.82–0.98	0.0451	0.021 *
Decrease in SpO_2 (%)	1.0	1.1	1.0–1.3	0.0528	0.029 *
Walk distance (m)	10.0	0.95	0.90–0.99	0.00241	0.032 *
Serum biomarker					
CRP (mg/dL)	1.0	1.1	0.42–3.0	0.458	0.82
KL-6 (IU/mL)	100.0	1.008	0.95–1.1	0.000265	0.75
LDH (IU/L)	10.0	1.1	1.0–1.2	0.00508	0.055
Monocyte count (/uL)	10.0	1.02	0.99–1.05	0.00137	0.22
CAT	5.0	1.3	0.99–1.7	0.0268	0.065
Immunosuppressant use		0.57	0.14–2.0	0.331	0.39

Table 3. *Cont.*

	Change in Variables	OR	95% CI	S.E.	*p* Value
		(B)			
mMRC scale 0 (without dyspnea)		0.17	0.045–0.67	0.343	0.011 *
Age (years)	5.0				N.S.
Male gender					N.S.
IPF					N.S.
6 min walk distance (m)	10.0				N.S.
Lowest SpO_2 (%)	1.0				N.S.
Decrease in SpO_2 (%)	1.0				N.S.
FVC (%)	10.0				N.S.
D_{LCO} (%)	10.0				N.S.
		(C)			
mMRC scale 0 (without dyspnea)		0.14	0.022–0.83	0.463	0.031 *
Age (years)	5.0	0.90	0.61–1.3	0.0379	0.58
Male gender		0.64	0.15–2.7	0.367	0.54
IPF		4.4	1.1–16.6	0.341	0.031 *
6 min walk distance (m)	10.0	0.98	0.91–1.04	0.00330	0.45
Lowest SpO_2 (%)	1.0	0.99	0.73–1.3	0.151	0.98
Decrease in SpO_2 (%)	1.0	1.01	0.97–1.1	0.168	0.60
FVC (%)	10.0	0.81	0.56–1.1	0.0178	0.24
D_{LCO} (%)	10.0	1.1	0.75–1.7	0.0203	0.56

(**A**) OR, odds ratio; SE, standard error; confidence interval; FILD, fibrosing interstitial lung disease; ILD, interstitial lung disease; IPF, idiopathic pulmonary fibrosis; UC-ILD, unclassifiable interstitial lung disease; HP, hypersensitivity pneumonia; CTD, connective tissue disease; mMRC, modified Medical Research Council; GAP, gender–age–physiology; UIP, usual interstitial pneumonia; CT, computed tomography; FVC, forced vital capacity; D_{LCO}, diffusing capacity of the lung for carbon monoxide; 6MWT, 6 min walk test; SpO_2, saturation of percutaneous oxygen; CRP, C-reactive protein; KL-6, Krebs von den Lungen-6; LDH, lactate dehydrogenase; CAT, chronic obstructive pulmonary disease assessment test. ORs are the values when explanatory variables fluctuate within the range of change. * $p < 0.05$ is regarded as statistically significant. (**B**) OR, odds ratio; SE, standard error; confidence interval; FILD, fibrosing interstitial lung disease; mMRC, modified Medical Research Council; IPF, idiopathic pulmonary fibrosis; SpO_2, saturation of percutaneous oxygen; FVC, forced vital capacity; D_{LCO}, diffusing capacity of the lung for carbon monoxide; ORs are the values when explanatory variables fluctuate within the range of change. * $p < 0.05$ is regarded as statistically significant. (**C**) OR, odds ratio; SE, standard error; confidence interval; FILD, fibrosing interstitial lung disease; mMRC, modified Medical Research Council; IPF, idiopathic pulmonary fibrosis; SpO_2, saturation of percutaneous oxygen; FVC, forced vital capacity; D_{LCO}, diffusing capacity of the lung for carbon monoxide; ORs are the values when explanatory variables fluctuate within the range of change. * $p < 0.05$ is regarded as statistically significant.

3.4. Tolerability of Nintedanib Therapy in Dyspnea and Non-Dyspnea Groups

The results of the analysis of tolerability of nintedanib are shown in Table 4. The comparison of the nintedanib therapeutic period between the two groups is shown in Figure 4C.

Among the 76 patients, the incidences of discontinuing nintedanib for all causes and because of side effects were 26 (34%) and 20 (26%) patients throughout the overall period. Similarly, annual discontinuation was experienced in 10 (13%) patients after starting nintedanib and was due to side effects in all of these patients. Interruption and dose reduction in nintedanib were experienced in 27 (36%) and 52 (68%) patients throughout the overall period. Causes of discontinuing nintedanib were worsening FILD in seven (9%) patients, diarrhea in nine (12%), liver toxicity in three (4%), nausea in three (4%), and appetite loss, fatigue, worsening performance status, thrombocytosis, proteinuria, pulmonary hypertension, and edema in one (1%) each. The incidences of discontinuation, interruption, and dose reduction and the therapeutic period showed no significant differences between patients with and without dyspnea. The present study showed no difference in the tolerability of nintedanib therapy according to the presence of dyspnea in patients with FILD.

Table 4. Comparison of tolerability for nintedanib therapy with or without dyspnea.

	Overall	Non-Dyspnea Group	Dyspnea Group	*p* Value
Number	76	18 (24%)	58 (74%)	
Discontinuation				
Overall period/all cause	26 (34%)	6 (33%)	20 (34%)	0.78
Overall period/due to side effect	20 (26%)	4 (22%)	16 (28%)	0.77
For 1 year/all cause	10 (13%)	1 (6%)	9 (16%)	0.44
For 1 year/due to side effect	10 (13%)	1 (6%)	9 (16%)	0.44
Interruption	27 (36%)	8 (44%)	19 (33%)	0.41
Dose reduction	52 (68%)	15 (83%)	37 (64%)	0.15
Cause of discontinuation				
Worsening ILD	7 (9%)	2 (11%)	5 (9%)	
Diarrhea	9 (12%)	2 (11%)	7 (12%)	
Liver toxicity	3 (4%)	1 (6%)	2 (4%)	
Nausea	3 (4%)	1 (6%)	2 (4%)	
Appetite loss	1 (1%)	0	1 (2%)	
Fatigue	1 (1%)	0	1 (2%)	
Worsening of PS	1 (1%)	0	1 (2%)	
Thrombocytopenia	1 (1%)	0	1 (2%)	
Proteinuria	1 (1%)	0	1 (2%)	
Developing PH	1 (1%)	0	1 (2%)	
Edema	1 (1%)	0	1 (2%)	

OR, odds ratio; SE, standard error; CI, confidence interval; IPF, idiopathic pulmonary fibrosis; mMRC, modified Medical Research Council; SpO_2, saturation of percutaneous oxygen; FVC, forced vital capacity; D_{LCO}, diffusing capacity of the lung for carbon monoxide; CAT, chronic obstructive pulmonary disease assessment test.

4. Discussion

This study demonstrated that a substantial proportion of asymptomatic patients with FILD who require nintedanib therapy have significant exercise-induced oxygen desaturation. The outcomes after nintedanib therapy were better in patients without than with dyspnea, as evidenced by a lower incidence of progression, a slower decline in pulmonary function, and better survival of FILD even after adjustment for covariates.

Among the 18 patients with FILD without dyspnea, 4 (24%) showed a decrease in SpO_2 to <90%, and 12 (71%) showed a decrease in SpO_2 of >4% during the 6MWT. These cut-off levels of desaturation were associated with survival in patients with FILD [17,18]. Similarly, 6 (40%) of 18 patients who had FILD without dyspnea showed a CAT score of >10 as a prognostic factor for COPD [28]. The CAT score was reported as a predictor of OS in patients receiving oxygen therapy (i.e., patients with non-early-stage disease) in a previous report [27], but this finding has not been revealed in patients without dyspnea. The present study showed that asymptomatic patients with FILD have potential exercise-induced oxygen desaturation and high CAT scores. Moreover, in the comparative analyses adjusted for covariates as prognostic factors of FILD, patients without dyspnea had better outcomes after nintedanib therapy than those with dyspnea. These findings demonstrate that antifibrotic drugs can benefit asymptomatic patients with FILD and should not be avoided merely because of the absence of dyspnea. The mechanisms underlying the differences in outcomes after nintedanib therapy between patients with and without dyspnea are unknown. In the subgroup analysis of the SENSCIS phase 3 trial, there was no difference in the decrease over 1 year between the non-dyspnea and dyspnea placebo groups with SSc-ILD. These findings suggest that nintedanib can slow the decline in pulmonary function in patients who have FILD without dyspnea [15]. By contrast, the non-dyspnea group had a numerically smaller extent of fibrotic area and lower pulmonary function at baseline in this subgroup study [15]. The results of the present study, which show that patients without dyspnea have better outcomes after nintedanib therapy than those with dyspnea, might be associated with the possibility that patients with dyspnea have fewer established fibrotic lesions resistant to drug therapy. Moreover, initiating antifibrotic drugs for all asymptomatic patients with FILD may lead to excessive side effects and an economic burden for patients. Therefore, further research is needed to identify biomarkers to select asymptomatic patients with FILD who are suitable for early intervention with antifibrotic drugs. These issues should be addressed in future studies.

Although blood biomarkers, including C-reactive protein, KL-6, lactate dehydrogenase (LDH), and the monocyte count, were not associated with annual progression of FILD in the present study, they have been reported as biomarkers for predicting mortality, progression, and the development of AE [31–35]. Huang et al. [31] reported that high baseline plasma KL-6 levels are a risk factor for death, AE, and liver damage in IPF patients treated with nintedanib. Additionally, in our retrospective study, the effectiveness of nintedanib in suppressing a decline in D_{LCO} in patients with IPF was higher in patients with higher than lower serum KL-6 or LDH levels [32]. Further studies are needed to clarify serum biomarkers that predict the effectiveness of antifibrotic drugs in patients with FILD.

Although the diagnosis of IPF and a definite UIP pattern on chest computed tomography have been reported as prognostic factors of FILD [1–4,36], neither was associated with annual progression of FILD in our study. This result may be associated with the possibility that patients with progression were selected for nintedanib therapy. A previous study showed that OS was not significantly different between patients with progressive pulmonary fibrosis and those with IPF [6]. Another study showed that among patients with IPF, there was no significant difference in OS between those showing a definite UIP pattern and those showing a probable UIP pattern [36].

In the present study, there was no difference in nintedanib tolerability between patients with and without dyspnea, as demonstrated by comparable discontinuation rates and therapeutic period. This suggests that the presence of dyspnea may not be associated with the tolerability of nintedanib. Previous retrospective studies in Japan have identified higher age, lower body mass index, and worse performance status as risk factors for lower tolerability and safety of nintedanib, which could be mitigated by dose reduction from 300 to 200 mg/day [37–39]. The results of our study may have been influenced by the fact that there were no significant differences in age, body mass index, or percentage of patients with a reduced starting dose of nintedanib, because nintedanib therapy for patients with FILD tends to be started at an early disease stage in our hospital. Further studies involving more patients with severe disease may be needed to clarify the difference in tolerability between patients with and without dyspnea.

The present study had several limitations. First, the sample size was relatively small, and larger population studies are needed to validate these findings. Second, this was a retrospective, single-arm study. Although a randomized controlled trial would be the most appropriate design for evaluating the effectiveness and tolerability of nintedanib, conducting such a trial would be challenging. Nevertheless, the present study provides a rationale for planning future randomized controlled trials.

5. Conclusions

We showed that patients who had FILD without dyspnea have severe exercise-induced oxygen desaturation and better outcomes after nintedanib therapy than those with dyspnea, but there was no difference in tolerability of this therapy between the two groups. Treatment with antifibrotic drugs should not be avoided solely because of an absence of symptoms.

Author Contributions: Conceptualization, M.O., T.Y., A.K. and T.H.; methodology, M.O., T.Y. and A.K.; validation, M.O., T.Y., K.F., T.C., K.T., Y.Z., M.T., A.S., Y.N., N.M., T.N., S.M., A.K. and T.H.; formal analysis, A.K.; writing—original draft preparation, M.O.; writing—review and editing, All authors; supervision, A.K. and T.H.; funding acquisition, M.O. All authors have read and agreed to the published version of the manuscript.

Funding: This work was supported by research funds from the Department of Respirology at the NHO Kyushu Medical Center.

Institutional Review Board Statement: This study complied with all applicable laws regarding subject privacy and received approval for all procedures from the Institutional Review Board (IRB) of NHO Kyushu Medical Center. The IRB approval number for our study is 22C080, granted on 21 December 2022. All research was conducted in accordance with relevant guidelines and regulations.

Informed Consent Statement: Informed consent was obtained from all patients using an opt-out methodology.

Data Availability Statement: The datasets used and/or analyzed during the current study are available from the corresponding author on reasonable request.

Acknowledgments: We thank Natsuko Shibata, M.T. of the Department of Respirology, NHO Kyushu Medical Center, for sorting the medical data.

Conflicts of Interest: Masaki Okamoto, Toyoshi Yanagihara, and Tomoaki Hoshino received more than JPY 1,000,000 as research funding from Nippon Boehringer-Ingelheim, Co., Ltd. Kiminori Fujimoto received more than JPY 1,000,000 as research funding from Micron KK. Masaki Okamoto and Yoshiaki Zaizen received more than JPY 500,000 as honoraria from Nippon Boehringer-Ingelheim, Co., Ltd. The other co-authors have no potential conflicts of interest.

References

1. Raghu, G.; Remy-Jardin, M.; Richeldi, L.; Thomson, C.C.; Inoue, Y.; Johkoh, T.; Kreuter, M.; Lynch, D.A.; Maher, T.M.; Martinez, F.J.; et al. Idiopathic Pulmonary Fibrosis (an Update) and Progressive Pulmonary Fibrosis in Adults: An Official ATS/ERS/JRS/ALAT Clinical Practice Guideline. *Am. J. Respir. Crit. Care Med.* **2022**, *205*, e18–e47. [CrossRef] [PubMed]
2. Raghu, G.; Remy-Jardin, M.; Myers, J.L.; Richeldi, L.; Ryerson, C.J.; Lederer, D.J.; Behr, J.; Cottin, V.; Danoff, S.K.; Morell, F.; et al. Diagnosis of Idiopathic Pulmonary Fibrosis. An Official ATS/ERS/JRS/ALAT Clinical Practice Guideline. *Am. J. Respir. Crit. Care Med.* **2018**, *198*, e44–e68. [CrossRef] [PubMed]
3. Raghu, G.; Collard, H.R.; Egan, J.J.; Martinez, F.J.; Behr, J.; Brown, K.K.; Colby, T.V.; Cordier, J.F.; Flaherty, K.R.; Lasky, J.A.; et al. An Official ATS/ERS/JRS/ALAT Statement: Idiopathic Pulmonary Fibrosis: Evidence-based Guidelines for Diagnosis and Management. *Am. J. Respir. Crit. Care Med.* **2011**, *183*, 788–824. [CrossRef] [PubMed]
4. Travis, W.D.; Costabel, U.; Hansell, D.M.; King, T.E., Jr.; Lynch, D.A.; Nicholson, A.G.; Ryerson, C.J.; Ryu, J.H.; Selman, M.; Wells, A.U.; et al. An official American Thoracic Society/European Respiratory Society statement: Update of the international multidisciplinary classification of the idiopathic interstitial pneumonias. *Am. J. Respir. Crit. Care Med.* **2013**, *188*, 733–748. [CrossRef]
5. Natsuizaka, M.; Chiba, H.; Kuronuma, K.; Otsuka, M.; Kudo, K.; Mori, M.; Bando, M.; Sugiyama, Y.; Takahashi, H. Epidemiologic survey of Japanese patients with idiopathic pulmonary fibrosis and investigation of ethnic differences. *Am. J. Respir. Crit. Care Med.* **2014**, *190*, 773–779. [CrossRef] [PubMed]
6. Khor, Y.H.; Farooqi, M.; Hambly, N.; Kolb, M.; Ryerson, C.J.; Austin ILD Registry and CARE-PF Investigators. Patient Characteristics and Survival for Progressive Pulmonary Fibrosis Using Different Definitions. *Am. J. Respir. Crit. Care Med.* **2013**, *207*, 102–105. [CrossRef] [PubMed]
7. Richeldi, L.; du Bois, R.M.; Raghu, G.; Azuma, A.; Brown, K.K.; Costabel, U.; Cottin, V.; Flaherty, K.R.; Hansell, D.M.; Inoue, Y.; et al. Efficacy and safety of nintedanib in idiopathic pulmonary fibrosis. *N. Engl. J. Med.* **2014**, *370*, 2071–2082. [CrossRef] [PubMed]
8. King, T.E., Jr.; Bradfor, W.Z.; Castro-Bernardini, S.; Fagan, E.A.; Glaspole, I.; Glassberg, M.K.; Gorina, E.; Hopkins, P.M.; Kardatzke, D.; Lancaster, L.; et al. A phase 3 trial of pirfenidone in patients with idiopathic pulmonary fibrosis. *N. Engl. J. Med.* **2014**, *370*, 2083–2092. [CrossRef]
9. Petnak, T.; Lertjitbanjong, P.; Thongprayoon, C.; Moua, T. Impact of Antifibrotic Therapy on Mortality and Acute Exacerbation in Idiopathic Pulmonary Fibrosis: A Systematic Review and Meta-Analysis. *Chest* **2021**, *160*, 1751–1763. [CrossRef] [PubMed]
10. Flaherty, K.R.; Wells, A.U.; Cottin, V.; Devaraj, A.; Walsh, S.L.F.; Inoue, Y.; Richeldi, L.; Kolb, M.; Tetzlaff, K.; Stowasser, S.; et al. Nintedanib in Progressive Fibrosing Interstitial Lung Diseases. *N. Engl. J. Med.* **2019**, *381*, 1718–1727. [CrossRef]
11. Homma, S.; Bando, M.; Azuma, A.; Sakamoto, S.; Sugino, K.; Ishii, Y.; Izumi, S.; Inase, N.; Inoue, Y.; Ebina, M.; et al. Japanese guideline for the treatment of idiopathic pulmonary fibrosis. *Respir. Investig.* **2018**, *56*, 268–291. [CrossRef]
12. Maher, T.M.; Stowasser, S.; Nishioka, Y.; White, E.S.; Cottin, V.; Noth, I.; Selman, M.; Rohr, K.B.; Michael, A.; Ittrich, C.; et al. Biomarkers of extracellular matrix turnover in patients with idiopathic pulmonary fibrosis given nintedanib (INMARK study): A randomised, placebo-controlled study. *Lancet Respir. Med.* **2019**, *7*, 771–779. [CrossRef]
13. Kolb, M.; Flaherty, K.R.; Silva, R.S.; Prasse, A.; Vancheri, C.; Mueller, H.; Sroka-Saidi, K.; Wells, A.U.; INBUILD trial investigators. Effect of Nintedanib in Patients with Progressive Pulmonary Fibrosis in Subgroups with Differing Baseline Characteristics. *Adv. Ther.* **2023**, *40*, 5536–5546. [CrossRef]
14. Nishiyama, O.; Taniguchi, H.; Kondoh, H.; Kimura, T.; Kato, K.; Kataoka, K.; Ogawa, T.; Watanabe, F.; Arizono, S. A simple assessment of dyspnoea as a prognostic indicator in idiopathic pulmonary fibrosis. *Eur. Respir. J.* **2010**, *36*, 1067–1072. [CrossRef]

15. Volkmann, E.R.; Kreuter, M.; Hoffmann-Vold, A.M.; Wijsenbeek, M.; Smith, V.; Khanna, D.; Denton, C.P.; Wuyts, W.A.; Miede, C.; Alves, M.; et al. Dyspnoea and cough in patients with systemic sclerosis-associated interstitial lung disease in the SENSCIS trial. *Rheumatology* **2022**, *61*, 4397–4408. [CrossRef]
16. Lama, V.N.; Flaherty, K.R.; Toews, G.B.; Colby, T.V.; Travis, W.D.; Long, Q.; Murray, S.; Kazerooni, E.A.; Gross, B.H.; Lynch, J.P., 3rd; et al. Prognostic value of desaturation during a 6-minute walk test in idiopathic interstitial pneumonia. *Am. J. Respir. Crit. Care Med.* **2003**, *168*, 1084–1090. [CrossRef] [PubMed]
17. Lederer, D.J.; Arcasoy, S.M.; Wilt, J.S.; D'Ovidio, F.; Sonett, J.R.; Kawut, S.M. Six-minute-walk distance predicts waiting list survival in idiopathic pulmonary fibrosis. *Am. J. Respir. Crit. Care Med.* **2006**, *174*, 659–664. [CrossRef]
18. Kondoh, Y.; Taniguchi, H.; Kataoka, K.; Furukawa, T.; Ando, M.; Murotani, K.; Mishima, M.; Inoue, Y.; Ogura, T.; Bando, M.; et al. Disease severity staging system for idiopathic pulmonary fibrosis in Japan. *Respirology* **2017**, *22*, 1609–1614. [CrossRef] [PubMed]
19. Sugino, K.; Ono, H.; Watanabe, N.; Ando, M.; Tsuboi, E.; Homma, S.; Kishi, K. Efficacy of early antifibrotic treatment for idiopathic pulmonary fibrosis. *BMC Pulm. Med.* **2021**, *21*, 218. [CrossRef]
20. Nishiyama, O.; Taniguchi, H.; Kondoh, Y.; Kimura, T.; Kato, K.; Ogawa, T.; Watanabe, F.; Arizono, S. Dyspnoea at 6-min walk test in idiopathic pulmonary fibrosis: Comparison with COPD. *Respir. Med.* **2007**, *101*, 833–838. [CrossRef] [PubMed]
21. van den Hoogen, F.; Khanna, D.; Fransen, J.; Johnson, S.R.; Baron, M.; Tyndall, A.; Matucci-Cerinic, M.; Naden, R.P.; Medsger, T.A., Jr.; Carreira, P.E.; et al. 2013 Classification criteria for systemic sclerosis: An American College of Rheumatology/European League against rheumatism collaborative initiative. *Arthritis Rheum.* **2013**, *65*, 2737–2747. [CrossRef]
22. Bohan, A.; Peter, J.B. Polymyositis and dermatomyositis (first of two parts). *N. Engl. J. Med.* **1975**, *292*, 344–347. [CrossRef]
23. Aletaha, D.; Neogi, T.; Silman, A.J.; Funovits, J.; Felson, D.T.; Bingham, C.O., 3rd; Birnbaum, N.S.; Burmester, G.R.; Bykerk, V.P.; Cohen, M.D.; et al. 2010 Rheumatoid arthritis classification criteria: An American College of Rheumatology/European League Against Rheumatism collaborative initiative. *Arthritis Rheum.* **2010**, *62*, 2569–2581. [CrossRef]
24. Shiboski, C.H.; Shiboski, S.C.; Seror, R.; Criswell, L.A.; Labetoulle, M.; Lietman, T.M.; Rasmussen, A.; Scofield, H.; Vitali, C.; Bowman, S.J.; et al. 2016 American College of Rheumatology/European League Against Rheumatism classification criteria for primary Sjogren's syndrome: A consensus and data-driven methodology involving three international patient cohorts. *Ann. Rheum. Dis.* **2017**, *76*, 9–16. [CrossRef]
25. Collard, H.R.; Moore, B.B.; Flaherty, K.R.; Brown, K.K.; Kaner, R.J.; King, T.E., Jr.; Lasky, J.A.; Loyd, J.E.; Noth, I.; Olman, M.A.; et al. Acute exacerbations of idiopathic pulmonary fibrosis. *Am. J. Respir. Crit. Care Med.* **2007**, *176*, 636–643. [CrossRef]
26. Ryerson, C.J.; Vittinghoff, E.; Ley, B.; Lee, J.S.; Mooney, J.J.; Jones, K.D.; Elicker, B.M.; Wolters, P.J.; Koth, L.L.; King, T.E., Jr.; et al. Predicting survival across chronic interstitial lung disease: The ILD-GAP model. *Chest* **2014**, *145*, 723–728. [CrossRef]
27. Kataoka, K.; Oda, K.; Takizawa, H.; Ogura, T.; Miyamoto, A.; Inoue, Y.; Akagawa, S.; Hashimoto, S.; Kishaba, T.; Sakamoto, K.; et al. Cohort study to evaluate prognostic factors in idiopathic pulmonary fibrosis patients introduced to oxygen therapy. *Sci. Rep.* **2023**, *13*, 13664. [CrossRef] [PubMed]
28. Venkatesan, P. GOLD COPD report: 2024 update. *Lancet Respir. Med.* **2024**, *12*, 15–16. [CrossRef]
29. Miller, M.R.; Hankinson, J.; Brusasco, V.; Burgos, F.; Casaburi, R.; Coates, A.; Crapo, R.; Enright, P.; van der Grinten, C.P.; Gustafsson, P.; et al. Standardization of spirometry. *Eur. Respir. J.* **2005**, *26*, 319–338. [CrossRef]
30. ATS Committee on Proficiency Standards for Clinical Pulmonary Function Laboratories. ATS statement: Guidelines for the six-minute walk test. *Guidel. Am. J. Respir. Crit. Care Med.* **2002**, *166*, 111–117. [CrossRef]
31. Huang, T.H.; Kuo, C.W.; Chen, C.W.; Tseng, Y.L.; Wu, C.L.; Lin, S.H. Baseline plasma KL-6 level predicts adverse outcomes in patients with idiopathic pulmonary fibrosis receiving nintedanib: A retrospective real-world cohort study. *BMC Pulm. Med.* **2021**, *21*, 165.
32. Okamoto, M.; Fujimoto, K.; Johkoh, T.; Kawaguchi, A.; Mukae, H.; Sakamoto, N.; Ogura, T.; Ikeda, S.; Kondoh, Y.; Yamano, Y.; et al. A prospective cohort study of periostin as a serum biomarker in patients with idiopathic pulmonary fibrosis treated with nintedanib. *Sci. Rep.* **2023**, *13*, 22977. [CrossRef]
33. Stock, C.J.W.; Bray, W.G.; Kouranos, V.; Jacob, J.; Kokosi, M.; George, P.M.; Chua, F.; Wells, A.U.; Sestini, P.; Renzoni, E.A. Serum C-reactive protein is associated with earlier mortality across different interstitial lung diseases. *Respirology* **2024**, *29*, 228–234. [CrossRef] [PubMed]
34. Kreuter, M.; Lee, J.S.; Tzouvelekis, A.; Oldham, J.M.; Molyneaux, P.L.; Weycker, D.; Atwood, M.; Kirchgaessler, K.U.; Maher, T.M. Monocyte Count as a Prognostic Biomarker in Patients with Idiopathic Pulmonary Fibrosis. *Am. J. Respir. Crit. Care Med.* **2021**, *204*, 74–81. [CrossRef] [PubMed]
35. Zinellu, A.; Fois, A.G.; Pirina, P.; Carru, C.; Mangoni, A.A. A Systematic Review and Meta-analysis of Clinical, Respiratory, and Biochemical Risk Factors for Acute Exacerbation of idiopathic Pulmonary Fibrosis. *Arch. Med. Res.* **2023**, *54*, 319–331. [CrossRef] [PubMed]
36. Adegunsoye, A.; Oldham, J.M.; Bellam, S.K.; Montner, S.; Churpek, M.M.; Noth, I.; Vij, R.; Strek, M.E.; Chung, J.H. Computed tomography honeycombing identifies a progressive fibrotic phenotype with increased mortality across diverse interstitial lung diseases. *Ann. Am. Thorac. Soc.* **2019**, *16*, 580–588. [CrossRef]
37. Uchida, Y.; Ikeda, S.; Sekine, A.; Katano, T.; Tabata, E.; Oda, T.; Okuda, R.; Kitamura, H.; Baba, T.; Komatsu, S.; et al. Tolerability and safety of nintedanib in elderly patients with idiopathic pulmonary fibrosis. *Respir. Investig.* **2021**, *59*, 99–105. [CrossRef] [PubMed]

38. Ikeda, S.; Sekine, A.; Baba, T.; Yamanaka, Y.; Sadoyama, S.; Yamakawa, H.; Oda, T.; Okuda, R.; Kitamura, H.; Okudela, K.; et al. Low body surface area predicts hepatotoxicity of nintedanib in patients with idiopathic pulmonary fibrosis. *Sci. Rep.* **2017**, *7*, 10811. [CrossRef] [PubMed]
39. Kato, M.; Sasaki, S.; Nakamura, T.; Kurokawa, K.; Yamada, T.; Ochi, Y.; Ihara, H.; Takahashi, F.; Takahashi, K. Gastrointestinal adverse effects of nintedanib and the associated risk factors in patients with idiopathic pulmonary fibrosis. *Sci. Rep.* **2019**, *9*, 12062. [CrossRef] [PubMed]

Journal of
Clinical Medicine

MDPI

Review

Examining Cough's Role and Relief Strategies in Interstitial Lung Disease

Chee Yao Lim [1,2,*], Sanam Wasim Khan [3], Tarek Alsibai [1,2] and Gayathri Sathiyamoorthy [1,2]

[1] Corewell Health, Grand Rapids, MI 49503, USA; tarek.alsibai@corewellhealth.org (T.A.); gayathri.sathiyamoorthy@corewellhealth.org (G.S.)
[2] College of Human Medicine, Michigan State University, East Lansing, MI 48824, USA
[3] CMH Lahore Medical College, Lahore 54810, Pakistan; sanamhumayun13@gmail.com
* Correspondence: cheeyao.lim@corewellhealth.org; Tel.: +1-(929)-507-9325

Abstract: Chronic cough is a distressing and prevalent symptom in interstitial lung disease (ILD), significantly impairing quality of life (QoL) and contributing to disease progression, particularly in idiopathic pulmonary fibrosis (IPF). It is associated with physical discomfort, psychological distress, and social isolation and is often refractory to conventional therapies. The pathophysiology of cough in ILD is complex and multifactorial, involving neural hypersensitivity, structural lung changes, inflammatory processes, and comorbid conditions such as gastroesophageal reflux disease (GERD). Evaluating cough in ILD relies on subjective and objective tools to measure its severity, frequency, and impact on daily life, although standardization of these measures remains challenging. Management strategies span pharmacological interventions, including neuromodulators such as opiates, antifibrotic agents, pharmacologic and surgical GERD treatments, and non-pharmacological approaches like behavioral therapies, cough suppression techniques, and pulmonary rehabilitation and physiotherapy. Emerging treatments, such as P2X3 receptor antagonists and airway hydration therapies, offer promising avenues but require further investigation through robust clinical trials. This review aims to demonstrate the importance of addressing cough in ILD as a significant symptom and present objective and subjective methods of quantifying coughs, while providing insights into effective and emerging therapeutic options. By highlighting these potential therapies, we hope to guide healthcare practitioners in considering them through a thorough evaluation of benefits and risks on a case-by-case basis, with relevance both in the U.S. and internationally.

Keywords: cough; interstitial lung disease; idiopathic pulmonary fibrosis; treatment; update

1. Cough in ILD

Interstitial lung disease (ILD) encompasses a heterogeneous group of pulmonary disorders that are marked by inflammation and fibrosis of the lung interstitium, leading to progressive respiratory dysfunction, which includes chronic cough. Chronic cough, a prevalent and debilitating symptom in ILD, significantly impacts quality of life [1–3] and contributes to physical discomfort, psychological distress, and social isolation, all of which pose substantial clinical management challenges [4]. Chronic cough in ILD is a significant outcome measure of the management of ILD [3], which is often refractory to conventional therapeutic interventions. The cough severity was found to be higher in patients with idiopathic pulmonary fibrosis (IPF) compared to non-IPF fibrotic ILD, and the baseline cough severity was independently associated with disease progression and reduced transplant-free survival [5,6].

The pathophysiology of cough in ILD is multifactorial and only partially understood. It involves complex interactions between mechanical alterations in the lung architecture, the activation of neural pathways, and inflammatory processes. Factors such as fibrotic remodeling, increased airway sensitivity, and coexistent conditions like gastroesophageal reflux disease (GERD) and upper airway cough syndrome further complicate the clinical picture.

Current treatment approaches for cough in ILD are often empirical and yield variable results, highlighting a significant unmet clinical need [7]. Therapeutic options range from pharmacological interventions, including antitussives, neuromodulators, and anti-inflammatory agents, to non-pharmacological measures, such as pulmonary rehabilitation and cough suppression techniques. Recent advances in developing antifibrotic therapies and targeted neuromodulators offer promising avenues for improved symptom control. The efficacy and safety profiles of these treatments necessitate further exploration through robust clinical trials.

This review aims to elucidate the current understanding of cough's epidemiology, pathophysiology, and impact on ILD, while emphasizing the need for standardizing the approach to diagnosing coughing that is specific to ILD/IPF, distinguishing it from chronic coughs of other etiologies. Furthermore, it highlights advancements in measuring and monitoring cough in ILD patients and explores updated and solidified treatment options. By synthesizing the contemporary evidence, this review provides a comprehensive resource to guide clinicians and researchers in improving the management of cough and enhancing patient outcomes in ILD. Figures 1 and 2 illustrate a systematic approach to the diagnosis and investigation of patients presenting with subacute and chronic cough [8].

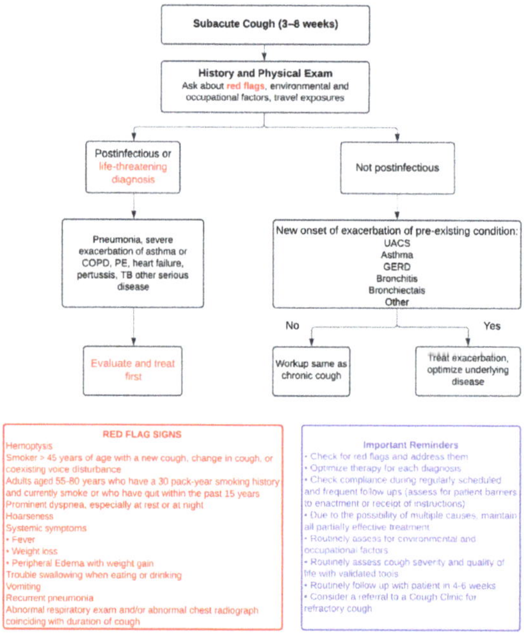

Figure 1. The figure illustrates a systematic approach to diagnosing subacute cough (3–8 weeks), beginning with a comprehensive history and physical examination to identify "red flags" such as hemoptysis, significant weight loss, recurrent pneumonia, or abnormal imaging findings, while also

considering environmental, occupational, and travel exposures. Postinfectious or life-threatening conditions, including pneumonia, severe asthma or COPD exacerbations, pulmonary embolism, or tuberculosis, require immediate evaluation and treatment. For non-postinfectious causes, such as exacerbations of chronic conditions like upper airway cough syndrome (UACS), asthma, or GERD, management focuses on optimizing the underlying disease. In cases without exacerbation, the workup follows that of chronic cough. Red flag signs are clues to potential life-threatening conditions. Adapted from: Irwin RS et al., 2017 [8].

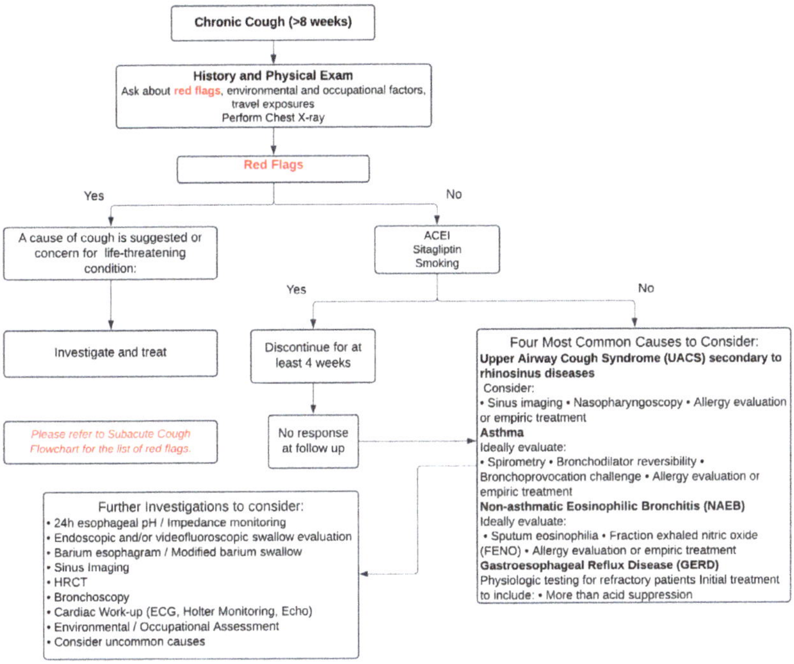

Figure 2. The figure presents a structured approach to the evaluation and management of chronic cough (≥8 weeks), beginning with a detailed history, physical examination, and chest X-ray to identify potential "red flags" suggestive of life-threatening or serious conditions, which warrant immediate investigation and treatment. In the absence of red flags, common causes such as upper airway cough syndrome (UACS), asthma, gastroesophageal reflux disease (GERD), or non-asthmatic eosinophilic bronchitis (NAEB) should be systematically considered and managed. For unresolved cases after 4 weeks of treatment, further investigations such as 24-h pH monitoring, spirometry, allergy testing, and HRCT may be necessary. It emphasizes a stepwise evaluation to address underlying causes while minimizing unnecessary interventions. Adapted from: Irwin RS et al., 2017 [8].

2. Measuring Cough in ILD

The assessment of cough, particularly in terms of its severity, frequency, and impact on health-related quality of life (HRQOL), is essential in clinical practice and research. Among the key tools that are used to evaluate cough in ILD patients are the Leicester Cough Questionnaire (LCQ), the Cough Quality of Life Questionnaire (CQLQ), and the Cough Visual Analog Scale (VAS).

The LCQ is a widely accepted measure of cough severity and its impact on quality of life [9]. It is a 19-item, self-administered questionnaire that assesses cough in three physical, psychological, and social domains [Appendix A]. The LCQ has been particularly valuable in patients with ILD, because it captures the multidimensional impact of chronic cough, which often worsens over time in progressive diseases like IPF [10]. By providing a reliable measure of cough severity and its effect on everyday activities, the LCQ is used to track disease progression and evaluate the effectiveness of interventions [11]. Improvements in LCQ scores have been associated with a reduction in cough severity, reflecting an overall improvement in HRQOL. Similarly, a lower LCQ score is independently linked to an increased risk of respiratory hospitalization, death, and the need for lung transplantation [11].

Similarly, the CQLQ focuses on how chronic cough affects a patient's daily life. This tool delves into different aspects of well-being, including physical discomfort, emotional health, and the social implications of persistent cough [Appendix B] [12]. In ILD, where cough is often refractory to treatment, the CQLQ is a valuable outcome measure to determine how well therapeutic interventions address cough-related symptoms and their psychosocial burden. Clinicians and researchers use this tool to gauge the symptom burden and understand the treatment response more holistically by assessing changes in HRQOL.

The VASc is another tool that is used to assess cough in ILD, especially for its simplicity and ease of use. It is a unidimensional scale, where patients rate their perceived cough severity on a continuum, usually a 100 mm line ranging from "no cough" to "worst cough imaginable" [Appendix C]. The VASc is quick to administer and can be highly useful in clinical settings for both initial assessments and follow-up visits. The cough VAS can be applied in ILD patients alongside more detailed, objective tools like the LCQ and CQLQ to provide a rapid snapshot of symptom severity [13]. It is often employed to monitor treatment responses over time, as shifts in VASc scores can indicate changes in cough severity that correlate with HRQOL improvements [14]. A recent study looked into the VASc in predicting survival and identified significant quality of life differences in patients with IPF, with a clinically meaningful cutoff score of 30 mm [15]. More studies would be helpful to validate the VASc among ILD patients [16].

The St. George's Respiratory Questionnaire (SGRQ) assesses HRQOL in patients with chronic respiratory diseases, including ILD [Appendix D] [17,18]. While it has been validated and utilized in various studies involving ILD patients, the SGRQ only partially addresses cough. Cough is included as part of its broader assessment of respiratory symptoms rather than being a central focus. As a result, the SGRQ provides insight into how cough may contribute to the overall symptom burden. Still, it does not explicitly measure cough severity or its detailed impact on quality of life.

The Living with Pulmonary Fibrosis (L-PF) questionnaire is a relatively new patient-reported outcome (PRO) measure, developed to assess symptoms and quality of life in patients with progressive fibrosing ILD (PF-ILDs) [Appendix E]. The L-PF is an adaptation of the original Living with Pulmonary Fibrosis (L-IPF) questionnaire and includes two modules: Symptoms and Impacts. It focuses on crucial symptom domains, such as dyspnea, cough, and fatigue, and uses a 24 h recall period to capture daily fluctuations in these symptoms. Validation studies have confirmed the relevance of the L-PF for patients with various forms of PF-ILDs, demonstrating good face validity and responsiveness to change. This makes it a valuable tool for both clinical research and potentially for routine clinical practice, providing insights into the symptom burden and quality of life impacts for patients [19,20].

These tools—the LCQ, CQLQ, SGRQ, and cough VASc—offer complementary approaches to measuring cough and its impact on patients with ILD. While the LCQ and CQLQ provide a more comprehensive assessment of cough's multidimensional effects, the

VAS offers a straightforward and immediate measure of the symptom severity, allowing for a detailed understanding of the patient's experience and tracking of the treatment efficacy.

The measures discussed are subjective patient-reported outcomes, which primarily focus on how cough symptoms affect quality of life [21]. Attempts at validating the tools have been made and correlate well with the objective cough severity [13]. A limitation of these tools is that they do not directly measure cough severity but address it indirectly through their impact on daily functioning. This distinction is important, because improvements in a patient's perception of their cough may result from actual cough suppression but also from the central neuromodulatory effects of treatments. These treatments could include opioids, pregabalin, and gabapentin, which reduce the unpleasantness of the cough experience [7].

Several modern objective cough measuring tools such as the Leicester Cough Monitor (LCM) and VitaloJAK™ are commercially available. These are primarily used in clinical trials to validate subjective cough measurements across various disease-specific cough conditions [22]. Although direct comparisons between these tests are lacking, their results are relatively consistent [22].

3. GERD and Cough in ILD

Over the past 10–15 years, evidence has highlighted the complex relationship between GERD and cough in ILD [23,24]. GERD is commonly observed in patients with ILD, particularly in those with idiopathic pulmonary fibrosis (IPF), where the prevalence of reflux can be as high as 90% [24,25]. The connection between GERD and cough in ILD is thought to stem from silent microaspiration of gastric contents into the lower airways. This causes or exacerbates lung inflammation, which may worsen the underlying disease and contribute to a chronic, persistent cough [24].

Several studies have suggested that GERD may act as both a trigger and perpetrator of cough in ILD patients. Aggressive GERD management, including lifestyle changes or using proton pump inhibitors (PPIs) or Histamine 2 receptor blockers, may help control cough and potentially slow the disease progression [26,27]. However, the benefit of antireflux therapies in improving overall ILD outcomes remains controversial, with some studies showing improvement in cough symptoms but limited evidence of a clear impact on long-term disease progression or survival [28].

One key study by Raghu et al. (2006) [29] explored the high prevalence of GERD in patients with IPF and suggested that antireflux treatment could reduce chronic cough, but randomized controlled trials have not consistently confirmed a clear therapeutic benefit. Additionally, non-acid reflux and silent aspiration—conditions where patients experience reflux without typical GERD symptoms—complicate the diagnosis and management of cough in ILD [30]. These forms of reflux may still contribute to cough and disease progression but are more challenging to detect and treat. Thus, conventional GERD therapies alone may not be sufficient for all ILD patients with cough [31].

Moreover, in recent years, the role of surgical interventions, such as fundoplication, has been investigated as a more definitive approach to controlling GERD in ILD patients [32]. Although the causal relationship is not well established, risk factors include cough, and an association with aspiration and the worsening of IPF is a suggested theory [32,33]. There are limited data stating that repairing hiatal hernia would improve outcomes among patients in IPF or symptomatic controls [34]. We believe that with cough as a predictor of mortality among patients with IPF, treating cough effectively by means of acid suppression and surgical correction of anatomical anomalies such as hiatal hernia would be a conjugate of mortality benefit. More studies would need to be carried out. While some studies suggest that surgical intervention may help reduce the incidence of reflux-related cough and microaspiration [35], the risks associated with surgery, particularly in patients with advanced lung disease, remain a concern. More research is needed to determine which subsets of ILD patients are most likely to benefit from GERD management strategies, both pharmacological and surgical.

4. Opiates as Antitussive Treatment in ILD-Associated Cough

Opiates have long been recognized for their potent antitussive (cough-suppressing) properties. They work by directly suppressing the cough reflex through mu receptors in the brainstem. Their use in treating chronic refractory cough, including cough associated with ILD, has received significant attention in recent years.

In ILD, where chronic cough can be debilitating, low-dose opioids have been explored as a therapeutic option to improve quality of life. Morphine decreased the cough frequency, improved patients' comfort, and reduced the distress associated with persistent coughing. Other studies have supported these findings, indicating that low-dose opioids (5 mg controlled-release morphine sulfate (MST)) can be a valuable adjunct for symptom control in refractory cough when other options are ineffective [36]. In a randomized, double-blind, placebo-controlled crossover trial, a nalbuphine extended-release tablet (NAL ER) was shown to significantly reduce cough in IPF [37]. This drug is currently not available in the United States. Table 1 provides an overview of studies evaluating the role and efficacy of opioid therapy in managing cough among patients with IPF.

Table 1. Studies evaluating the role and efficacy of opioid therapy in managing cough among patients with IPF.

Author	Article	Journal	Year	Result	Intervention
Zhe Wu, et al. [36]	PACIFY COUGH	*The Lancet Respiratory Medicine*	2024	In patients with cough related to IPF, low-dose controlled-release morphine significantly reduced objective cough counts over 14 days compared to placebo.	5 mg oral morphine twice daily.
Toby M. Maher, et al. [37]	Nalbuphine Tablets for Cough in Patients with IPF	*NEJM Evidence*	2023	NAL ER reduced cough in individuals with IPF.	Nalbuphine ER 27 mg once daily, up-titrated to 162 mg twice daily on day 16.

Despite the potential benefits, the use of opiates in ILD patients is not without challenges. Although low-dose morphine has a good safety profile, it does carry a risk of side effects, including nausea, vomiting, constipation, and, importantly, respiratory depression, which can be particularly concerning in patients with already impaired lung function [36,38]. This risk requires careful consideration and monitoring when prescribing opioids to ILD patients, particularly those with more advanced disease and age. As a result, opiates are often reserved for patients with severe cough who have not responded to other therapeutic options.

Codeine, a weaker opioid, is sometimes used to manage chronic cough but tends to be less effective than morphine in controlling severe cases. While it is more commonly prescribed due to its milder side effect profile, its efficacy in ILD-related cough is less well established [39]. The balance between symptom relief and minimizing side effects remains a crucial consideration in the use of any opioid for cough management in ILD.

5. Role of Neuromodulators in Cough Associated with ILD

In recent years, neuromodulators such as gabapentin and pregabalin have emerged as potential therapeutic options for treating refractory cough. Since cough in ILD can be refractory, there has been significant research interest in exploring novel approaches targeting the neural pathways that are involved in cough reflex hypersensitivity. Gabapentin and pregabalin, traditionally used to treat neuropathic pain, are believed to modulate the excitability of sensory nerves that trigger cough, offering relief in cases where other treatments have failed.

Gabapentin, in particular, has been studied more extensively for its role in reducing chronic cough. Several randomized controlled trials, including studies conducted in non-ILD populations, have shown that gabapentin can significantly minimize the cough frequency and severity by suppressing the heightened sensitivity of the cough reflex. These findings have led to its off-label use in patients with ILD who experience debilitating coughs. A notable study by Ryan et al. (2012) demonstrated that gabapentin reduced cough symptoms in patients with chronic cough of various etiologies, including those related to lung disease [40]. However, the specific evidence relating to ILD remains limited, and more research is needed to fully understand its efficacy in this population.

Pregabalin, a related neuromodulator, has also been explored as a treatment for chronic cough [41]. Like gabapentin, pregabalin works by reducing neuronal excitability and has shown promise in reducing the cough frequency in small trials. While the available data on pregabalin in ILD-related cough are sparse, its similar mechanism of action suggests that it could be a viable option for patients who do not respond to other treatments [42]. Both drugs are typically well tolerated, although side effects such as drowsiness, dizziness, and fatigue may limit their use in some patients. Starting at a lower dose and titrating up can overcome these side effects and improve tolerance.

Duloxetine is a serotonin norepinephrine reuptake inhibitor that is used for various psychiatric conditions and chronic pain. There is currently an active trial evaluating the role of duloxetine in refractory chronic cough by inhibiting the activity of the transient receptor potential vanilloid 1 (TRPV1) channel [43]. The study aims to investigate duloxetine's efficacy in reducing cough by modulating central hypersensitivity pathways, potentially offering a novel therapeutic option for this challenging condition.

6. Macrolides

Macrolides, particularly azithromycin, have been studied for their potential to treat chronic cough in various respiratory conditions, including IPF and chronic productive cough. In IPF, a randomized controlled trial found no significant improvement in cough related quality of life or objective cough frequency after 12 weeks of azithromycin therapy compared to a placebo, despite its known anti-inflammatory effects [44]. However, in patients with chronic productive cough of unknown origin, azithromycin demonstrated a marked improvement in cough-related quality of life (LCQ scores), sputum volume, and sputum color after a 12-week course of treatment, especially in those with neutrophilic airway inflammation [45]. These findings suggest that macrolides may benefit specific chronic cough subgroups, but their efficacy in IPF-related cough remains uncertain.

7. Inhaled Corticosteroids

Oral and inhaled corticosteroids are widely used to treat a variety of lung conditions and their symptoms. A small non-randomized study looked into the positive effect of corticosteroids in controlling cough in IPF patients and showed a significant reduction in VAS score [46]. However, there are no studies to date that improve the quality of life or survival among patients with cough in IPF [47]. The small benefit of improved symptoms needs to be weighed against the larger side effect profile of chronic steroid use. Among patients with Sjogren Syndrome-related ILD, such as nonspecific interstitial pneumonia (NSIP) and lymphocytic interstitial pneumonia (LIP), corticosteroids are not beneficial in improving the course of disease, nor in reducing cough [48].

Inhaled corticosteroids (ICSs), like budesonide and fluticasone, have been used as alternatives or adjuncts to oral steroids, particularly in patients with milder disease or airway hyperreactivity. Although some studies suggest that ICSs can reduce cough and improve quality of life in subset of ILD patients (sarcoidosis), their efficacy in improving lung function or preventing long-term disease progression is limited [49–51]. Inhaled corticosteroids (ICSs) have been evaluated for their effectiveness in treating chronic cough associated with COVID-19. A study published in March 2024 investigated the use of ICSs in patients experiencing persistent cough following COVID-19 infection during the Omicron variant outbreak. The findings indicated that while ICS treatment did not significantly alleviate cough symptoms, it did improve impaired the lung function in these individuals [52].

8. Pirfenidone in IPF and Other ILDs

Pirfenidone is an antifibrotic and anti-inflammatory agent that inhibits the TGF-B and TNF-a pathways; it is used for the treatment of IPD to slow disease progression [53]. It has demonstrated potential in managing cough associated with IPF and fibrosis related to COVID-19. In an international multicenter study, pirfenidone reduced the objective 24 h cough frequency by 34% after 12 weeks, showing both objective improvements in cough counts and subjective enhancements in cough-related QoL measures [54,55]. Another study further supported these findings, reporting improvement in patient-reported symptoms, including cough and general well-being, after 12 months of treatment with pirfenidone, making it a promising option for cough management in fibrotic lung diseases [56,57].

Both the RELIEF trial and Maher et al.'s 2019 study explored the efficacy of pirfenidone in treating patients with progressive fibrosing interstitial lung diseases (PF-ILD). In both trials, there were no significant differences in quality of life improvements, as measured by the SGRQ. Despite promising to slow the decline of the forced vital capacity (FVC), the studies did not demonstrate substantial improvements in symptom relief, particularly regarding cough or overall respiratory symptoms, as captured by the SGRQ [58,59].

9. Nintedanib in IPF and PPF

Nintedanib is a tyrosine kinase inhibitor targeting the vascular endothelial growth factor, platelet-derived growth factor, and fibroblast growth factor pathways and is approved for treating IPF and slowing the disease progression [60]. In studies evaluating the role of nintedanib in IPF, connective-tissue-disease-associated interstitial lung disease (CTD-ILD), and progressive pulmonary fibrosis (PPF), cough-related parameters such as those measured by the SGRQ, L-PF, and LCQ were primary and secondary outcomes, respectively. These studies focused on slowing lung function decline, but improvements in respiratory-related quality of life, including cough, were also observed. While nintedanib's main impact was a reduction in the rate of forced vital capacity (FVC) decline, the secondary analysis of SGRQ scores demonstrated improvements in the overall symptom burden, including cough, with modest enhancements in LCQ scores, indicating a positive effect on cough-related quality of life [61–63].

10. Novel Therapies for Intractable Cough

Two novel therapies targeting cough in ILD and IPF are P2X3 receptor antagonist/inhibitor and humidified high-flow therapy (HHFT). P2X3 receptor antagonists (Gefapixant, Filapixant, Silopixant) [64,65] were evaluated in a trial, where they reduced the cough frequency but with variable degrees of significant taste-related side effects, including dysgeusia and ageusia [66]. Gefapixant was approved in some countries but was not approved by the FDA by 2023. Long-term HHFT, though less studied, showed substantial improvement in cough severity in small case reports, with immediate effect upon commencement of treatment, by reducing the cough intensity through airway hydration and mucociliary clearance, with minimal side effects [67]. Both therapies offer promise but require further validation.

11. IPF Treatments That Worsened/Did Not Improve Cough

11.1. *Sodium Cromoglycate*

Inhaled sodium cromoglycate, once considered for treating chronic cough in various conditions, has shown mixed results in recent studies, particularly for IPF. Earlier research suggested the potential benefits of sodium cromoglycate in conditions like ACE-inhibitor cough and chronic lung diseases by inhibiting mast cell degranulation and reducing afferent C-fiber activity [68,69]. However, recent trials, such as the SCENIC trial, failed to demonstrate any significant efficacy of inhaled sodium cromoglycate (RVT-1601) in reducing the cough frequency in IPF patients [70,71]. This highlights its limited role in IPF-related cough management despite previous evidence in other respiratory conditions.

11.2. *Phosphodiesterase 4B Inhibitor*

In two recent studies, the phosphodiesterase 4B inhibitor BI 1015550 was evaluated for its impact on lung function and symptoms in patients with IPF. In a Phase 2 trial, BI 1015550 positively prevented the decline in forced vital capacity (FVC) over 12 weeks. Cough was monitored as a secondary outcome, but no significant changes in cough parameters were noted during this short-term study [72]. The Phase 3 FIBRONEER-IPF trial, which is currently active, will assess BI 1015550's long-term impact, including changes in cough-related symptoms, as measured by the L-PF questionnaire [73].

11.3. *Recombinant Human Pentraxin-2*

In a long-term evaluation of recombinant human pentraxin-2 (rhPTX-2) for IPF, while the primary focus was on forced vital capacity (FVC) and 6 min walk distance (6MWD), cough was also monitored as a secondary outcome. Cough was one of the more frequently reported treatment-emergent adverse events (TEAEs), occurring in 27% of patients during the open-label extension period. The study noted no significant changes in cough-related outcomes as measured by the LCQ over time, with the LCQ total score showing little change from baseline to Week 128 [74].

11.4. *Lysophosphatidic Acid 1 Antagonist*

In a study on Admilparant, an LPA1 antagonist, cough was noted as a treatment-emergent adverse event (TEAE). In the IPF cohort, cough occurred in 10.8% of patients receiving 60 mg of Admilparant, while in the PPF cohort, it occurred in 11.9% of those receiving the same dose. These rates were slightly higher than those observed in the placebo group (5.4% for IPF and 9.8% for PPF). As the study moves into Phase 3 trials, further evaluation of cough as a TEAE is expected to continue alongside the primary endpoints related to lung function, particularly given the role of cough in affecting patients' quality of life [74]. Table 2 outlines potential novel therapeutic approaches for the management of cough in patients with chronic cough, with ILD and IPF included.

Table 2. Potential novel therapeutic approaches for the management of cough in patients with chronic cough, ILD and IPF.

Author	Article	Journal	Year	Result	Intervention
Aiko Niimi, et al. [64]	Randomised Trial of the P2X3 Receptor Antagonist Sivopixant for Refractory Chronic Cough	*ERS Publications*	2022	Sivopixant reduced objective cough frequency and improved HRQoL	Sivopixant 150 mg for 2 weeks
Christian Friedrich, et al. [65]	The P2X3 Receptor Antagonist Filapixant in Patients with Refractory Chronic Cough: An RCT	*BMC Respiratory Research*	2023	Filapixant significantly reduced cough frequency and severity and improved cough HRQoL	Filapixant doses ≥ 80 mg
Fernando J. Martinez, et al. [66]	Treatment of Persistent Cough in Subjects with IPD with Gefapixant, a P2X3 Antagonist, in a Randomized, Placebo-Controlled Clinical Trial	*Springer Nature*	2021	Gefapixant did not demonstrate a significant reduction versus placebo in cough by day 14	
Matthew Bricknell, et al. [67]	A Novel Therapy for Intractable Cough	*Respiralogy Case Reports*	2024	Case series of humidified high-flow therapy (HHFT) treatment of intractable chronic cough with IPF/ILD	
Fernando J. Martinez, et al. [70]	Phase 2B study of RVT-1601 for Chronic Cough in IPF (SCENIC Trial)	*American Journal of Respiratory and Critical Care Medicine*	2021	Treatment with inhaled RVT-1601 did not provide benefit over placebo for treatment of chronic cough in patients with IPF	Cromolyn Sodium 10, 40 and 80 mg
Luca Richeldi, et al. [71]	Trial of a Preferential PDE 4B Inhibitor for IPF (FIBRONEER-IPF)	*BMJ Open Respiratory Research*	2023	BI 1015550 (PDE4B inhibitor) prevented a decrease in lung function in patients with IPF	BI 1015550 9 mg BID, 18 mg BID

11.5. Cough Suppression Techniques

Cough suppression techniques have garnered increasing attention as a non-pharmacological intervention for managing chronic cough, particularly in conditions like ILD. Although research on cough suppression in ILD is more limited than in other respiratory conditions, the evidence supports the efficacy of behavioral therapies in reducing cough frequency and the improving quality of life of these patients.

A pivotal study by Vertigan et al. (2006) explored speech pathology interventions, including cough suppression techniques, in patients with chronic refractory cough and demonstrated significant improvements in cough-related quality of life and reductions in cough frequency [75]. Although this study primarily focused on chronic cough that is not related to ILD, it provided a foundation for applying these techniques to ILD populations. Cough suppression techniques focus on managing the mechanisms of cough reflex hypersensitivity. Cough suppression physiotherapy, consisting of education, counselling, and cough suppression techniques, aims to retrain this reflex through controlled breathing, relaxation exercises, and vocal cord training. These interventions can help reduce the frequency and severity of cough by addressing the heightened sensitivity of the airways, as shown in ref. [76], including in patients with ILD who suffer from chronic refractory cough [77,78].

A pertinent example comes from a recent case report on an 83-year-old female with hypersensitivity pneumonitis with a chronic cough for 18 months, where non-pharmacological cough control therapy was initiated as part of the treatment plan. She participated in a 4-week biweekly session facilitated by a physiotherapist and a speech–language pathologist. The sessions included an introduction and overview of chronic cough and cough suppression techniques, followed by breathing exercises, vocal exercises, and laryngeal relaxation techniques. This was the first case report exploring non-pharmacological cough control therapy in an ILD patient. Improvement was noted in the HRQOL questionnaire, in addition to cough severity and intensity.

Although it may not benefit all patients, the risk of harm with therapy is minimal to none and could thus be a key adjunct to the comprehensive management in motivated patients.

12. Conclusions

Chronic cough in ILD remains a challenging symptom to evaluate and manage due to its multifactorial nature and significant impact on quality of life and disease outcomes. The current assessment relies on patient-reported tools such as the LCQ, CQLQ, and VAS, which, while valuable, require further validation for ILD-specific use. Therapeutic options, including neuromodulators, antifibrotic agents, and GERD management, provide variable benefits but often fall short of achieving comprehensive symptom control. Emerging treatments like P2X3 receptor antagonists and behavioral interventions, including cough suppression techniques, offer promising avenues for improvement. An individualized treatment focusing on a multidisciplinary approach that integrates robust evaluation tools and a combination of pharmacological and non-pharmacological strategies is essential for advancing the care of patients with ILD-related chronic refractory cough. This review not only highlights the potential updated treatment options that are available for managing cough in ILD/IPF but also underscores the lack of robust evidence supporting these approaches. There is a need for longer-term studies on opiates, which have shown strong short-term therapeutic potential, exploring the role of duloxetine in ILD/IPF cough, as well as larger RCTs exploring pharmacological and surgical treatments for GERD associated with ILD/IPF. Additionally, research specifically focusing on the role of physiotherapy in ILD/IPF patients is warranted. We eagerly anticipate the development and evaluation of novel agents targeting cough in ILD/IPF patients.

Author Contributions: Conceptualization, C.Y.L. and G.S.; methodology, C.Y.L. and G.S.; software, C.Y.L.; validation, C.Y.L., T.A., S.W.K. and G.S.; resources, C.Y.L., T.A., S.W.K. and G.S.; writing—original draft preparation, C.Y.L., writing—review and editing, C.Y.L., S.W.K. and G.S.; visualization, C.Y.L. and G.S.; supervision, G.S.; project administration, G.S. All authors have read and agreed to the published version of the manuscript.

Funding: This research received no external funding.

Institutional Review Board Statement: Not applicable.

Informed Consent Statement: Not applicable.

Data Availability Statement: Not applicable.

Conflicts of Interest: The authors declare no conflicts of interest.

Appendix A

This questionnaire is designed to assess the impact of cough on various aspects of your life. Read each question carefully and answer by CIRCLING the response that best applies to you. Please answer ALL questions, as honestly as you can.

1. In the last 2 weeks, have you had chest or stomach pains as a result of your cough?

1	2	3	4	5	6	7
All of the time	Most of the time	A good bit of the time	Some of the time	A little of the time	Hardly any of the time	None of the time

2. In the last 2 weeks, have you been bothered by sputum (phlegm) production when you cough?

1	2	3	4	5	6	7
Every time	Most times	Several times	Some times	Occasionally	Rarely	Never

3. In the last 2 weeks, have you been tired because of your cough?

1	2	3	4	5	6	7
All of the time	Most of the time	A good bit of the time	Some of the time	A little of the time	Hardly any of the time	None of the time

4. In the last 2 weeks, have you felt in control of your cough?

1	2	3	4	5	6	7
None of the time	Hardly any of the time	A little of the time	Some of the time	A good bit of the time	Most of the time	All of the time

5. How often during the last 2 weeks have you felt embarrassed by your coughing?

1	2	3	4	5	6	7
All of the time	Most of the time	A good bit of the time	Some of the time	A little of the time	Hardly any of the time	None of the time

6. In the last 2 weeks, my cough has made me feel anxious

1	2	3	4	5	6	7
All of the time	Most of the time	A good bit of the time	Some of the time	A little of the time	Hardly any of the time	None of the time

7. In the last 2 weeks, my cough has interfered with my job, or other daily tasks

1	2	3	4	5	6	7
All of the time	Most of the time	A good bit of the time	Some of the time	A little of the time	Hardly any of the time	None of the time

8. In the last 2 weeks, I felt that my cough interfered with the overall enjoyment of my life

1	2	3	4	5	6	7
All of the time	Most of the time	A good bit of the time	Some of the time	A little of the time	Hardly any of the time	None of the time

9. In the last 2 weeks, exposure to paints or fumes has made me cough

1	2	3	4	5	6	7
All of the time	Most of the time	A good bit of the time	Some of the time	A little of the time	Hardly any of the time	None of the time

10. In the last 2 weeks, has your cough disturbed your sleep?

1	2	3	4	5	6	7
All of the time	Most of the time	A good bit of the time	Some of the time	A little of the time	Hardly any of the time	None of the time

11. In the last 2 weeks, how many times a day have you had coughing bouts?

1	2	3	4	5	6	7
All of the time (continuously)	Most times during the day	Several times during the day	Some times during the day	Occasionally through the day	Rarely	None

12. In the last 2 weeks, my cough has made me feel frustrated

1	2	3	4	5	6	7
All of the time	Most of the time	A good bit of the time	Some of the time	A little of the time	Hardly any of the time	None of the time

13. In the last 2 weeks, my cough has made me feel fed up

1	2	3	4	5	6	7
All of the time	Most of the time	A good bit of the time	Some of the time	A little of the time	Hardly any of the time	None of the time

14. In the last 2 weeks, have you suffered from a hoarse voice as a result of your cough?

1	2	3	4	5	6	7
All of the time	Most of the time	A good bit of the time	Some of the time	A little of the time	Hardly any of the time	None of the time

15. In the last 2 weeks, have you had a lot of energy?

1	2	3	4	5	6	7
None of the time	Hardly any of the time	A little of the time	Some of the time	A good bit of the time	Most of the time	All of the time

16. In the last 2 weeks, have you worried that your cough may indicate serious illness?

1	2	3	4	5	6	7
All of the time	Most of the time	A good bit of the time	Some of the time	A little of the time	Hardly any of the time	None of the time

17. In the last 2 weeks, have you been concerned that other people think something is wrong with you, because of your cough?

1	2	3	4	5	6	7
All of the time	Most of the time	A good bit of the time	Some of the time	A little of the time	Hardly any of the time	None of the time

18. In the last 2 weeks, my cough has interrupted conversation or telephone calls

1	2	3	4	5	6	7
Every time	Most times	A good bit of the time	Some of the time	A little of the time	Hardly any of the time	None of the time

19. In the last 2 weeks, I feel that my cough has annoyed my partner, family or friends

1	2	3	4	5	6	7
Every time I cough	Most times when I cough	Several times when I cough	Some times when I cough	Occasionally when I cough	Rarely	Never

Thank you for completing this questionnaire.

Figure A1. An example of the Leicester Cough Questionnaire. Available at LCQ. Published with permission.

Appendix B

The Cough-Specific Quality-of-Life Questionnaire (CQLQ) ©

NAME (OPTIONAL): ______________________ STUDY RECORD #: ______________ DATE: ________

Please indicate below how your *cough currently* affects you. Circle the answer that best describes your agreement with each item. Please respond to every item. Thank you for your help.

1. **During the past week, family and or close friends can't tolerate my cough any more.**	**STRONGLY DISAGREE**	**DISAGREE**	**AGREE**	**STRONGLY AGREE**
2. During the past week, I have experienced prolonged absences from important activities such as work, school, or volunteer services because of my cough.	STRONGLY DISAGREE	DISAGREE	AGREE	STRONGLY AGREE
3. **During the past week, I have been completely prevented from engaging in important activities such as work, school, or volunteer services because of my cough.**	**STRONGLY DISAGREE**	**DISAGREE**	**AGREE**	**STRONGLY AGREE**
4. During the past week, I have lost my appetite because of my cough.	STRONGLY DISAGREE	DISAGREE	AGREE	STRONGLY AGREE
5. **During the past week, I am sick to my stomach and vomit because of my cough.**	**STRONGLY DISAGREE**	**DISAGREE**	**AGREE**	**STRONGLY AGREE**
6. During the past week, I retch (dry heaves) because of my cough.	STRONGLY DISAGREE	DISAGREE	AGREE	STRONGLY AGREE
7. **During the past week, I have a fear that I might have AIDS or tuberculosis because of my cough.**	**STRONGLY DISAGREE**	**DISAGREE**	**AGREE**	**STRONGLY AGREE**
8. During the past week, I have headaches because of my cough.	STRONGLY DISAGREE	DISAGREE	AGREE	STRONGLY AGREE
9. **During the past week, I am concerned that I have cancer because of my cough.**	**STRONGLY DISAGREE**	**DISAGREE**	**AGREE**	**STRONGLY AGREE**
10. During the past week, I am dizzy because of my cough.	STRONGLY DISAGREE	DISAGREE	AGREE	STRONGLY AGREE
11. **During the past week, I wet my pants because of my cough.**	**STRONGLY DISAGREE**	**DISAGREE**	**AGREE**	**STRONGLY AGREE**

Figure A2. *Cont.*

12. During the past week, I soil my pants because of my cough.	STRONGLY DISAGREE	DISAGREE	AGREE	STRONGLY AGREE
13. During the past week, I sweat because of my cough.	**STRONGLY DISAGREE**	**DISAGREE**	**AGREE**	**STRONGLY AGREE**
14. During the past week, I am hoarse because of my cough.	STRONGLY DISAGREE	DISAGREE	AGREE	STRONGLY AGREE
15. During the past week, it hurts when I breathe because of my cough.	**STRONGLY DISAGREE**	**DISAGREE**	**AGREE**	**STRONGLY AGREE**
16. During the past week, I broke a rib because of my cough.	STRONGLY DISAGREE	DISAGREE	AGREE	STRONGLY AGREE
17. During the past week, I cannot sleep at night because of my cough.	**STRONGLY DISAGREE**	**DISAGREE**	**AGREE**	**STRONGLY AGREE**
18. During the past week, I have difficulty speaking on the phone because of my cough.	STRONGLY DISAGREE	DISAGREE	AGREE	STRONGLY AGREE
19. During the past week, I can no longer sing, for instance in church, because of my cough.	**STRONGLY DISAGREE**	**DISAGREE**	**AGREE**	**STRONGLY AGREE**
20. During the past week, I have stopped going to social activities such as movies, plays, town meetings because of my cough.	STRONGLY DISAGREE	DISAGREE	AGREE	STRONGLY AGREE
21. During the past week, I have had to change my lifestyle because of my cough.	**STRONGLY DISAGREE**	**DISAGREE**	**AGREE**	**STRONGLY AGREE**
22. During the past week, I ache all over because of my cough.	STRONGLY DISAGREE	DISAGREE	AGREE	STRONGLY AGREE
23. During the past week, I am exhausted because of my cough.	**STRONGLY DISAGREE**	**DISAGREE**	**AGREE**	**STRONGLY AGREE**
24. During the past week, I am embarrassed because of my cough.	STRONGLY DISAGREE	DISAGREE	AGREE	STRONGLY AGREE
25. During the past week, I am upset by people thinking that I have something wrong with me because of my cough.	**STRONGLY DISAGREE**	**DISAGREE**	**AGREE**	**STRONGLY AGREE**

Figure A2. *Cont.*

26. During the past week, I want to be reassured that I do not have anything seriously the matter with me because of my cough.	STRONGLY DISAGREE	DISAGREE	AGREE	STRONGLY AGREE
27. During the past week, I am self conscious because of my cough.	**STRONGLY DISAGREE**	**DISAGREE**	**AGREE**	**STRONGLY AGREE**
28. During the past week, I am concerned that I have something seriously the matter with me because of my cough.	STRONGLY DISAGREE	DISAGREE	AGREE	STRONGLY AGREE

Figure A2. Cough Quality of Life Questionnaire. Available at CQLQ.

Appendix C

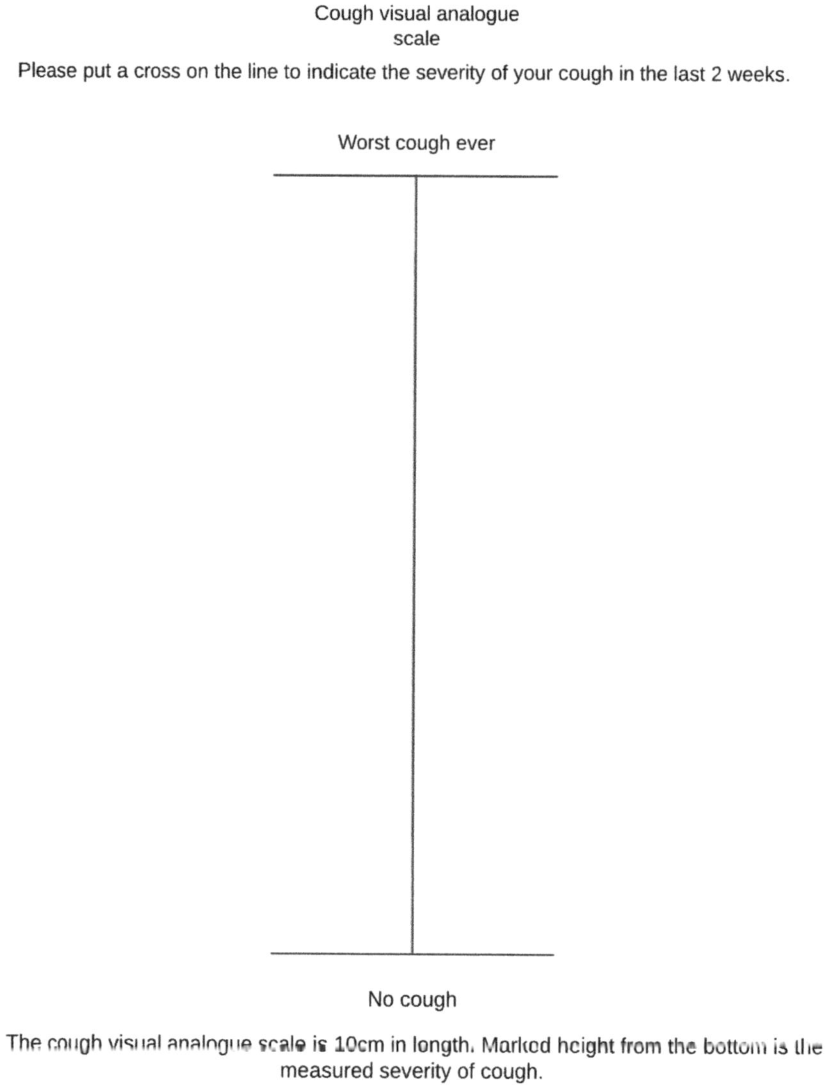

Figure A3. Cough Visual Analogue Scale. The vertical line should be 100 mm in length.

Appendix D

THE ST GEORGE'S RESPIRATORY QUESTIONNAIRE
IDIOPATHIC PULMONARY FIBROSIS VERSION
The SGRQ-I

This questionnaire is designed to help us learn much more about how your breathing is troubling you and how it affects your life. We are using it to find out which aspects of your illness cause you most problem, rather than what the doctors and nurses think your problems are.

Please read the instructions carefully and ask if you do not understand anything. Do not spend too long deciding about your answers.

Name: .... Date: ....

ID Number: ....

Age: .... Sex: Male/Female

Please tick in one box to show how you describe your current health:-

Very good	Good	Fair	Poor	Very poor
☐	☐	☐	☐	☐

P.W. Jones, PhD FRCP
Professor of Respiratory Medicine,
St. George's University of London,
Jenner Wing,
Cranmer Terrace,
London SW17 ORE, UK.
Tel. +44 (0) 20 8725 5371
Fax +44 (0) 20 8725 5955

SGRQ-I Current Health Status
Version 1.0 August 2012

Figure A4. *Cont.*

Part 1

Questions about how much chest trouble you currently have. Please tick in one box for each question.

	Almost every day	Only with chest infections	Not at all
1. I cough:	☐	☐	☐
2. I bring up phlegm (sputum):	☐	☐	☐
3. I have shortness of breath:	☐	☐	☐
4. I have attacks of wheezing:	☐	☐	☐

5. In a typical week how many attacks of chest trouble do you have? Please tick (✓) one:

More than 1 attack ☐

No attacks ☐

6. In a typical week how often do you have good days? Please tick (✓) one:

None ☐

A few days ☐

Every day is a good day ☐

SGRQ-I Current health status 2
Version 1.0 August 2012

Figure A4. *Cont.*

Part 2

Section 1:
If you have ever had paid employment:

Please tick (✓) one:

My lung condition interferes or made me stop work ☐

My lung problem does not affect my job ☐

Section 2: ***Questions about what activities usually make you feel breathless. Please tick in each box that applies to you <u>these days</u>.***

Please tick (✓) in *each box* that applies to you *these days*:

		True	False
1.	Getting washed or dressed	☐	☐
2.	Walking around the home	☐	☐
3.	Walking outside on the level	☐	☐
4.	Walking up a flight of stairs	☐	☐
5.	Playing sports or games	☐	☐

Section 3: ***Some more questions about your cough and breathlessness. Please tick in each box that applies to you <u>these days</u>.***

Please tick (✓) in *each box* that applies to you *these days*:

		True	False
1.	My cough hurts	☐	☐
2.	My cough makes me tired	☐	☐
3.	I am breathless when I talk	☐	☐
4.	I am breathless when I bend over	☐	☐
5.	My cough or breathing disturbs my sleep	☐	☐
6.	I get exhausted easily	☐	☐

Section 4: ***Questions about other effects that your chest trouble may have on you. Please tick in each box that applies to you <u>these days</u>.***

Please tick (✓) in *each box* that applies to you *these days*:

		True	False
1.	My cough or breathing is embarrassing in public	☐	☐
2.	My chest trouble is a nuisance to my family, friends or neighbours	☐	☐
3.	I get afraid or panic when I cannot get my breath	☐	☐
4.	I feel that I am not in control of my chest problem	☐	☐
5.	Exercise is not safe for me	☐	☐
6.	Everything seems too much of an effort	☐	☐

SGRQ-I Current health status 3
Version 1.0 August 2012

Figure A4. *Cont.*

Section 5: These are questions about how your activities might be affected by your breathing. Please tick in each box which you think applies to you because of your breathing

	True	False
1. Jobs such as housework take a long time, or I have to stop for rests	☐	☐
2. If I walk up one flight of stairs, I have to go slowly or stop	☐	☐
3. If I hurry or walk fast, I have to stop or slow down	☐	☐
4. My breathing makes it difficult to do things such as walk up hills, carrying things up stairs, light gardening such as weeding, dance, play bowls or play golf	☐	☐
5. My breathing makes it difficult to do things such as very heavy manual work, run, cycle, swim fast or play competitive sports	☐	☐

Section 6: We would like to know how your chest usually affects your daily life. Please tick in each box that applies to you because of your chest trouble

	True	False
1. I cannot play sports or games	☐	☐
2. I cannot go out of the house to do the shopping	☐	☐
3. I cannot do housework	☐	☐
4. I cannot move far from my bed or chair	☐	☐

Now, would you tick in the box (one only) which you think best describes how your chest affects you:-

It does not stop me doing anything I would like to do	☐
It stops me doing one or two things I would like to do	☐
It stops me doing most of the things I would like to do	☐
It stops me doing everything I would like to do	☐

SGRQ-I Current health status 4
Version 1.0 August 2012

Figure A4. St. George's Respiratory Questionnaire for IPF patients (document consists of four (4) pages). Published with permission from SGRQ.

Appendix E

Instructions for Completing the Living with L-IPF Symptoms Questionnaire

Complete this questionnaire every evening, to assess the symptoms you may have experienced from Idiopathic Pulmonary Fibrosis (IPF) over the last 24 hours.

Keep in mind:

- you are not being asked to compare yourself to anyone else
- you are not being asked to compare how you are now with any time in the past

---

Items 1-6: The first 6 items ask about your symptoms in relation to physical activities, some of which you may not have done in the **last 24 hours.** If you did not perform an activity, we would like to know whether it was because you did not have the opportunity to do it (for example, maybe your home doesn't have stairs, so you did not walk up a flight of stairs), or whether you avoided the activity because it was too difficult.

If you did the stated activity, then reflect on the last 24 hours, and consider whether, on average, doing the activity at your usual pace or intensity level made you short of breath—and if so, how much.

If you normally use oxygen when you perform a given activity, then consider your response as if you were using supplemental oxygen.

Please select the box that best describes your experience.

1. Did you walk up one flight of stairs in the last 24 hours?

[Yes] How short of breath did walking up one flight of stairs make you?

Not at all [0] [1] [2] [3] [4] **Extremely**

[No] I did not walk up one flight of stairs in the last 24 hours because:

[A] I avoided this activity because it was too difficult to perform

[B] Not applicable, because I did not want or have the opportunity to do it

L-IPF Symptoms – United States/English
L-IPF_Symptoms_AU2.0_eng-USori.docx

Figure A5. *Cont.*

2. Over the last 24 hours, how short of breath have you been while sitting down, relaxing, reading, or watching TV?

Not at all [0] [1] [2] [3] [4] **Extremely**

3. Did you perform a grooming activity (e.g., brush teeth, shave, fix hair) in the last 24 hours?

[Yes] How short of breath did grooming make you?

Not at all [0] [1] [2] [3] [4] **Extremely**

[No] I did not perform a grooming activity in the last 24 hours because:

[A] I avoided this activity because it was too difficult to perform

[B] Not applicable, because I did not want or have the opportunity to do it

4. Did you walk outside on a level surface (approximately 150 feet/45 meters, or the distance of half a typical city block) in the last 24 hours?

[Yes] How short of breath did walking outside on a level surface make you?

Not at all [0] [1] [2] [3] [4] **Extremely**

[No] I did not walk outside on a level surface in the last 24 hours because:

[A] I avoided this activity because it was too difficult to perform

[B] Not applicable, because I did not want or have the opportunity to do it

L-IPF Symptoms – United States/English
L-IPF_Symptoms_AU2.0_eng-USori.docx

Figure A5. *Cont.*

5. Did you bathe or shower in the last 24 hours?

[Yes] How short of breath did bathing or showering make you?

Not at all [0] [1] [2] [3] [4] Extremely

[No] I did not bathe or shower in the last 24 hours because:

[A] I avoided this activity because it was too difficult to perform

[B] Not applicable, because I did not want or have the opportunity to do it

6. Did you lift and carry a light load (e.g., less than 10 lbs) a short distance (e.g., from one room to another) in the last 24 hours?

[Yes] How short of breath did lifting and carrying a light load make you?

Not at all [0] [1] [2] [3] [4] Extremely

[No] I did not lift or carry a light load a short distance in the last 24 hours because:

[A] I avoided this activity because it was too difficult to perform

[B] Not applicable, because I did not want or have the opportunity to do it

L-IPF Symptoms – United States/English
L-IPF_Symptoms_AU2.0_eng-USori.docx

Figure A5. *Cont.*

Items 7-9: Each item focuses on cough. Again, reflect on the last 24 hours as you consider where you are on the scale between the two statements.

7. Over the last 24 hours, how often did you cough?

Not at all [0] [1] [2] [3] [4] Constantly

If you chose "0", please skip to item 10.

8. Over the last 24 hours, how often did you cough when you took a deep breath?

Not at all [0] [1] [2] [3] [4] Constantly

9. Over the last 24 hours, how often did you cough when you over-exerted yourself?

Not at all [0] [1] [2] [3] [4] Constantly

10. Over the last 24 hours, how often did you feel an annoying tickle in your throat?

Not at all [0] [1] [2] [3] [4] Constantly

L-IPF Symptoms – United States/English

Figure A5. *Cont.*

Items 11-15: These items primarily focus on your energy level. Again, reflect on the last 24 hours as you consider where you are on the scale between the two statements.

11. Over the last 24 hours, how was your energy level?

Extremely low [0] [1] [2] [3] [4] Excellent

12. Over the last 24 hours, of all that you wanted to get done, how much did you actually get done?

Nothing [0] [1] [2] [3] [4] Everything

13. Over the last 24 hours, how much energy did you have to do all the things you like to do?

No energy [0] [1] [2] [3] [4] A lot

14. Over the last 24 hours, how much did coughing have a negative effect on your energy?

No energy [0] [1] [2] [3] [4] A lot

15. Did you become short of breath in the last 24 hours?

[Yes] How long did it take you to recover when you became short of breath?

No time at all [0] [1] [2] [3] [4] An extremely long time

[No] Please continue to the next page

L-IPF Symptoms – United States/English
L-IPF_Symptoms_AU1.1_eng-USori.docx

Figure A5. *Cont.*

Finally, we would like to ask you 5 questions about your supplemental oxygen use.

Oxygen Question 1. Do you ever use supplemental oxygen?
(Place an "X" in one box)

Yes	→→	proceed to Oxygen Question #2.
No	→→	skip Oxygen Questions 2-5

Oxygen Question 2. I use supplemental oxygen...
(Place an "X" in one box)

1	→→	only when I sleep (answer Oxygen Question #3)
2	→→	only when I perform a physical activity (such as getting dressed or walking) (answer Oxygen Question #4)
3	→→	when I sleep or perform a physical activity (such as getting dressed or walking) but not at rest (answer Oxygen Questions #3 and #4)
4	→→	all the time (answer Oxygen Questions #3-5)

Oxygen Question 3. When I sleep, I most often use an oxygen flow rate of ___ L/min.
(Place an "X" in one box)

0.5	1.0	1.5	2.0	2.5	3.0	3.5	4.0	4.5	5	6	7	8	9	10	11	12	>12

Oxygen Question 4. When I perform a physical activity (such as getting dressed or walking), I most often use an oxygen flow rate of L/min.
(Place an "X" in one box)

0.5	1.0	1.5	2.0	2.5	3.0	3.5	4.0	4.5	5	6	7	8	9	10	11	12	>12

Oxygen Question 5. At rest, I most often use an oxygen flow rate of ___ L/min.
(Place an "X" in one box)

0.5	1.0	1.5	2.0	2.5	3.0	3.5	4.0	4.5	5	6	7	8	9	10	11	12	>12

Thank you for taking the time to complete the L-IPF Symptoms Questionnaire.

L-IPF Symptoms – United States/English
L-IPF_Symptoms_AU2.0_eng-USori.docx

Figure A5. Living with Pulmonary Fibrosis Questionnaire, available at L-IPF.

References

1. Aronson, K.I.; Suzuki, A. Health Related Quality of Life in Interstitial Lung Disease: Can We Use the Same Concepts Around the World? *Front. Med.* **2021**, *8*, 745908. [CrossRef] [PubMed]
2. Birring, S.S.; Kavanagh, J.E.; Irwin, R.S.; Keogh, K.A.; Lim, K.G.; Ryu, J.H. Treatment of Interstitial Lung Disease Associated Cough. *Chest* **2018**, *154*, 904–917. [CrossRef] [PubMed]
3. Lammi, M.R.; Baughman, R.P.; Birring, S.S.; Russell, A.-M.; Ryu, J.H.; Scholand, M.B.; Distler, O.; LeSage, D.; Sarver, C.; Antoniou, K.; et al. Outcome Measures for Clinical Trials in Interstitial Lung Diseases. *Curr. Respir. Med. Rev.* **2015**, *11*, 163–174. [CrossRef] [PubMed]
4. Gallacher, K.; May, C.R.; Montori, V.M.; Mair, F.S. Understanding Patients' Experiences of Treatment Burden in Chronic Heart Failure Using Normalization Process Theory. *Ann. Fam. Med.* **2011**, *9*, 235–243. [CrossRef]
5. Khor, Y.H.; Johannson, K.A.; Marcoux, V.; Fisher, J.; Assayag, D.; Manganas, H.; Khalil, N.; Kolb, M.; Ryerson, C.J.; CARE-PF Investigators. Epidemiology and Prognostic Significance of Cough in Fibrotic Interstitial Lung Disease. *Am. J. Respir. Crit. Care Med.* **2024**, *210*, 1035–1044. [CrossRef]

6. Mann, J.M.V.; Holland, A.E.; Goh, N.S.L.; Khor, Y.H. Understanding patient experience of chronic cough in interstitial lung disease. *ERJ Open Res.* **2023**, *9*, 00039–02023. [CrossRef]
7. Sanchez-Ramirez, D.C.; Kosowan, L.; Singer, A. Management of cough in patients with idiopathic interstitial lung diseases in primary care. *Chron. Respir. Dis.* **2022**, *19*, 14799731221089319. [CrossRef]
8. Irwin, R.S.; Chang, A.B.; Altman, K.W.; Adams, T.M.; Azoulay, E.; Barker, A.F.; Birring, S.S.; Blackhall, F.; Bolser, D.C.; Boulet, L.-P.; et al. Classification of Cough as a Symptom in Adults and Management Algorithms. *Chest* **2017**, *153*, 196–209. [CrossRef]
9. Saunders, P.; Wu, Z.; Fahy, W.A.; Stewart, I.D.; Saini, G.; Smith, D.J.F.; Braybrooke, R.; Stock, C.; Renzoni, E.A.; Johnson, S.R.; et al. The Burden and Impact of Cough in Patients with Idiopathic Pulmonary Fibrosis: An Analysis of the Prospective Observational PROFILE Study. *Ann. Am. Thorac. Soc.* **2023**, *20*, 1267–1273. [CrossRef]
10. Birring, S.S. Development of a symptom specific health status measure for patients with chronic cough: Leicester Cough Questionnaire (LCQ). *Thorax* **2003**, *58*, 339–343. [CrossRef]
11. Lee, J.; White, E.; Freiheit, E.; Scholand, M.B.; Strek, M.E.; Podolanczuk, A.J.; Patel, N.M.; on behalf of the Pulmonary Fibrosis Foundation. Cough-Specific Quality of Life Predicts Disease Progression Among Patients with Interstitial Lung Disease. *Chest* **2022**, *162*, 603–613. [CrossRef] [PubMed]
12. French, C.T.; Irwin, R.S.; Fletcher, K.E.; Adams, T.M. Evaluation of a Cough-Specific Quality-of-Life Questionnaire. *Chest* **2002**, *121*, 1123–1131. [CrossRef] [PubMed]
13. Key, A.L.; Holt, K.; Hamilton, A.; Smith, J.A.; Earis, J.E. Objective cough frequency in Idiopathic Pulmonary Fibrosis. *Cough* **2010**, *6*, 4. [CrossRef] [PubMed]
14. Channick, J.E.; Swigris, J. Cough in Fibrotic Interstitial Lung Disease: Effects and Implications. *Am. J. Respir. Crit. Care Med.* **2024**, *210*, 975–976. [CrossRef]
15. Yates, H.; Adamali, H.I.; Maskell, N.; Barratt, S.; Sharp, C. Visual analogue scales for interstitial lung disease: A prospective validation study. *QJM Int. J. Med.* **2018**, *111*, 531–539. [CrossRef]
16. Wu, Z.; Smith, D.J.F.; Yazbeck, L.; Saunders, P.; Smith, J.A.; Maher, T.M.; Molyneaux, P.L. Cough Severity Visual Analog Scale Assesses Cough Burden and Predicts Survival in Idiopathic Pulmonary Fibrosis. *Am. J. Respir. Crit. Care Med.* **2024**, *209*, 1165–1167. [CrossRef]
17. Suzuki, A.; Kondoh, Y.; Swigris, J.J.; Ando, M.; Kimura, T.; Kataoka, K.; Yamano, Y.; Furukawa, T.; Numata, M.; Sakamoto, K.; et al. Performance of the St George's Respiratory Questionnaire in patients with connective tissue disease-associated interstitial lung disease. *Respirology* **2018**, *23*, 851–859. [CrossRef]
18. Swigris, J.J.; Brown, K.K.; Behr, J.; du Bois, R.M.; King, T.E.; Raghu, G.; Wamboldt, F.S. The SF-36 and SGRQ: Validity and first look at minimum important differences in IPF. *Respir. Med.* **2010**, *104*, 296–304. [CrossRef]
19. Swigris, J.J.; Bushnell, D.M.; Rohr, K.; Mueller, H.; Baldwin, M.; Inoue, Y. Responsiveness and meaningful change thresholds of the Living with Pulmonary Fibrosis (L-PF) questionnaire Dyspnoea and Cough scores in patients with progressive fibrosing interstitial lung diseases. *BMJ Open Respir. Res.* **2022**, *9*, e001167. [CrossRef]
20. Swigris, J.; Cutts, K.; Male, N.; Baldwin, M.; Rohr, K.B.; Bushnell, D.M. The Living with Pulmonary Fibrosis questionnaire in progressive fibrosing interstitial lung disease. *ERJ Open Res.* **2021**, *7*, 00145–02020. [CrossRef]
21. Kum, E.; Guyatt, G.H.; Devji, T.; Devji, T.; Wang, Y.; Bakaa, L.; Lan, L.; Liu, E.; Mastrolonardo, A.; Couban, R.; et al. Cough symptom severity in patients with refractory or unexplained chronic cough: A systematic survey and conceptual framework. *Eur. Respir. Rev.* **2021**, *30*, 210104. [CrossRef] [PubMed]
22. Hall, J.I.; Lozano, M.; Estrada-Petrocelli, L.; Birring, S.; Turner, R. The present and future of cough counting tools. *J. Thorac. Dis.* **2020**, *12*, 5207–5223. [CrossRef] [PubMed]
23. Baqir, M.; Vasirreddy, A.; Vu, A.N.; Moua, T.; Chamberlain, A.M.; Frank, R.D.; Ryu, J.H. Idiopathic pulmonary fibrosis and gastroesophageal reflux disease: A population-based, case-control study. *Respir. Med.* **2021**, *178*, 106309. [CrossRef] [PubMed]
24. Allaix, M.E.; Fisichella, P.M.; Noth, I.; Herbella, F.A.; Borraez Segura, B.; Patti, M.G. Idiopathic Pulmonary Fibrosis and Gastroesophageal Reflux. Implications for Treatment. *J. Gastrointest. Surg.* **2014**, *18*, 100–105. [CrossRef]
25. Hoppo, T.; Komatsu, Y.; Jobe, B.A. Gastroesophageal reflux disease and patterns of reflux in patients with idiopathic pulmonary fibrosis using hypopharyngeal multichannel intraluminal impedance: IPF and laryngopharyngeal reflux. *Dis. Esophagus.* **2014**, *27*, 530–537. [CrossRef]
26. Lee, C.M.; Lee, D.H.; Ahn, B.K.; Hwang, J.J.; Yoon, H.; Shin, C.M.; Park, Y.S.; Kim, N. Protective Effect of Proton Pump Inhibitor for Survival in Patients with Gastroesophageal Reflux Disease and Idiopathic Pulmonary Fibrosis. *J. Neurogastroenterol. Motil.* **2016**, *22*, 444–451. [CrossRef]
27. Dutta, P.; Funston, W.; Mossop, H.; Ryan, V.; Jones, R.; Forbes, R.; Sen, S.; Pearson, J.; Michael Griffin, S.; Smith, J.A.; et al. Randomised, double-blind, placebo-controlled pilot trial of omeprazole in idiopathic pulmonary fibrosis. *Thorax* **2019**, *74*, 346–353. [CrossRef]

28. Johannson, K.A.; Strâmbu, I.; Ravaglia, C.; Grutters, J.C.; Valenzuela, C.; Mogulkoc, N.; Luppi, F.; Richeldi, L.; Wells, A.U.; Vancheri, C.; et al. Antacid therapy in idiopathic pulmonary fibrosis: More questions than answers? *Lancet Respir. Med.* **2017**, *5*, 591–598. [CrossRef]
29. Raghu, G. High prevalence of abnormal acid gastro-oesophageal reflux in idiopathic pulmonary fibrosis. *Eur. Respir. J.* **2006**, *27*, 136–142. [CrossRef]
30. Kilduff, C.E.; Counter, M.J.; Thomas, G.A.; Harrison, N.K.; Hope-Gill, B.D. Effect of acid suppression therapy on gastroesophageal reflux and cough in idiopathic pulmonary fibrosis: An intervention study. *Cough* **2014**, *10*, 4. [CrossRef]
31. Ghebre, Y.T.; Raghu, G. Idiopathic Pulmonary Fibrosis: Novel Concepts of Proton Pump Inhibitors as Antifibrotic Drugs. *Am. J. Respir. Crit. Care Med.* **2016**, *193*, 1345–1352. [CrossRef] [PubMed]
32. Sweet, M.P.; Herbella, F.A.; Leard, L.; Hoopes, C.; Golden, J.; Hays, S.; Patti, M.G. The prevalence of distal and proximal gastroesophageal reflux in patients awaiting lung transplantation. *Trans. Meet. Am. Surg. Assoc.* **2006**, *124*, 156–162. [CrossRef] [PubMed]
33. Sweet, M.P.; Patti, M.G.; Leard, L.E.; Golden, J.A.; Hays, S.R.; Hoopes, C.; Theodore, P.R. Gastroesophageal reflux in patients with idiopathic pulmonary fibrosis referred for lung transplantation. *J. Thorac. Cardiovasc. Surg.* **2007**, *133*, 1078–1084. [CrossRef]
34. Ruaro, B.; Pozzan, R.; Confalonieri, P.; Tavano, S.; Hughes, M.; Cerinic, M.M.; Baratella, E.; Zanatta, E.; Lerda, S.; Geri, P.; et al. Gastroesophageal reflux disease in idiopathic pulmonary fibrosis: Viewer or actor? To treat or not to treat? *Pharmaceuticals* **2022**, *15*, 1033. [CrossRef]
35. Raghu, G.; Pellegrini, C.A.; Yow, E.; Flaherty, K.R.; Meyer, K.; Noth, I.; Scholand, M.B.; Cello, J.; Ho, L.A.; Pipavath, S.; et al. Laparoscopic anti-reflux surgery for the treatment of idiopathic pulmonary fibrosis (WRAP-IPF): A multicentre, randomised, controlled phase 2 trial. *Lancet Respir. Med.* **2018**, *6*, 707–714. [CrossRef]
36. Wu, Z.; Spencer, L.G.; Banya, W.; Westoby, J.; Tudor, V.A.; Rivera-Ortega, P.; Chaudhuri, N.; Jakupovic, I.; Patel, B.; Thillai, M.; et al. Morphine for treatment of cough in idiopathic pulmonary fibrosis (PACIFY COUGH): A prospective, multicentre, randomised, double-blind, placebo-controlled, two-way crossover trial. *Lancet Respir. Med.* **2024**, *12*, 273–280. [CrossRef]
37. Maher, T.M.; Avram, C.; Bortey, E.; Hart, S.P.; Hirani, N.; Molyneux, P.L.; Porter, J.C.; Smith, J.A.; Sciascia, T. Nalbuphine Tablets for Cough in Patients with Idiopathic Pulmonary Fibrosis. *NEJM Evid.* **2023**, *2*, EVIDoa2300083. [CrossRef]
38. Bajwah, S.; Davies, J.M.; Tanash, H.; Currow, D.C.; Oluyase, A.O.; Ekström, M. Safety of benzodiazepines and opioids in interstitial lung disease: A national prospective study. *Eur. Respir. J.* **2018**, *52*, 1801278. [CrossRef]
39. Madison, J.M.; Irwin, R.S. Chronic cough in adults with interstitial lung disease. *Curr. Opin. Pulm. Med.* **2005**, *11*, 412–416. [CrossRef]
40. Ryan, N.M.; Birring, S.S.; Gibson, P.G. Gabapentin for refractory chronic cough: A randomised, double-blind, placebo-controlled trial. *Lancet* **2012**, *380*, 1583–1589. [CrossRef]
41. Vertigan, A.E.; Kapela, S.L.; Ryan, N.M.; Birring, S.S.; McElduff, P.; Gibson, P.G. Pregabalin and Speech Pathology Combination Therapy for Refractory Chronic Cough. *Chest* **2016**, *149*, 639–648. [CrossRef] [PubMed]
42. Saint-Pierre, M.D. Pregabalin for Interstitial Lung Disease-related Cough: A Single-center Experience. In *A39. Management of Interstitial Lung Disease and Its Co-Morbidities*; American Thoracic Society: New York, NY, USA, 2023; p. A1517. [CrossRef]
43. Wang, S.; Li, S.; Wu, H.; Zhang, T.; Chen, Y.; Zhu, Y.; Wen, S.; Shi, C.; Yu, L.; Xu, X. A randomized, double-blinded, placebo-controlled clinical trial of duloxetine hydrochloride enteric-coated tablets in the treatment of refractory chronic cough. *BMC Pulm. Med.* **2023**, *23*, 282. [CrossRef] [PubMed]
44. Guler, S.A.; Clarenbach, C.; Brutsche, M.; Guler, S.A.; Clarenbach, C.; Brutsche, M.; Hosteller, K.; Brill, A.-K.; Schertel, A.; Geiser, T.K.; et al. Azithromycin for the Treatment of Chronic Cough in Idiopathic Pulmonary Fibrosis: A Randomized Controlled Crossover Trial. *Ann. Am. Thorac. Soc.* **2021**, *18*, 2018–2026. [CrossRef] [PubMed]
45. Martin, M.J.; Lee, H.; Clayton, C.; Pointon, K.; Soomro, I.; Shaw, D.E.; Harrison, T.W. Idiopathic chronic productive cough and response to open-label macrolide therapy: An observational study. *Respirology* **2019**, *24*, 558–565. [CrossRef]
46. Paramothayan, N.S.; Lasserson, T.J.; Jones, P. Corticosteroids for pulmonary sarcoidosis. *Cochrane Database Syst. Rev.* **2005**, *2010*, CD001114. [CrossRef]
47. Gerke, A.K. Treatment of Sarcoidosis: A Multidisciplinary Approach. *Front. Immunol.* **2020**, *11*, 545413. [CrossRef]
48. Van Manen, M.J.G.; Birring, S.S.; Vancheri, C.; Cottin, V.; Renzoni, E.A.; Russel, A.-M.; Wijsenbeek, M.S. Cough in idiopathic pulmonary fibrosis. *Eur. Respir. Rev.* **2016**, *25*, 278–286. [CrossRef]
49. Hope-Gill, B.D.M.; Hilldrup, S.; Davies, C.; Newton, R.P.; Harrison, N.K. A Study of the Cough Reflex in Idiopathic Pulmonary Fibrosis. *Am. J. Respir. Crit. Care Med.* **2003**, *168*, 995–1002. [CrossRef]
50. Flament, T.; Bigot, A.; Chaigne, B.; Henique, H.; Diot, E.; Marchand-Adam, S. Pulmonary manifestations of Sjögren's syndrome. *Eur. Respir. Rev.* **2016**, *25*, 110–123. [CrossRef]

51. Ohno, S.; Nakazawa, S.; Kobayashi, A.; Yamasawa, H.; Bando, M.; Sugiyama, Y. Inhaled Corticosteroid Rapidly Improved Pulmonary Sarcoidosis. *Intern. Med.* **2005**, *44*, 1276–1279. [CrossRef]
52. Xie, P.P.; Zhang, Y.; Niu, W.K.; Tu, B.; Yang, N.; Fang, Y.; Shi, Y.-H.; Wang, F.-S.; Yuan, X. Clinical characteristics and effects of inhaled corticosteroid in patients with post-COVID-19 chronic cough during the Omicron variant outbreak. *BMC Pulm. Med.* **2024**, *24*, 156. [CrossRef] [PubMed]
53. King, T.E.; Bradford, W.Z.; Castro-Bernardini, S.; Fagan, E.A.; Glaspole, I.; Glassberg, M.K.; Gorina, E.; Hopkins, P.M.; Kardatzke, D.; Lancaster, L.; et al. A Phase 3 Trial of Pirfenidone in Patients with Idiopathic Pulmonary Fibrosis. *N. Engl. J. Med.* **2014**, *370*, 2083–2092. [CrossRef] [PubMed]
54. Van Manen, M.J.G.; Birring, S.S.; Vancheri, C.; Vindigni, V.; Renzoni, E.; Russel, A.-M.; Wapenaar, M.; Cottin, V.; Wijsenbeek, M.S. Effect of pirfenidone on cough in patients with idiopathic pulmonary fibrosis. *Eur. Respir. J.* **2017**, *50*, 1701157. [CrossRef] [PubMed]
55. Jastrzębski, D.; Kostorz-Nosal, S.; Galle, D.; Gałeczka-Turkiewicz, A.; Warzencha, J.; Majerski, S.; Piotrowski, W.J.; Ziora, D. Expectations, symptoms, and quality of life before and after 1 year of Pirfenidone treatment in patients with idiopathic pulmonary fibrosis: A single-arm, open-label nonrandomized study. *Health Sci. Rep.* **2023**, *6*, e1449. [CrossRef]
56. Kang, M.; Gupta, S.; Tu, Y.H.; Raimundo, K.; Patel, A.M.; Flaherty, K.R. Impact of Pirfenidone on Patient-Reported Outcomes in Patients with Idiopathic Pulmonary Fibrosis from the Pulmonary Fibrosis Foundation Patient Registry. *CHEST Pulm.* **2024**, *2*, 100082. [CrossRef]
57. Schreiber, J.; Schütte, W.; Koerber, W.; Seese, B.; Koschel, D.; Neuland, K.; Grohe, C. Clinical course of mild-to-moderate idiopathic pulmonary fibrosis during therapy with pirfenidone: Results of the non-interventional study AERplus. *Pneumologie* **2024**, *78*, 236–243. [CrossRef]
58. Maher, T.M.; Corte, T.J.; Fischer, A.; Keruter, M.; Lederer, D.J.; Molina-Molina, M.; Axmann, J.; Kirshgaessler, K.-U.; Samara, K.; Gilberg, F.; et al. Pirfenidone in patients with unclassifiable progressive fibrosing interstitial lung disease: A double-blind, randomised, placebo-controlled, phase 2 trial. *Lancet Respir. Med.* **2020**, *8*, 147–157. [CrossRef]
59. Behr, J.; Prasse, A.; Kreuter, M.; Johow, J.; Rabe, K.F.; Bonella, F.; Bonnet, R.; Grohe, C.; Held, M.; Wilkens, H.; et al. Pirfenidone in patients with progressive fibrotic interstitial lung diseases other than idiopathic pulmonary fibrosis (RELIEF): A double-blind, randomised, placebo-controlled, phase 2b trial. *Lancet Respir. Med.* **2021**, *9*, 476–486. [CrossRef]
60. Richeldi, L.; Du Bois, R.M.; Raghu, G.; Azuma, A.; Brown, K.K.; Costabel, U.; Cottin, V.; Flaherty, K.R.; Hansell, D.M.; Inoue, Y.; et al. Efficacy and safety of nintedanib in idiopathic pulmonary fibrosis. *N. Engl. J. Med.* **2014**, *370*, 2071–2082. [CrossRef]
61. Distler, O.; Highland, K.B.; Gahlemann, M.; Azuma, A.; Fischer, A.; Mayes, M.D.; Raghu, G.; Sauter, W.; Girard, M.; Alves, M.; et al. Nintedanib for Systemic Sclerosis–Associated Interstitial Lung Disease. *N. Engl. J. Med.* **2019**, *380*, 2518–2528. [CrossRef]
62. Raman, L.; Stewart, I.; Barratt, S.L.; Chua, F.; Chaudhuri, N.; Crawshaw, A.; Gibbons, M.; Hogben, C.; Hoyles, R.; Kouranos, V.; et al. Nintedanib for non-IPF progressive pulmonary fibrosis: 12-month outcome data from a real-world multicentre observational study. *ERJ Open Res.* **2023**, *9*, 00423–02022. [CrossRef] [PubMed]
63. Wijsenbeek, M.; Swigris, J.J.; Inoue, Y.; Kreuter, M.; Maher, T.M.; Suda, T.; Baldwin, M.; Mueller, H.; Rohr, K.B.; Flaherty, K.R.; et al. Effects of nintedanib on symptoms in patients with progressive pulmonary fibrosis. *Eur. Respir. J.* **2024**, *63*, 2300752. [CrossRef] [PubMed]
64. Niimi, A.; Saito, J.; Kamei, T.; Shinkai, M.; Ishihara, H.; Machida, M.; Miyazaki, S. Randomised trial of the $P2X_3$ receptor antagonist sivopixant for refractory chronic cough. *Eur. Respir. J.* **2022**, *59*, 2100725. [CrossRef] [PubMed]
65. Friedrich, C.; Francke, K.; Birring, S.S.; van den Berg, J.W.K.; Mardsen, P.A.; McGarvey, L.; Turner, A.M.; Wielders, P.; Gashaw, I.; Klein, S.; et al. The P2X3 receptor antagonist filapixant in patients with refractory chronic cough: A randomized controlled trial. *Respir. Res.* **2023**, *24*, 109. [CrossRef] [PubMed]
66. Martinez, F.J.; Afzal, A.S.; Smith, J.A.; Ford, A.P.; Li, J.J.; Li, Y.; Kitt, M.M.; Chronic Cough in IPF Study Group. Treatment of Persistent Cough in Subjects with Idiopathic Pulmonary Fibrosis (IPF) with Gefapixant, a P2X3 Antagonist, in a Randomized, Placebo-Controlled Clinical Trial. *Pulm. Ther.* **2021**, *7*, 471–486. [CrossRef]
67. Bricknell, M.; Zhao, C.Z.; Smallwood, N.; Goh, N. A novel therapy for intractable chronic cough. *Respirol. Case Rep.* **2024**, *12*, e01323. [CrossRef]
68. Birring, S.S.; Wijsenbeek, M.S.; Agrawal, S.; van den Berg, J.W.K.; Stone, H.; Maher, T.M.; Tutuncu, A.; Morice, A.H. A novel formulation of inhaled sodium cromoglicate (PA101) in idiopathic pulmonary fibrosis and chronic cough: A randomised, double-blind, proof-of-concept, phase 2 trial. *Lancet Respir. Med.* **2017**, *5*, 806–815. [CrossRef]
69. Moroni, M.; Porta, C.; Gualtieri, G.; Nastasi, G.; Tinelli, C. Inhaled sodium cromoglycate to treat cough in advanced lung cancer patients. *Br. J. Cancer.* **1996**, *74*, 309–311. [CrossRef]

70. Martinez, F.J.; Wijsenbeek, M.S.; Raghu, G.; Flaherty, K.R.; Maher, T.M.; Wuyts, W.A.; Kreuter, M.; Kolb, M.; Chambers, D.C.; Fogarty, C.; et al. Phase 2B Study of Inhaled RVT-1601 for Chronic Cough in Idiopathic Pulmonary Fibrosis: A Multicenter, Randomized, Placebo-controlled Study (SCENIC Trial). *Am. J. Respir. Crit. Care Med.* **2022**, *205*, 1084–1092. [CrossRef]
71. Richeldi, L.; Azuma, A.; Cottin, V.; Hesslinger, C.; Stowasser, S.; Valenzuela, C.; Wijsenbeek, M.S.; Zoz, D.F.; Voss, F.; Maher, T.M.; et al. Trial of a Preferential Phosphodiesterase 4B Inhibitor for Idiopathic Pulmonary Fibrosis. *N. Engl. J. Med.* **2022**, *386*, 2178–2187. [CrossRef]
72. Richeldi, L.; Azuma, A.; Cottin, V.; Kreuter, M.; Maher, T.M.; Martinez, F.J.; Oldham, J.M.; Valenzuela, C.; Gordat, M.; Liu, Y.; et al. Design of a phase III, double-blind, randomised, placebo-controlled trial of BI 1015550 in patients with idiopathic pulmonary fibrosis (FIBRONEER-IPF). *BMJ Open Respir Res.* **2023**, *10*, e001563. [CrossRef] [PubMed]
73. Raghu, G.; Hamblin, M.J.; Brown, A.W.; Golden, J.A.; Ho, L.A.; Wijsenbeek, M.S.; Vasakova, M.; Pesci, A.; Antin-Ozerkis, D.E.; Meyer, K.C.; et al. Long-term evaluation of the safety and efficacy of recombinant human pentraxin-2 (rhPTX-2) in patients with idiopathic pulmonary fibrosis (IPF): An open-label extension study. *Respir. Res.* **2022**, *23*, 129. [CrossRef] [PubMed]
74. Corte, T.J.; Behr, J.; Cottin, V.; Glassberg, M.K.; Kreuter, M.; Martinez, F.J.; Ogura, T.; Suda, T.; Wijsenberk, M.; Berkowitz, E.; et al. Efficacy and Safety of Admilparant, an LPA $_1$ Antagonist in Pulmonary Fibrosis: A Phase 2 Randomized Clinical Trial. *Am. J. Respir. Crit. Care Med.* **2024**, rccm.202405-0977OC. [CrossRef] [PubMed]
75. Vertigan, A.E.; Theodoros, D.G.; Gibson, P.G.; Winkworth, A.L. Efficacy of speech pathology management for chronic cough: A randomised placebo controlled trial of treatment efficacy. *Thorax* **2006**, *61*, 1065–1069. [CrossRef]
76. Hirons, B.; Rhatigan, K.; Wright, L.; Kesavan, H.; Mackay, E.; Cho, P.S.P.; Birring, S.S.; Myall, K.J. Patient Perception of Cough in Interstitial Lung Disease; Impact of Cough Hypersensitivity. *Lung* **2024**, *202*, 425–430. [CrossRef]
77. Patel, A.S.; Watkin, G.; Willig, B.; Mutalithas, K.; Bellas, H.; Garrod, R.; Pavord, I.D.; Birring, S.S. Improvement in health status following cough-suppression physiotherapy for patients with chronic cough. *Chron. Respir. Dis.* **2011**, *8*, 253–258. [CrossRef]
78. Chamberlain Mitchell, S.A.F.; Garrod, R.; Clark, L.; Douiri, A.; Parker, S.M.; Ellis, J.; Fowler, S.J.; Ludlow, S.; Hull, J.H.; Chung, K.F.; et al. Physiotherapy, and speech and language therapy intervention for patients with refractory chronic cough: A multicentre randomised control trial. *Thorax* **2017**, *72*, 129–136. [CrossRef]

Journal of
Clinical Medicine

MDPI

Review

Beyond the Graft: Recurrence of Interstitial Lung Diseases Post Transplant

Prince Ntiamoah [1] and Atul C. Mehta [2,*]

[1] Department of Interventional Pulmonology, Advocate Aurora Health, Green Bay, WI 54311, USA; prince.ntiamoah@aah.org
[2] Department of Pulmonary Medicine, Respiratory Institute, Cleveland Clinic Foundation, Cleveland, OH 44195, USA
* Correspondence: mehtaa1@ccf.org; Tel.: +1-216-444-2911; Fax: +1-216-445-8160

Abstract: Interstitial lung diseases (ILDs) represent a heterogenous group of lung disorders marked by inflammation and/or fibrosis of the lung parenchyma, often leading to progressive shortness of breath and end-stage respiratory failure. In the U.S., ILDs affect approximately 650,000 individuals and cause approximately 25,000–30,000 deaths annually. Lung transplantation (LTx) offers definitive treatment for advanced ILD, with improved survival attributed to advancements in immunosuppression, organ preservation, surgical techniques, and postoperative care. However, disease recurrence in transplanted lungs remains a significant concern. Understanding the risk factors and mechanisms underlying recurrence is critical for refining recipient selection and improving outcomes. This review examines ILD recurrence post LTx and its implications for lung transplantation success.

Keywords: interstitial lung disease; idiopathic pulmonary fibrosis; lung transplantation; connective tissue disease; bronchoscopy; primary disease recurrence; lymphangioleiomyomatosis; sarcoidosis; pulmonary Langerhans cell histiocytosis; hard metal lung disease

1. Methodology for Study Selection

This narrative review was conducted to synthesize the current body of evidence on the recurrence of interstitial lung disease (ILD) after lung transplantation. A systematic approach was followed to ensure the comprehensiveness and accuracy of the review while adhering to established guidelines for narrative reviews. A comprehensive search of the literature was performed using the following electronic databases: PubMed, Scopus, Web of Science, and Embase. Keywords and Medical Subject Headings (MeSH) terms related to ILD recurrence after lung transplantation were employed, including but not limited to "interstitial lung disease", "lung transplantation", "recurrence", "graft survival", and "post-transplant outcomes". Boolean operators (e.g., AND, OR) were utilized to combine terms and refine results. The search results were imported into reference management software to remove duplicates.

2. Introduction

Lung transplantation (LTx) has evolved over the past 40 years into a standard treatment for patients with end-stage lung diseases. Since the inception of the International Society for Heart and Lung Transplantation (ISHLT) registry, approximately 70,000 adult LTx procedures have been recorded, with a median survival of 6.2 years for recipients [1,2]. The true number of lung transplants is likely higher, as the ISHLT Registry is voluntary and does not capture all transplant centers worldwide.

To be eligible for LTx, patients must meet strict criteria, including a greater than 50% two-year mortality risk without transplantation, a more than 80% probability of surviving at least 90 days post-transplant, and an equally high likelihood of five-year survival with adequate graft function. Re-transplants make up around 5% of all lung transplants [1,3,4].

Progressive pulmonary fibrosis develops in about 30% to 40% of individuals with ILD, typically leading to respiratory failure and a median survival of 2.5 to 3.5 years without treatment [5,6]. Two anti-fibrotic drugs have shown promise in slowing disease progression and reducing the rate of forced vital capacity (FVC) decline in patients with confirmed or probable usual interstitial pneumonia (UIP) [7–9].

ILDs encompass a variety of diffuse parenchymal lung conditions that share common clinical, radiographic, and pathological features. Idiopathic pulmonary fibrosis (IPF), which is the most prevalent, also has the worst prognosis [1]. While the term "interstitial" points to the focus on the interstitium in ILD pathology, this term is somewhat misleading, as most ILDs also involve extensive alterations in alveolar and airway architecture.

Common causes of ILD include occupational and environmental exposures, such as organic or inorganic dust, drug-induced toxicity, and radiation-related lung injury. ILDs are also associated with connective tissue diseases (CTDs) [5,10]. Idiopathic causes are also extensive [11,12].

Treatment generally focuses on addressing the underlying causes; however, progressive cases often lead to fibrosis and necessitate lung transplantation.

ILD-related cases account for 21% of LTx worldwide, with IPF being the leading cause [13]. However, the recurrence of ILD post LTx remains a significant challenge to long-term success. Genetic factors, such as TSC and TTR mutations, and host immune responses have been increasingly recognized as contributing to post-transplant outcomes [14,15].

This review explores disease-specific recurrence patterns and highlights strategies to improve management and outcomes in LTx recipients.

3. Disease-Specific Recurrence Patterns

3.1. Interstitial Lung Diseases

In 2018, ILD accounted for 60% of all lung transplants performed in the United States, a substantial increase from 20.4% in 2006 [4,16]. Idiopathic pulmonary fibrosis (IPF), the most common ILD, carries the worst prognosis. According to the 2019 report by the International Society for Heart and Lung Transplantation, the median survival after lung transplantation for idiopathic interstitial pneumonias, including IPF, was 5.2 years, compared to 6.7 years for other ILDs and 6.2 years across all lung transplant recipients [3,4]. While bilateral LTx is generally favored, studies suggest it does not confer a survival advantage over SLT [17,18]. The primary goals of LTx are to extend survival and improve quality of life, but the recurrence of ILDs in transplanted lungs remains a significant concern. Factors such as age, sex, EGFR mutations, and the underlying disease play a role in recurrence risk, underscoring the importance of personalized post-transplant care [1].

The recurrence rates of ILDs following LTx vary depending on the specific subtype. DIP is the most frequently reported. King et al. described a case of DIP recurrence as early as one month post LTx, which resulted in patient death [19]. Verleden and Kotecha reported cases of recurrence at 12 and 14 months, respectively, with both patients recovering fully [20,21]. Atypical bacteria, viral, and fungal infections may have contributed to disease recurrence.

Bhatt et al. documented NSIP recurrence in a middle-aged female post bilateral LTx, with histology showing recipient-origin macrophages progressing to interstitial fibrosis as early as two months post transplant [22]. This highlights the role of host factors in recurrence. Similarly, Kern et al. reported a case of hypersensitivity pneumonitis recurring three years post LTx due to continued antigen exposure [23] Table 1.

Table 1. Features of recurrence of various ILDs following lung transplantation.

Reference	Primary Disease	Number of Patients with Recurrence	Type of Transplant	Patient Age (in Years), Mean	Post-Transplant Immunosuppressive Medications	Post-Transplant Complications	Outcomes
Martel S et al. [24]	Sarcoidosis	One	Single LTx	25	Patient was started on steroids, AZA and cyclosporine	Acute rejection occurred within the first year of LTx	There was primary disease recurrence 1 year 10 months post transplant
Nunley DR et al. [25]	Sarcoidosis	Five	Single LTx	44	Patients were on AZA, steroids, cyclosporin, or tacrolimus		The earliest primary disease recurrence was noted at 3 weeks. Four patients died from refractory acute rejection and opportunistic infections
Walker S et al. [26]	Sarcoidosis	Three	Single LTx		Steroids, AZA, and cyclosporine		Granulomas were found at 5-, 6- and 56 months post transplant. There was 56% survival at 5 years
Carre P et al. [27]	Sarcoidosis	One	Single	25	Steroids, AZA, and cyclosporine	Acute rejection	
Bjørtuft et al. [28]	Sarcoidosis	One	Single LTx	46		Acute rejection, CMV	Interestingly, recurrence occurred 26 weeks post transplant. After re-transplant, there was recurrence again at 46 weeks
Milman N et al. [29]	Sarcoidosis	Three	Single LTx	51	Steroids, AZA, and cyclosporine	Bronchiolitis obliterans	Recurrence occurred one to 6 months post transplant
Martinez et al. [30]	Sarcoidosis	One	Bilateral LTx	40			Disease recurred 13 months post transplant
Le Pavec et al. [31]	Sarcoidosis	Eleven	Bilateral LTx	52		Most of the patients developed CLAD	Recurrence occurred without 24 months. Three of the patients underwent re-transplant
Nine JS et al. [32]	LAM	One	Single lung transplant	45	Steroids, tacrolimus, and inhaled cyclosporine	Bronchiolitis Obliterans	Patient died from disseminated fungal infection. At autopsy, LAM recurrence was confirmed—3 years post transplant
Bittmann et al. [33]	LAM	One	Single lung transplant	34		Acute rejection	Patient died 2 years post transplant. Disease recurrence was confirmed on autopsy

Table 1. *Cont.*

Reference	Primary Disease	Number of Patients with Recurrence	Type of Transplant	Patient Age (in Years), Mean	Post-Transplant Immunosuppressive Medications	Post-Transplant Complications	Outcomes
O'Brien et al. [34]	LAM	One	Single LTx	42	Steroids, AZA, and cyclosporine	Acute rejection	Patient died from cholecystectomy complications. Recurrence was detected on autopsy—2 years post transplant
Sugimoto et al. [35]	LAM	One	Bilateral LTx	23	Steroids, AZA, and tacrolimus		Patient had worsening lung function 5 years post transplant. Imaging was suggestive of possible disease recurrence. Improved symptoms after sirolimus was started
Karbowniczek et al. [36]	LAM	One	Single LTx	44	Steroids, AZA, and cyclosporine		Patient died from invasive aspergillosis. LAM recurrence noted on autopsy—22 months post transplant
Taveira-Da Silva et al. [37]	LAM	One	Bilateral LTx	26		Fungal pneumonia	LAM recurred 36 months post transplant.
Zaki et al. [38]	LAM	One	Bilateral LTx	66	Steroids, mycophenolate, and tacrolimus	Multiple pneumonias from pseudomonas, chronic rejection	Patient developed disease recurrence on biopsies 9 years post transplant
Habib et al. [39]	PLCH	One	Bilateral LTx	28	Steroids, AZA, and cyclosporine	CMV pneumonia	Recurrence occurred 11 months post transplant
Gabbay et al. [40]	PLCH	One	Bilateral LTx	32	Steroids, AZA, and cyclosporine		Disease recurrence at 2 years post transplant
Dauriat et al. [41]	PLCH	Eight	Seven bilateral LTx One single LTx	31			The average time to recurrence was 28 months, with the earliest being 5 months post transplant. Three of these patients resumed smoking prior to recurrence. Four of the eight patients died
Etienne et al. [42]	PLCH	Two	Single LTx	26	Steroids, AZA, and cyclosporine	CMV pneumonia	Recurrence occurred 12 months post transplant
Tarabichi et al. [43]	Hard metal disease	One	Single LTx	45		Acute rejection	Patient had relapse and died after 2.4 years post transplant

Table 1. *Cont.*

Reference	Primary Disease	Number of Patients with Recurrence	Type of Transplant	Patient Age (in Years), Mean	Post-Transplant Immunosuppressive Medications	Post-Transplant Complications	Outcomes
Frost et al. [44]	Hard metal disease	One	Single LTx				Patient had recurrence after 2 years post transplant. Died
Ntiamoah et al. [45]	Hard metal disease	One	Bilateral LTx	40	Steroids, tacrolimus, and mycophenolate	Grade 3 PGD	Recurrence in native, transplanted, and retransplanted lung. Patient still alive 11 years post initial transplant
Takaki et al. [46]	Pulmonary Alveolar Proteinosis	One	Bilateral LTx	36			Disease recurred 16 months post transplant. Died
Santamaria et al. [47]	Pulmonary Alveolar Proteinosis	One	Bilateral LTx	3		EBV pneumonia	Recurrence occurred after 18 months. Patient died 26 months post transplant
Parker et al. [48]	Pulmonary Alveolar Proteinosis	One	Bilateral LTx	41		Bronchiolitis obliterans	Disease recurred 3 years post transplant
Kern et al. [23]	Hypersensitivity pneumonitis	One	Bilateral LTx	49			Primary disease recurrence after 3 years
Arboleda et al. [49]	Polymyositis-ILD	One	Bilateral LTx	15			Disease recurred after 9 months. Died.
Bhatt et al. [22]	Nonspecific interstitial pneumonia	One	Bilateral LTx	42		Grade 3 PGD	Primary disease recurrence several months post transplant
Kotecha et al. [20]	Desquamative interstitial pneumonia	One	Bilateral LTx	59		CMV pneumonia with AMR	Primary disease recurred 1 year 2 months post transplant
Scallan et al. [50]	Fibrotic Nonspecific interstitial pneumonia	One	Bilateral LTx	52		Developed Grade A2 rejection	Primary disease recurred 2.5 years post transplant

Table 1. *Cont*

Reference	Primary Disease	Number of Patients with Recurrence	Type of Transplant	Patient Age (in Years), Mean	Post-Transplant Immunosuppressive Medications	Post-Transplant Complications	Outcomes
King et al. [19]	Desquamative interstitial pneumonia	One	Single LTx	52		Opportunistic infections (Nocardia, CMV)	Primary disease recurred just 4 weeks post transplant. Died.
Verleden et al. [21]	Desquamative interstitial pneumonia	One	Single LTx	51		PJP pneumonia, Acute rejection	Primary disease recurred 12 months post transplant.

AZA: azathioprine, CMV: cytomegalovirus, EBV Epstein–Barr virus, LAM: lymphangioleiomyomatosis, LTx: lung transplant, PGD: primary graft dysfunction, PLCH: pulmonary Langerhans cell histiocytosis, PJP: pneumocystis pneumonia

There have been reported instances of recurrence of CTD-related ILDs following LTx. One such case involved a 15-year-old patient with polymyositis who underwent bilateral LTx but experienced disease recurrence. Postmortem examination revealed pulmonary fibrosis consistent with usual interstitial pneumonia [49]. Additionally, Scallan et al. described a unique case of fibrotic NSIP (NSIP-F) recurrence after bilateral LTx, which manifested as de novo antisynthetase syndrome (anti-SS) more than 2 years after transplantation. This case represents the first documented instance of such an occurrence [50]. The recurrence may be attributed to the development of tissue-specific autoantibodies, potentially triggered by an episode of acute rejection occurring one month post transplant, despite the absence of connective tissue disease in the donor [50,51]. More research is essential to identify the risk factors contributing to ILD recurrence post LTX and to refine preventive and management strategies.

3.2. *Impact of Telomere Length on Lung Transplantation for Interstitial Lung Disease*

Advancements in precision genomic medicine have greatly improved the ability to associate clinical phenotypes with abnormal cellular pathways and their underlying genetic mutations. Telomeres—repetitive nucleotide sequences at chromosome ends—serve to protect against chromosomal degradation [52,53]. Telomere dysfunction has been linked to idiopathic pulmonary fibrosis (IPF), impaired alloreactive immune responses, and poorer outcomes after lung transplantation. A heritable, age-adjusted short telomere (ST) length, defined as below the 10th percentile, has been strongly associated with IPF onset [14,53,54]. As many as one-third of individuals with familial IPF exhibit shortened telomeres or harbor mutations in telomere-related genes, while telomere-related mutations are found in approximately 10% of those with sporadic IPF [55]. Regardless of ILD subtype, individuals with short telomeres or known telomere-related mutations tend to experience faster disease progression and a reduced time to lung transplantation or death [55]. For example, transplant recipients with *TERC* mutations have been found to have a higher risk of bone marrow dysfunction [56].

Due to the connection between telomere-related mutations and ILD, along with the possibility of extrapulmonary organ dysfunction and immune system disturbances, there is increasing attention within the lung transplant community paid to refining the evaluation and the management of such patients. In some ILD programs, telomere length measurement has become routine; however, most U.S. transplant centers have yet to widely adopt this practice for evaluating lung transplant candidates with IPF [57]. Studies comparing transplant recipients with ST to those with normal telomere length have yielded mixed results regarding survival and graft function. While some studies report higher incidences of PGD, leukopenia, and reduced CLAD-free survival, others find no significant link between ST and outcomes such as PGD, ACR, time to CLAD, or long-term post-transplant survival [54–56,58,59]. These inconsistencies likely arise from variations in how ST is defined across studies. Findings from a single-center study by Newton et al. suggested that ILD recipients with telomeres below the 10th percentile experienced increased rates of severe primary graft dysfunction, a shorter time to developing CLAD, and reduced survival [56]. Additionally, various studies have shown mixed results on how donor telomere length affects lung transplant function [56,58]. Pathologic analysis of lung tissue from recipients with CLAD showed that their telomeres are shorter compared to age-matched controls (lungs from unused donors). However, it is still uncertain whether this shortened telomere length is due to a genetic predisposition from the donor's telomere length or if the telomeres specifically shorten in the lung tissue of recipients as a result of CLAD [60].

Although lung transplantation mitigates the effects of telomere dysfunction in the lung parenchyma, systemic effects may still influence immune function. Lung transplant recipients with IPF and ST (IPF-LTRs) face an elevated risk of complications, including infections like cytomegalovirus and Epstein–Barr virus, post-transplant lymphoproliferative disease, and a higher prevalence of rare mutations in key telomere-related genes [53,57]. Given these risks, individuals with ILD being evaluated for lung transplantation should undergo telomere length screening if they have a personal history of early graying (before the age of 30), strong family history of pulmonary fibrosis, or signs of extrapulmonary organ dysfunction linked to short telomere syndrome [14,55]. For transplant recipients with telomere-related mutations, immunosuppression regimens should be carefully tailored based on bone marrow reserve. If feasible, T-cell-depleting agents like antithymocyte globulin should be avoided, since these have been linked to telomere shortening and reduced telomerase activity in real transplant patients [61].

Despite these findings, the effects of shortened telomeres on post-transplant outcomes remain inconclusive. Gaining a deeper insight into how telomere-related mutations influence ILD in the context of lung transplantation will aid in optimizing post-transplant management and refine individual care strategies for these patients, and possibly prevent retransplantation.

3.3. *Sarcoidosis*

Sarcoidosis is a multisystem disorder characterized by the formation of noncaseating granulomas and an exaggerated T-cell-mediated immune response [62–64]. While spontaneous remission occurs in a significant number of cases (approximately 80% for stage I, 60% for stage II, and 30% for stage III), 10–15% of patients progress to end-stage lung disease, with respiratory failure being the leading cause of mortality (1–6%) [62,65–68].

Lung transplantation (LTx) is a recognized treatment option for advanced sarcoidosis, particularly in cases with pulmonary hypertension, chronic respiratory failure, or resting hypoxemia [31,69]. Between 1995 and 2018, 1540 lung transplants (2.4% of all procedures) were performed for sarcoidosis, with 5-year survival rates ranging from 47% to 69% [26,31,70].

Among interstitial lung diseases, sarcoidosis is the most likely to recur following LTx, with reported recurrence rates between 14% and 47% [31]. Typically, granulomas reappear within 6–12 months post transplant, originate from the recipient's immune cells, and rarely compromise graft function [71,72]. Through DNA analysis, Ionescu et al. confirmed that granulomas in the transplanted lungs are recipient derived [73]. The first case series documenting recurrent sarcoidosis appeared in 1993, describing recurrences occurring as early as two weeks and as late as two years post transplant [24,73,74]. Bilateral LTx may reduce the risk of recurrence compared to single LTx by offering increased functional reserve and mitigating infections linked to persistent bronchiectasis [28,31] Table 1.

Recurrent sarcoidosis often manifests with milder symptoms compared to the initial disease, likely due to the effects of immunosuppressive therapies. It can present as solitary or miliary nodules [24–26,28–31,72,74–77]. Because granulomas may appear in scattered or localized patterns, a negative biopsy does not definitely exclude recurrent sarcoidosis. Transplanted organs in recipients with pre-existing sarcoidosis are prone to developing sarcoid granulomas, while grafts from donors with known sarcoidosis rarely exhibit significant disease progression when transplanted into recipients without sarcoidosis. "Donor-acquired sarcoidosis" refers to cases where recipients presumed naïve develop the condition after receiving organs from donors not known to have active sarcoidosis [73].

Although the exact cause of sarcoidosis remains unclear, it is believed to result from a combination of genetic susceptibility and exposure to environmental or microbial triggers, such as *Mycobacterium tuberculosis* or *Propionibacterium acnes* [78]. Granulomas in transplanted lungs may reflect the infectious nature of the disease, as documented cases have shown transmission from donors to recipients [78–80]. A decline in recurrence rates since 2013 coincides with the increased use of mTOR inhibitors, which are thought to suppress granuloma formation [31,81,82]. Additionally, the switch from cyclosporine to tacrolimus in the early 2010s may have contributed to improved outcomes, although this hypothesis requires further investigation [31].

While granulomas in transplanted lungs are a potential marker of disease recurrence, they rarely impair graft function or survival and are generally managed with corticosteroids [72,73]. In cases where recurrence of sarcoidosis leads to respiratory failure, retransplantation may be considered, but this decision should account for the risks and benefits of the procedure. It is essential to rule out extrapulmonary involvement before proceeding. Further research is required to validate the long-term effectiveness of evolving therapies in preventing recurrence.

3.4. *Lymphangioleiomyomatosis (LAM)*

LAM is a rare, slowly progressive systemic disease characterized by cystic lung destruction and chylous fluid accumulation due to abnormal smooth muscle-like cell infiltration [83]. Primarily affecting women, LAM is associated either with tuberous sclerosis complex (TSC-LAM) or with sporadic TSC2 mutations (sporadic LAM) [36,84,85]. Common symptoms include progressive dyspnea and recurrent Pneumothoraces, which contribute significantly to morbidity and often necessitate repeated medical interventions [84,86,87].

The disease course of LAM is highly variable, ranging from mild symptoms to severe respiratory failure. In some cases, median survival exceeds 20 years [88]. Histological analysis reveals that LAM cells express both melanoma-related and smooth muscle antigens, which aid in diagnosis [87,89]. Management primarily focuses on symptom control complication management. Sirolimus, an MTOR1 inhibitor, has been shown to stabilize lung function, reduce serum VEGF-D levels, and improve quality of life, although its discontinuation often leads to disease progression [87]. Everolimus, another mTORC1 inhibitor, has also demonstrated efficacy in multiple trials [90,91].

For patients with end-stage LAM, lung transplantation (LTx) remains the definitive treatment, offering better post-transplant survival compared to other advanced lung diseases [1,86,92]. The use of MTOR inhibitors has reduced the need for lung transplantation in some LAM patients; however, LTX is still indicated for those with severely reduced lung function (<30%), significant exertional dyspnea (NYHA class III or IV), or resting hypoxemia [1]. The first reported LTx for LAM was a combined heart–lung transplant in 1984 [93]. By 2019, 582 LTx procedures for LAM had been performed worldwide [3]. Survival after LTx is generally favorable, with one study reporting a median survival of 12 years post transplant, including survival rates of 94% at one year, 73% at five years, and 55% at ten years [94]. The recurrence of LAM following lung transplant is rare, with rates of 6–7% and only 23 reported cases [32–36,38,76,77,87,91,95–101], Table 1. Recurrence can occur as early as two months post transplant, but survival outcomes remain excellent.

Genetic studies suggest that LAM recurrence in the allograft results from metastatic LAM cells, potentially driven by immunosuppression and genetic predisposition [36,84,87,88,102]. Effective management requires careful balancing of the benefits of mTOR inhibitors, such as reduced recurrence risk, against potential complications like bronchial dehiscence, particularly during the immediate postoperative period [103,104]. Premature discontinuation of sirolimus prior to transplantation has been associated with rapid declines in lung function [104–106]. Since bronchial dehiscence typically occurs 4–6 weeks post transplantation, some centers opt to continue sirolimus up to the time of surgery or switch to everolimus, a shorter-acting mTORC1 inhibitor, to maintain pre-transplant stability while minimizing post-surgical complications [105,106].

Retransplantation in LAM is rare, with only five cases documented, including two due to graft failure and one resulting from bronchiolitis obliterans syndrome. Notably, no cases of retransplantation have been specifically attributed to LAM recurrence [86,107,108]. It remains unclear whether mTOR inhibitors or hormonal therapies could prevent or delay recurrence in the transplanted lung [38,109].

The rarity of LAM presents challenges for conducting large, randomized trials, limiting the evidence base for optimal management. Nonetheless, sirolimus is recommended as a primary therapy for LAM, either alone or in combination with calcineurin inhibitors (CNI) [38]. Alternative regimens may include second-line antiproliferative agents, such as everolimus, or substitutions like mycophenolate or azathioprine. The long-term benefits of lifelong mTOR inhibitor therapy remain an area for further research.

3.5. Pulmonary Langerhans Cell Histiocytosis (PLCH)

PLCH is a rare cystic lung disease strongly associated with smoking, primarily affecting young adults and potentially leading to pulmonary hypertension and respiratory failure. This disease arises from a myeloid dendritic cell disorder and accounts for 3–5% of adult diffuse parenchymal lung diseases, with over 90% of cases linked to cigarette smoking [10,110]. The typical age of onset is between 20 and 40 years, with an equal incidence among males and females, although women tend to present at older ages [10]. There are no known occupational or geographic predispositions; however, nearly all affected individuals have a history of current or prior smoking [111,112].

Langerhans cells, normally present in small quantities in the dermis, reticuloendothelial system, lungs, and pleura, play a central role in PLCH pathogenesis. Smoking is believed to drive the accumulation of CD1a-positive dendritic cells that harbor oncogenic mutations, such as BRAF, V600E, and MAPK2K1 [113]. These mutations activate the MAPK pathway, a key mechanism underlying disease progression. Diagnosis is supported by the detection of CD1a- and CD207-positive cells in the bronchoalveolar lavage (BAL) samples [114,115].

In asymptomatic or mild cases, smoking cessation and regular monitoring are often sufficient. For progressive disease, systemic glucocorticoids provide limited benefits, while refractory cases may require treatment with cytotoxic agents such as cladribine or cytarabine, which necessitate careful monitoring for cytopenias and infection risks [116].

Lung transplantation (LTx) is a therapeutic option for patients with advanced, progressive PLCH and constitutes approximately 0.4% of adult transplants [117]. Post-transplant survival rates are 77% at one year and 54% at ten years [118]. Recurrence of PLCH in the transplanted lung is rare, occurring in roughly 10% of cases, typically within 5–60 months post transplant [39–42,119]. Risk factors for recurrence include resumption of smoking and preoperative extrapulmonary involvement [41].

The first documented case of PLCH recurrence was reported in a 32-year-old non-smoker who underwent bilateral LTx and experienced recurrence two years later [40]. Subsequent reports, such as those by Etienne et al., describe recurrence following single LTx in patients who resumed smoking after surgery [42] Table 1. Recurrence may be driven by extrapulmonary factors or the local proliferation of abnormal Langerhans cells, which may exhibit neoplastic-like behavior [39]. The tendency of PLCH to recur in similar pulmonary distributions before and after transplantation remains poorly understood.

A multicenter study of 39 patients found that PLCH recurrence occurred in 10% of cases, with no significant impact on survival [41,118]. Extrapulmonary involvement, however, was a significant risk factor for recurrence. Management typically includes smoking cessation and corticosteroids, with pulse steroid therapy often providing symptom relief and resolution of pulmonary infiltrates [119]. Retransplantation for PCLH is rare and has been performed for bronchiolitis obliterans syndrome rather than for disease recurrence.

While recurrence of PLCH in the transplanted lung does not appear to significantly affect overall survival, preoperative extrapulmonary involvement remains a critical risk factor. Even in candidates for retransplantation, the potential for recurrence of the primary disease must be considered.

3.6. Pulmonary Alveolar Proteinosis

Pulmonary alveolar proteinosis (PAP) is a condition marked by the accumulation of lipoproteinaceous material within the alveoli, resulting from impaired surfactant clearance by alveolar macrophages [120,121]. It is classified into three types, genetic, secondary, and autoimmune, with the autoimmune variant being the most prevalent [122]. In autoimmune PAP, antibodies targeting granulocyte–macrophage colony-stimulating factor (GM-CSF) disrupt macrophage function, leading to defective surfactant processing [123]. The clinical presentation varies, ranging from asymptomatic cases to symptoms such as dyspnea, cough, fatigue, chest pain, fever, and hemoptysis. Diagnosis is supported by the identification of periodic acid–Schiff-positive eosinophilic granules within foamy macrophages [121].

The primary treatment for PAP is whole-lung lavage, which effectively clears accumulated surfactant in most patients. However, some individuals develop pulmonary fibrosis over time. In refractory cases, supplemental GM-CSF, rituximab, or plasmapheresis may be used [120,122,124]. For patients with end-stage disease, lung transplantation is a viable option, though disease recurrence after transplantation has been reported [124]. There have been three documented cases of recurrence, one associated with autoimmune PAP and two linked to genetic causes, occurring at 3-, 16-, and 26-months post-transplant [46–48]. Recurrence in genetic cases is thought to result from defective precursor macrophages originating from the bone marrow, raising the possibility that bone marrow transplantation could serve as an adjunct therapy to LTx in select patients.

Interestingly, PAP has also been identified in lung allografts of patients who underwent transplantation for unrelated conditions, including idiopathic Eisenmenger's syndrome, pulmonary fibrosis, and pulmonary hypertension [125–127]. Additionally, a case was reported in a patient who developed acute myeloid leukemia five years after LTx and subsequently developed PAP following chemotherapy [128]. These patients tested negative for GM-CSF autoantibodies, suggesting that secondary PAP in transplant recipients may be triggered by alveolar injury due to ischemia, infection, or immunosuppressive therapy (Table 1). Despite the presence of these potential mechanisms in many LTx recipients, only a small subset develops PAP, highlighting the need for further research to identify additional contributing factors.

3.7. Hard Metal Exposure

Hard metal lung disease (HMLD) arises from prolonged occupational exposure to cobalt and tungsten carbide. Its defining pathological feature is giant cell interstitial pneumonia (GIP), which is considered pathognomonic for the disease but has also been reported in cases without confirmed metal exposure [45,129]. Unlike many other occupational lung diseases, the development of HMLD does not depend on the cumulative level of exposure [119,130]. Histologically, GIP is characterized by the presence of multinucleated giant cells exhibiting emperipolesis, a phenomenon where neutrophils and lymphocytes are engulfed within the giant cells [131].

The primary approach to managing HMLD is the cessation of exposure to hard metals, which can lead to recovery in non-fibrotic cases. However, once fibrosis develops, the lung damage is generally irreversible. While corticosteroids and immunosuppressive therapies have been used in treatment, their effectiveness has not been definitely established [132, 133].

For patients with end-stage or progressive disease, LTx is a viable option. However, recurrence of the disease after transplantation has been reported, even in the absence of subsequent hard metal exposure [43,44]. Frost et al. described a case of single LTx with disease recurrence after two years, where autopsy findings revealed typical GIP changes in the allograft without evidence of inorganic particles [44]. Similarly, Tarabachi et al. documented recurrent lung injury characterized by multinucleated cells in the transplanted lung following single LTx [43]. Another notable case reported persistent GIP across native lungs, transplanted lungs, and re-transplanted lungs over an eight-year period in a patient without prior hard metal exposure (Table 1). This case suggests a potential autoimmune mechanism underlying disease recurrence [45]. Further research is needed to clarify the mechanisms driving recurrence in HMLD and to develop targeted strategies for post-transplant management and prevention of disease relapse.

4. Conclusions

The recurrence of interstitial lung diseases following transplantation is influenced by multiple factors, including recipient immune responses, persistent antigen exposure, donor–recipient immune interactions, and genetic predispositions such as short telomere syndromes. Understanding the pathophysiology and individual risk factors for recurrence has the potential to refine and guide personalized management strategies. Disease recurrence should be carefully evaluated as a potential cause of new-onset allograft dysfunction and must be excluded. Incorporating genetic screening into pre-transplant evaluations, particularly for high-risk patients with known telomere-related mutations, will be critical for optimizing long-term outcomes and advancing the field of lung transplantation.

Future Directions

Further research is needed to elucidate the mechanisms of disease recurrence after lung transplantation, particularly the role of genetic (short telomere) and immune factors and immune responses. Additionally, improving post-transplant management strategies, including optimizing immunosuppressive regimens and exploring novel therapies for refractory cases, is essential to enhance graft survival and patient outcomes.

Author Contributions: P.N., writing, editing, and submission of manuscript; A.C.M., writing and editing of manuscript. All authors have read and agreed to the published version of the manuscript.

Funding: This research received no external funding.

Conflicts of Interest: The authors declare no conflicts of interest.

References

1. Leard, L.E.; Holm, A.M.; Valapour, M.; Glanville, A.R.; Attawar, S.; Aversa, M.; Campos, S.V.; Christon, L.M.; Cypel, M.; Dellgren, G.; et al. Consensus document for the selection of lung transplant candidates: An update from the International Society for Heart and Lung Transplantation. *J. Heart Lung Transplant.* **2021**, *40*, 1349–1379. [CrossRef] [PubMed]
2. Perch, M.; Hayes, D.; Cherikh, W.S.; Zuckermann, A.; Harhay, M.O.; Hsich, E.; Potena, L.; Sadavarte, A.; Lindblad, K.; Singh, T.P.; et al. The International Thoracic Organ Transplant Registry of the International Society for Heart and Lung Transplantation: Thirty-ninth adult lung transplantation report—2022; focus on lung transplant recipients with chronic obstructive pulmonary disease. *J. Heart Lung Transplant.* **2022**, *41*, 1335–1347. [CrossRef] [PubMed]
3. Chambers, D.C.; Cherikh, W.S.; Harhay, M.O.; Hayes, D.; Hsich, E.; Khush, K.K.; Meiser, B.; Potena, L.; Rossano, J.W.; Toll, A.E.; et al. The International Thoracic Organ Transplant Registry of the International Society for Heart and Lung Transplantation: Thirty-sixth adult lung and heart–lung transplantation Report—2019; Focus theme: Donor and recipient size match. *J. Heart Lung Transplant.* **2019**, *38*, 1042–1055. [CrossRef]

4. Bos, S.; Vos, R.; Van Raemdonck, D.E.; Verleden, G.M. Survival in adult lung transplantation: Where are we in 2020? *Curr. Opin. Organ Transpl.* **2020**, *25*, 268–273. [CrossRef] [PubMed]
5. Maher, T.M. Interstitial Lung Disease: A Review. *JAMA* **2024**, *331*, 1655–1665. [CrossRef]
6. Oldham, J.M.; Lee, C.T.; Wu, Z.; Bowman, W.S.; Pugashetti, J.V.; Dao, N.; Tonkin, J.; Seede, H.; Echt, G.; Adegunsoye, A.; et al. Lung function trajectory in progressive fibrosing interstitial lung disease. *Eur. Respir. J.* **2022**, *59*, 2101396. [CrossRef] [PubMed]
7. Raghu, G.; Wells, A.U.; Nicholson, A.G.; Richeldi, L.; Flaherty, K.R.; Le Maulf, F.; Stowasser, S.; Schlenker-Herceg, R.; Hansell, D.M. Effect of nintedanib in subgroups of idiopathic pulmonary fibrosis by diagnostic criteria. *Am. J. Respir. Crit. Care Med.* **2017**, *195*, 78–85. [CrossRef] [PubMed]
8. Richeldi, L.; du Bois, R.M.; Raghu, G.; Azuma, A.; Brown, K.K.; Costabel, U.; Cottin, V.; Flaherty, K.R.; Hansell, D.M.; Inoue, Y.; et al. Efficacy and Safety of Nintedanib in Idiopathic Pulmonary Fibrosis. *New Engl. J. Med.* **2014**, *370*, 2071–2082. [CrossRef]
9. Wells, A.U.; Flaherty, K.R.; Brown, K.K.; Inoue, Y.; Devaraj, A.; Richeldi, L.; Moua, T.; Crestani, B.; Wuyts, W.A.; Stowasser, S.; et al. Nintedanib in patients with progressive fibrosing interstitial lung diseases—Subgroup analyses by interstitial lung disease diagnosis in the INBUILD trial: A randomised, double-blind, placebo-controlled, parallel-group trial. *Lancet Respir. Med.* **2020**, *8*, 453–460. [CrossRef]
10. Althobiani, M.A.; Russell, A.M.; Jacob, J.; Ranjan, Y.; Folarin, A.A.; Hurst, J.R.; Porter, J.C. Interstitial lung disease: A review of classification, etiology, epidemiology, clinical diagnosis, pharmacological and non-pharmacological treatment. *Front. Med.* **2024**, *11*, 1296890. [CrossRef] [PubMed]
11. Thomson, C.C.; Duggal, A.; Bice, T.; Lederer, D.J.; Wilson, K.C.; Raghu, G. 2018 Clinical practice guideline summary for clinicians: Diagnosis of idiopathic pulmonary fibrosis. *Ann. Am. Thorac. Soc.* **2019**, *16*, 285–290. [CrossRef]
12. Raghu, G.; Remy-Jardin, M.; Myers, J.L.; Richeldi, L.; Ryerson, C.J.; Lederer, D.J.; Behr, J.; Cottin, V.; Danoff, S.K.; Morell, F.; et al. Diagnosis of idiopathic pulmonary fibrosis An Official ATS/ERS/JRS/ALAT Clinical practice guideline. *Am. J. Respir. Crit. Care Med.* **2018**, *198*, e44–e68. [CrossRef]
13. Chambers, D.C.; Perch, M.; Zuckermann, A.; Cherikh, W.S.; Harhay, M.O.; Hayes, D.; Hsich, E.; Khush, K.K.; Potena, L.; Sadavarte, A.; et al. The International Thoracic Organ Transplant Registry of the International Society for Heart and Lung Transplantation: Thirty-eighth adult lung transplantation report—2021; Focus on recipient characteristics. *J. Heart Lung Transplant.* **2021**, *40*, 1060. [CrossRef] [PubMed]
14. Phillips-Houlbracq, M.; Mal, H.; Cottin, V.; Gauvain, C.; Beier, F.; de Fontbrune, F.S.; Sidali, S.; Mornex, J.F.; Hirschi, S.; Roux, A.; et al. Determinants of survival after lung transplantation in telomerase-related gene mutation carriers: A retrospective cohort. *Am. J. Transplant.* **2022**, *22*, 1236–1244. [CrossRef]
15. Armanios, M.Y.; Chen, J.J.L.; Cogan, J.D.; Alder, J.K.; Ingersoll, R.G.; Markin, C.; Lawson, W.E.; Xie, M.; Vulto, I.; Phillips, J.A.I.; et al. Telomerase Mutations in Families with Idiopathic Pulmonary Fibrosis. *New Engl. J. Med.* **2007**, *356*, 1317–1326. [CrossRef] [PubMed]
16. Valapour, M.; Lehr, C.J.; Skeans, M.A.; Smith, J.M.; Uccellini, K.; Goff, R.; Foutz, J.; Israni, A.K.; Snyder, J.J.; Kasiske, B.L. OPTN/SRTR 2018 Annual Data Report: Lung. *Am. J. Transplant.* **2020**, *20*, 427–508. [CrossRef] [PubMed]
17. Kim, C.; Cordova, F.; Toyoda, Y. Lung Transplantation in Interstitial Lung Disease. In *Pulmonary Hypertension and Interstitial Lung Disease*; Springer: Berlin/Heidelberg, Germany, 2017; pp. 85–102. [CrossRef]
18. De Oliveira, N.C.; Osaki, S.; Maloney, J.; Cornwell, R.D.; Meyer, K.C. Lung transplant for interstitial lung disease: Outcomes for single versus bilateral lung transplantation. *Interact. Cardiovasc. Thorac. Surg.* **2012**, *14*, 263–267. [CrossRef]
19. King, M.B.; Jessurun, J.; Hertz, M.I. Recurrence of Desquamative Interstitial Pneumonia after Lung Transplantation. *Am. J. Respir. Crit. Care Med.* **2012**, *156*, 2003–2005. [CrossRef]
20. Kotecha, A.; Balakrishnan, B.; Abu-Sayf, A.; Stagner, L.; Thavarajah, K. AN UNUSUAL CASE OF DESQUAMATIVE INTERSTITIAL PNEUMONIA RECURRENCE AFTER LUNG TRANSPLANT. *Chest* **2019**, *156*, A1233. [CrossRef]
21. Verleden, G.M. Recurrence of desquamative interstitial pneumonia after lung transplantation. *Am. J. Respir. Crit. Care Med.* **2012**, *157 Pt 4*, 1349–1350. [CrossRef]
22. Bhatt, S.P.; Parekh, K.R.; Geist, L.J.; Weydert, J.; Klesney-Tait, J.A. Rapid Recurrence of Interstitial Fibrosis Following Lung Transplantation. *Chest* **2010**, *138*, 44A. [CrossRef]
23. Kern, R.; Singer, J.; Jones, K.; Jasleen, K.; Golden, J.; Hays, S.; Lorriana, L.; Blanc, P. Recurrence of Hypersensitivity Pneumonitis After Lung Transplantation. *Chest* **2013**, *144*, 432A. [CrossRef]
24. Martel, S.; Carré, P.C.; Carrera, G.; Pipy, B.; Leophonte, P. Tumour necrosis factor-alpha gene expression by alveolar macrophages in human lung allograft recipient with recurrence of sarcoidosis. Toulouse Lung Transplantation Group. *Eur. Respir. J.* **1996**, *9*, 1087–1089. [CrossRef]
25. Nunley, D.R.; Hattler, B.; Keenan, R.J.; Iacono, A.T.; Yousem, S.; Ohori, N.P.; Dauber, J.H. Lung transplantation for end-stage pulmonary sarcoidosis. *Sarcoidosis Vasc. Diffuse Lung Dis.* **1999**, *16*, 93–100. Available online: https://europepmc.org/article/med/10207947 (accessed on 25 January 2025). [PubMed]

26. Walker, S.; Mikhail, G.; Banner, N.; Partridge, J.; Khaghani, A.; Burke, M.; Yacoub, M. Medium term results of lung transplantation for end stage pulmonary sarcoidosis. *Thorax* **1998**, *53*, 281. [CrossRef]
27. Carré, P.; Rouquette, I.; Durand, D.; Didier, A.; Dahan, M.; Fournial, G.; Léophonte, P. Recurrence of sarcoidosis in a human lung allograft. *Transplant Proc.* **1995**, *27*, 1686. [PubMed]
28. Bjortuft, O.; Foerster, A.; Boe, J.; Geiran, O. Single lung transplantation as treatment for end-stage pulmonary sarcoidosis: Recurrence of sarcoidosis in two different lung allografts in one patient. *J. Heart Lung Transplant.* **1994**, *13 Pt. 1*, 24–29.
29. Milman, N.; Hoffmann, A.L. Childhood sarcoidosis: Long-term follow-up. *Eur. Respir. J.* **2008**, *31*, 592–598. [CrossRef]
30. Martinez, F.J.; Orens, J.B.; Deeb, M.; Brunsting, L.A.; Flint, A.; Lynch, J.P. Recurrence of sarcoidosis following bilateral allogeneic lung transplantation. *Chest* **1994**, *106*, 1597–1599. [CrossRef] [PubMed]
31. Le Pavec, J.; Valeyre, D.; Gazengel, P.; Holm, A.M.; Schultz, H.H.; Perch, M.; Le Borgne, A.; Reynaud-Gaubert, M.; Knoop, C.; Godinas, L.; et al. Lung transplantation for sarcoidosis: Outcome and prognostic factors. *Eur. Respir. J.* **2021**, *58*, 2003358. [CrossRef]
32. Nine, J.S.; Yousem, S.A.; Paradis, I.L.; Keenan, R.; Griffith, B.P. Lymphangioleiomyomatosis: Recurrence after lung transplantation. *J. Heart Lung Transplant.* **1994**, *13*, 714–719. [PubMed]
33. Bittmann, I.; Dose, T.B.; Müller, C.; Dienemann, H.; Vogelmeier, C.; Lohrs, U. Lymphangioleiomyomatosis: Recurrence after single lung transplantation. *Hum. Pathol.* **1997**, *28*, 1420–1423. [CrossRef] [PubMed]
34. O'Brien, J.D.; Lium, J.H.; Parosa, J.F.; Deyoung, B.R.; Wick, M.R.; Trulock, E.P. Lymphangiomyomatosis recurrence in the allograft after single-lung transplantation. *Am. J. Respir. Crit. Care Med.* **1995**, *151*, 2033–2036. [CrossRef] [PubMed]
35. Sugimoto, R.; Nakao, A.; Yamane, M.; Toyooka, S.; Okazaki, M.; Aoe, M.; Seyama, K.; Date, H.; Oto, T.; Sano, Y. Sirolimus amelioration of clinical symptoms of recurrent lymphangioleiomyomatosis after living-donor lobar lung transplantation. *J. Heart Lung Transplant.* **2008**, *27*, 921–924. [CrossRef] [PubMed]
36. Karbowniczek, M.; Astrinidis, A.; Balsara, B.R.; Testa, J.R.; Lium, J.H.; Colby, T.V.; McCormack, F.X.; Henske, E.P. Recurrent lymphangiomyomatosis after transplantation: Genetic analyses reveal a metastatic mechanism. *Am. J. Respir. Crit. Care Med.* **2003**, *167*, 976–982. [CrossRef]
37. Taveira-DaSilva, A.M.; Steagall, W.K.; Moss, J. Lymphangioleiomyomatosis. *Cancer Control.* **2006**, *13*, 276–285. [CrossRef] [PubMed]
38. Zaki, K.S.; Aryan, Z.; Mehta, A.C.; Akindipe, O.; Budev, M. Recurrence of lymphangioleiomyomatosis: Nine years after a bilateral lung transplantation. *World J. Transplant.* **2016**, *6*, 249. [CrossRef]
39. Habib, S.B.; Congleton, J.; Carr, D.; Partridge, J.; Corrin, B.; Geddes, D.M.; Banner, N.; Yacoub, M.; Burke, M. Recurrence of recipient langerhans' cell histiocytosis following bilateral lung transplantation. *Thorax* **1998**, *53*, 323–325. [CrossRef] [PubMed]
40. Gabbay, E.; Dark, J.H.; Ashcroft, T.; Milne, D.; Gibson, G.J.; Healy, M.; A Corris, P. Recurrence of Langerhans' Cell Granulomatosis Following Lung Transplantation. *Thorax* **1998**, *53*, 326–327. [CrossRef] [PubMed]
41. Dauriat, G.; Mal, H.; Thabut, G.; Mornex, J.-F.; Bertocchi, M.; Tronc, F.; Leroy-Ladurie, F.; Dartevelle, P.; Reynaud-Gaubert, M.; Thomas, P.; et al. Lung transplantation for pulmonary Langerhans' cell histiocytosis: A multicenter analysis. *Transplantation* **2006**, *81*, 746–750. [CrossRef]
42. Etienne, B.; Bertocchi, M.; Gamondes, J.P.; Thévenet, F.; Boudard, C.; Wiesendanger, T.; Loire, R.; Brune, J. Case Reports Relapsing Pulmonary Langerhans Cell Histiocytosis after Lung Transplantation. *Am. J. Respir. Crit. Care Med.* **1998**, *157*, 288–291. [CrossRef] [PubMed]
43. Tarabichi, Y.; Saggar, R.; Wallace, W.D.; Lynch, J.P.; Saggar, R. Primary disease recurrence after single lung transplantation in a patient with prior hard metal exposure. *J. Heart Lung Transplant.* **2015**, *34*, 1216–1218. [CrossRef] [PubMed]
44. Frost, A.E.; Keller, C.A.; Brown, R.W.; Noon, G.P.; Short, H.D.; Abraham, J.L.; Pacinda, S.; Cagle, P.T. Giant cell interstitial pneumonitis. Disease recurrence in the transplanted lung. *Am. Rev. Respir. Dis.* **1993**, *148*, 1401–1404. [CrossRef] [PubMed]
45. Ntiamoah, P.; Mukhopadhyay, S.; Marshall, T.; You, J.Y.; Mehta, A.C. Giant Cell Interstitial Pneumonia In Native, Transplanted And Re-Transplanted Lungs 8 Years Apart Without Known Hard Metal Exposure. *Int. J. Surg. Pathol.* **2022**, *30*, 926–930. [CrossRef]
46. Takaki, M.; Tanaka, T.; Komohara, Y.; Tsuchihashi, Y.; Mori, D.; Hayashi, K.; Fukuoka, J.; Yamasaki, N.; Nagayasu, T.; Ariyoshi, K.; et al. Recurrence of pulmonary alveolar proteinosis after bilateral lung transplantation in a patient with a nonsense mutation in CSF2RB. *Respir. Med. Case Rep.* **2016**, *19*, 89–93. [CrossRef] [PubMed]
47. Santamaria, F.; Brancaccio, G.; Parenti, G.; Francalanci, P.; Squitieri, C.; Sebastio, G.; Dionisi-Vici, C.; D'Argenio, P.; Andria, G.; Parisi, F. Recurrent fatal pulmonary alveolar proteinosis after heart-lung transplantation in a child with lysinuric protein intolerance. *J. Pediatr.* **2004**, *145*, 268–272. [CrossRef]
48. Parker, L.A.; Novotny, D.B. Recurrent alveolar proteinosis following double lung transplantation. *Chest* **1997**, *111*, 1457–1458. [CrossRef] [PubMed]
49. Arboleda, R.; Gonzalez, O.; Cortes, M.; Perez-Cerda, F. Recurrent polymyositis-associated lung disease after lung transplantation. *Interact. Cardiovasc. Thorac. Surg.* **2015**, *20*, 560–562. [CrossRef] [PubMed]

50. Scallan, C.; Venado, A.; Han, L.; Xu, H.; Mulligan, M.; Raghu, G. Recurrent Pulmonary Fibrosis in a Lung Allograft Secondary to de Novo Antisynthetase Syndrome. *Ann. Am. Thorac. Soc.* **2020**, *17*, 901–904. [CrossRef] [PubMed]
51. Saini, D.; Weber, J.; Ramachandran, S.; Phelan, D.; Tiriveedhi, V.; Liu, M.; Steward, N.; Aloush, A.; Hachem, R.; Trulock, E.; et al. Alloimmunity-induced autoimmunity as a potential mechanism in the pathogenesis of chronic rejection of human lung allografts. *J. Heart Lung Transplant.* **2011**, *30*, 624–631. [CrossRef]
52. Wagner, C.L.; Hanumanthu, V.S.; Conover Talbot, C.; Abraham, R.S.; Hamm, D.; Gable, D.L.; Kanakry, C.G.; Applegate, C.D.; Siliciano, J.; Jackson, J.B.; et al. Short telomere syndromes cause a primary T cell immunodeficiency. *J. Clin. Investig.* **2018**, *128*, 5222–5234. [CrossRef] [PubMed]
53. Snyder, M.E.; Anderson, M.R.; Benvenuto, L.J.; Sutton, R.M.; Bondonese, A.; Koshy, R.; Burke, R.; Clifford, S.; Craig, A.; Iasella, C.J.; et al. Impact of age and telomere length on circulating T cells and rejection risk after lung transplantation for idiopathic pulmonary fibrosis. *J. Heart Lung Transplant.* **2023**, *42*, 1666–1677. [CrossRef] [PubMed]
54. Alder, J.K.; Sutton, R.M.; Iasella, C.J.; Nouraie, M.; Koshy, R.; Hannan, S.J.; Chan, E.G.; Chen, X.; Zhang, Y.; Brown, M.; et al. Lung transplantation for idiopathic pulmonary fibrosis enriches for individuals with telomere-mediated disease. *J. Heart Lung Transplant.* **2022**, *41*, 654–663. [CrossRef] [PubMed]
55. Courtwright, A.M.; El-Chemaly, S. Telomeres in interstitial lung disease: The short and the long of it. *Ann. Am. Thorac. Soc.* **2019**, *16*, 175–181. [CrossRef]
56. Newton, C.A.; Kozlitina, J.; Lines, J.R.; Kaza, V.; Torres, F.; Garcia, C.K. Telomere Length of Pulmonary Fibrosis Patients Associated with Chronic Lung Allograft Dysfunction and Post-Lung Transplantation Survival. *J. Heart Lung Transplant.* **2017**, *36*, 845. [CrossRef]
57. Kapse, B.; Budev, M.M.; Singer, J.P.; Greenland, J.R. Immune aging: Biological mechanisms, clinical symptoms, and management in lung transplant recipients. *Front. Transplant.* **2024**, *3*, 1356948. [CrossRef]
58. E Faust, H.; A Golden, J.; Rajalingam, R.; Wang, A.S.; Green, G.; Hays, S.R.; Kukreja, J.; Singer, J.P.; Wolters, P.J.; Greenland, J.R. Short lung transplant donor telomere length is associated with decreased CLAD-free survival. *Thorax* **2017**, *72*, 1052–1054. [CrossRef] [PubMed]
59. Courtwright, A.M.; Lamattina, A.M.; Takahashi, M.; Trindade, A.J.; Hunninghake, G.M.; Rosas, I.O.; Agarwal, S.; Raby, B.A.; Goldberg, H.J.; El-Chemaly, S. Shorter telomere length following lung transplantation is associated with clinically significant leukopenia and decreased chronic lung allograft dysfunction-free survival. *ERJ Open Res.* **2020**, *6*, 00003–02020. [CrossRef]
60. Everaerts, S.; Lammertyn, E.J.; Martens, D.S.; De Sadeleer, L.J.; Maes, K.; van Batenburg, A.A.; Goldschmeding, R.; van Moorsel, C.H.M.; Dupont, L.J.; Wuyts, W.A.; et al. The aging lung: Tissue telomere shortening in health and disease. *Respir. Res.* **2018**, *19*, 95. [CrossRef] [PubMed]
61. Crepin, T.; Carron, C.; Roubiou, C.; Gaugler, B.; Gaiffe, E.; Simula-Faivre, D.; Ferrand, C.; Tiberghien, P.; Chalopin, J.-M.; Moulin, B.; et al. ATG-induced accelerated immune senescence: Clinical implications in renal transplant recipients. *Am. J. Transplant.* **2015**, *15*, 1028–1038. [CrossRef]
62. Crouser, E.D.; Maier, L.A.; Wilson, K.C.; Bonham, C.A.; Morgenthau, A.S.; Patterson, K.C.; Abston, E.; Bernstein, R.C.; Blankstein, R.; Chen, E.S.; et al. Diagnosis and Detection of Sarcoidosis. An Official American Thoracic Society Clinical Practice Guideline. *Am. J. Respir. Crit. Care Med.* **2020**, *201*, E26–E51. [CrossRef] [PubMed]
63. Baughman, R.P.; Teirstein, A.S.; Judson, M.A.; Rossman, M.D.; Yeager, H., Jr.; Bresnitz, E.A.; DePalo, L.; Hunninghake, G.; Iannuzzi, M.C.; Johns, C.J.; et al. Clinical Characteristics of Patients in a Case Control Study of Sarcoidosis. *Am. J. Respir. Crit. Care Med.* **2012**, *164*, 1885–1889. [CrossRef] [PubMed]
64. Mañá, J.; Rubio-Rivas, M.; Villalba, N.; Marcoval, J.; Iriarte, A.; Molina-Molina, M.; Llatjos, R.; García, O.; Martínez-Yélamos, S.; Vicens-Zygmunt, V.; et al. Multidisciplinary approach and long-term follow-up in a series of 640 consecutive patients with sarcoidosis: Cohort study of a 40-year clinical experience at a tertiary referral center in Barcelona, Spain. *Medicine* **2017**, *96*, e7595. [CrossRef]
65. Kirkil, G.; Lower, E.E.; Baughman, R.P. Predictors of Mortality in Pulmonary Sarcoidosis. *Chest* **2018**, *153*, 105–113. [CrossRef]
66. Thillai, M.; Atkins, C.P.; Crawshaw, A.; Marcoval, J.; Iriarte, A.; Molina-Molina, M.; Llatjos, R.; García, O.; Martínez-Yélamos, S.; Vicens-Zygmunt, V.; et al. BTS Clinical Statement on pulmonary sarcoidosis. *Thorax* **2021**, *76*, 4–20. [CrossRef] [PubMed]
67. Drent, M.; Crouser, E.D.; Grunewald, J. Challenges of Sarcoidosis and Its Management. *N. Engl. J. Med.* **2021**, *385*, 1018–1032. [CrossRef] [PubMed]
68. Hunninghake, G.W.; Costabel, U.; Ando, M.; Marcoval, J.; Iriarte, A.; Molina-Molina, M.; Llatjos, R.; García, O.; Martínez-Yélamos, S.; Vicens-Zygmunt, V.; et al. Statement on Sarcoidosis. *Am. J. Respir. Crit. Care Med.* **2012**, *160*, 736–755. [CrossRef]
69. Zhang, S.; Tong, X.; Zhang, T.; Wang, D.; Liu, S.; Wang, L.; Fan, H. Prevalence of Sarcoidosis-Associated Pulmonary Hypertension: A Systematic Review and Meta-Analysis. *Front. Cardiovasc. Med.* **2022**, *8*, 809594. [CrossRef] [PubMed]
70. Taimeh, Z.; Hertz, M.I.; Shumway, S.; Pritzker, M. Lung transplantation for pulmonary sarcoidosis. Twenty-five years of experience in the USA. *Thorax* **2016**, *71*, 378–379. [CrossRef]

71. Schultz, H.H.; Andersen, C.B.; Steinbruuchel, D.; Perch, M.; Carlsen, J.; Iversen, M. Recurrence of sarcoid granulomas in lung transplant recipients is common and does not affect overall survival. *Sarcoidosis Vasc. Diffus. Lung Dis.* **2014**, *31*, 149–153.
72. Banga, A.; Sahoo, D.; Lane, C.R.; Farver, C.F.; Budev, M.M. Disease Recurrence and Acute Cellular Rejection Episodes during the First Year after Lung Transplantation among Patients with Sarcoidosis. *Transplantation* **2015**, *99*, 1940–1945. [CrossRef] [PubMed]
73. Ionescu, D.N.; Hunt, J.L.; Lomago, D.; Yousem, S.A. Recurrent sarcoidosis in lung transplant allografts: Granulomas are of recipient origin. *Diagn. Mol. Pathol.* **2005**, *14*, 140–145. [CrossRef] [PubMed]
74. Johnson, B.A.; Duncan, S.R.; Ohori, N.P.; Paradis, I.L.; Yousem, S.A.; Grgurich, W.F.; Dauber, J.H.; Griffith, B.P. Recurrence of Sarcoidosis in Pulmonary Allograft Recipients. *Am. Rev. Respir. Dis.* **2012**, *148*, 1373–1377. [CrossRef]
75. Kazerooni, E.A.; Jackson, C.; Cascade, P.N. Sarcoidosis: Recurrence of primary disease in transplanted lungs. *Radiology* **1994**, *192*, 461–464. [CrossRef]
76. Pigula, F.A.; Griffith, B.P.; Zenati, M.A.; Dauber, J.H.; Yousem, S.A.; Keenan, R.J. Lung Transplantation for Respiratory Failure Resulting From Systemic Disease. *Ann. Thorac. Surg.* **1997**, *64*, 1630–1634. [CrossRef] [PubMed]
77. Collins, J.; Hartman, M.J.; Warner, T.F.; Müller, N.L.; Kazerooni, E.A.; McAdams, H.P.; Slone, R.M.; Parker, L.A. Frequency and CT Findings of Recurrent Disease after Lung Transplantation1. *Radiology* **2001**, *219*, 503–509. [CrossRef]
78. Belperio, J.A.; Shaikh, F.; Abtin, F.G.; Müller, N.L.; Kazerooni, E.A.; McAdams, H.P.; Slone, R.M.; Parker, L.A. Diagnosis and Treatment of Pulmonary Sarcoidosis: A Review. *JAMA* **2022**, *327*, 856–867. [CrossRef]
79. Forman, J.D.; Klein, J.T.; Silver, R.F.; Liu, M.C.; Greenlee, B.M.; Moller, D.R. Selective activation and accumulation of oligoclonal V beta-specific T cells in active pulmonary sarcoidosis. *J. Clin. Investig.* **1994**, *94*, 1533–1542. [CrossRef] [PubMed]
80. Müller, C.; Briegel, J.; Haller, M.; Vogelmeier, C.; Bittman, I.; Welz, A.; Fürst, H.; Dienemann, H. Sarcoidosis recurrence following lung transplantation. *Transplantation.* **1996**, *61*, 1117–1119. [CrossRef] [PubMed]
81. Linke, M.; Pham, H.T.T.; Katholnig, K.; Schnöller, T.; Miller, A.; Demel, F.; Schütz, B.; Rosner, M.; Kovacic, B.; Sukhbaatar, N.; et al. Chronic signaling via the metabolic checkpoint kinase mTORC1 induces macrophage granuloma formation and marks sarcoidosis progression. *Nat. Immunol.* **2017**, *18*, 293–302. [CrossRef]
82. Pacheco, Y.; Lim, C.X.; Weichhart, T.; Valeyre, D.; Bentaher, A.; Calender, A. Sarcoidosis and the mTOR, Rac1, and Autophagy Triad. *Trends Immunol.* **2020**, *41*, 286–299. [CrossRef]
83. Warrior, K.; Dilling, D.F. Lung transplantation for lymphangioleiomyomatosis. *J. Heart Lung Transplant.* **2023**, *42*, 40–52. [CrossRef] [PubMed]
84. Kundu, N.; Holz, M.K. Lymphangioleiomyomatosis: A metastatic lung disease. *Am. J. Physiol. Cell Physiol.* **2023**, *324*, C320–C326. [CrossRef]
85. Moss, J.; Avila, N.A.; Barnes, P.M.; Litzenberger, R.A.; Bechtle, J.; Brooks, P.G.; Hedin, C.J.; Hunsberger, S.; Kristof, A.S. Prevalence and clinical characteristics of lymphangioleiomyomatosis (LAM) in patients with tuberous sclerosis complex. *Am. J. Respir. Crit. Care Med.* **2001**, *164*, 669–671. [CrossRef]
86. Esendagli, D.R.; Ntiamoah, P.; Kupeli, E.; Bhardwaj, A.; Ghosh, S.; Mukhopadhyay, S.; Mehta, A.C. Recurrence of primary disease following lung transplantation. *ERJ Open Res.* **2022**, 8. [CrossRef]
87. McCarthy, C.; Gupta, N.; Johnson, S.R.; Yu, J.J.; McCormack, F.X. Lymphangioleiomyomatosis: Pathogenesis, clinical features, diagnosis, and management. *Lancet Respir. Med.* **2021**, *9*, 1313–1327. [CrossRef]
88. Gupta, N.; Lee, H.S.; Ryu, J.H.; Taveira-DaSilva, A.M.; Beck, G.J.; Lee, J.-C.; McCarthy, K.; Finlay, G.A.; Brown, K.K.; Ruoss, S.J.; et al. The NHLBI LAM Registry: Prognostic Physiologic and Radiologic Biomarkers Emerge From a 15-Year Prospective Longitudinal Analysis. *Chest* **2019**, *155*, 288–296. [CrossRef]
89. Johnson, S.R.; Cordier, J.F.; Lazor, R.; Cottin, V.; Costabel, U.; Harari, S.; Reynaud-Gaubert, M.; Boehler, A.; Brauner, M.; Popper, H.; et al. European Respiratory Society guidelines for the diagnosis and management of lymphangioleiomyomatosis. *Eur. Respir. J.* **2010**, *35*, 14–26. [CrossRef]
90. Bee, J.; Fuller, S.; Miller, S.; Johnson, S.R. Lung function response and side effects to rapamycin for lymphangioleiomyomatosis: A prospective national cohort study. *Thorax* **2018**, *73*, 369–375. [CrossRef] [PubMed]
91. Ando, K.; Kurihara, M.; Kataoka, H.; Ueyama, M.; Togo, S.; Sato, T.; Doi, T.; Iwakami, S.-I.; Takahashi, K.; Seyama, K.; et al. Efficacy and safety of low-dose sirolimus for treatment of lymphangioleiomyomatosis. *Respir. Investig.* **2013**, *51*, 175–183. [CrossRef] [PubMed]
92. Oprescu, N.; McCormack, F.X.; Byrnes, S.; Kinder, B.W. Clinical predictors of mortality and cause of death in lymphangioleiomyomatosis: A population-based registry. *Lung* **2013**, *191*, 35–42. [CrossRef]
93. Estenne, M.; De Francquen, P.; Wellens, F.; Leclerc, J.-L.; Vanderhoeft, P.; Yernault, J.-C.; Primo, G. Combined heart-and-lung transplantation for lymphangioleiomyomatosis. *Lancet* **1984**, *1*, 275. [CrossRef] [PubMed]
94. Khawar, M.U.; Yazdani, D.; Zhu, Z.; Jandarov, R.; Dilling, D.F.; Gupta, N. Clinical outcomes and survival following lung transplantation in patients with lymphangioleiomyomatosis. *J. Heart Lung Transplant.* **2019**, *38*, 949–955. [CrossRef]
95. Kpodonu, J.; Massad, M.G.; Chaer, R.A.; Caines, A.; Evans, A.; Snow, N.J.; Geha, A.S. The US experience with lung transplantation for pulmonary lymphangioleiomyomatosis. *J. Heart Lung Transplant.* **2005**, *24*, 1247–1253. [CrossRef] [PubMed]

96. Benden, C.; Rea, F.; Behr, J.; Corris, P.A.; Reynaud-Gaubert, M.; Stern, M.; Speich, R.; Boehler, A. Lung Transplantation for Lymphangioleiomyomatosis: The European Experience. *J. Heart Lung Transplant.* **2009**, *28*, 1–7. [CrossRef] [PubMed]
97. Chen, F.; Bando, T.; Fukuse, T.; Omasa, M.; Aoyama, A.; Hamakawa, H.; Fujinaga, T.; Shoji, T.; Sakai, H.; Hanaoka, N.; et al. Recurrent lymphangioleiomyomatosis after living-donor lobar lung transplantation. *Transplant. Proc.* **2006**, *38*, 3151–3153. [CrossRef]
98. Johnson, S.R. Lymphangioleiomyomatosis. *Eur. Respir. J.* **2006**, *27*, 1056–1065. [CrossRef] [PubMed]
99. Pechet, T.T.; Meyers, B.F.; Guthrie, T.J.; Battafarano, R.J.; Trulock, E.P.; Cooper, J.D.; Patterson, G. Lung transplantation for lymphangioleiomyomatosis. *J. Heart Lung Transplant.* **2004**, *23*, 301–308. [CrossRef] [PubMed]
100. Reynaud-Gaubert, M.; Mornex, J.F.; Mal, H.; Treilhaud, M.; Dromer, C.; Quétant, S.; Leroy-Ladurie, F.; Guillemain, R.; Philit, F.; Dauriat, G.; et al. Lung transplantation for lymphangioleiomyomatosis: The french experience. *Transplantation* **2008**, *86*, 515–520. [CrossRef]
101. Ando, K.; Okada, Y.; Akiba, M.; Kondo, T.; Kawamura, T.; Okumura, M.; Chen, F.; Date, H.; Shiraishi, T.; Iwasaki, A.; et al. Lung Transplantation for Lymphangioleiomyomatosis in Japan. *PLoS ONE* **2016**, *11*, e0146749. [CrossRef] [PubMed]
102. Gupta, N.; Johnson, S.R. Lymphangioleiomyomatosis: No Longer Ultra-rare. *Am. J. Respir. Crit. Care Med.* **2024**, *209*, 358–359. [CrossRef]
103. Schmucki, K.; Gaisl, T.; Hofmann, P.; Hage, R.; Steinack, C.; Fehr, T.H.; Ulrich, S.; Schuurmans, M.M. mTOR inhibitors after lung transplantation: A real-life experience. *J. Thorac. Dis.* **2024**, *16*, 3007–3018. [CrossRef]
104. Groetzner, J.; Kur, F.; Spelsberg, F.; Behr, J.; Frey, L.; Bittmann, I.; Vogeser, M.; Ueberfuhr, P.; Meiser, B.; Hatz, R.; et al. Airway anastomosis complications in de novo lung transplantation with sirolimus-based immunosuppression. *J. Heart Lung Transplant.* **2004**, *23*, 632–638. [CrossRef]
105. Dilling, D.F.; Nair, A.; Gries, C.J.; Leard, L.; Fisher, A.; Johnson, S.; McCormack, F. Use of Sirolimus in Patients with Lymphangioleiomyomatosis (LAM) on Waiting Lists for Lung Transplant (LTX). *The J. Heart Lung Transplant.* **2018**, *37*, S457. [CrossRef]
106. El-Chemaly, S.; Goldberg, H.J.; Glanville, A.R. Should mammalian target of rapamycin inhibitors be stopped in women with lymphangioleiomyomatosis awaiting lung transplantation? *Expert. Rev. Respir. Med.* **2014**, *8*, 657–660. [CrossRef]
107. Wallinder, A.; Danielsson, C.; Magnusson, J.; Riise, G.C.; Dellgren, G. Outcomes and Long-term Survival After Pulmonary Retransplantation: A Single-Center Experience. *Ann. Thorac. Surg.* **2019**, *108*, 1037–1044. [CrossRef]
108. The First Lung Re-Transplantation in the Czech Republic. Available online: https://pubmed.ncbi.nlm.nih.gov/25754483/ (accessed on 28 November 2024).
109. Bittmann, I.; Rolf, B.; Amann, G.; Löhrs, U. Recurrence of lymphangioleiomyomatosis after single lung transplantation: New insights into pathogenesis. *Hum. Pathol.* **2003**, *34*, 95–98. [CrossRef]
110. Gaensler, E.A.; Carrington, C.B. Open Biopsy for Chronic Diffuse Infiltrative Lung Disease: Clinical, Roentgenographic, and Physiological Correlations in 502 Patients. *Ann. Thorac. Surg.* **1980**, *30*, 411–426. [CrossRef]
111. Wei, P.; Lu, H.W.; Jiang, S.; Fan, L.C.; Li, H.P.; Xu, J.F. Pulmonary langerhans cell histiocytosis: Case series and literature review. *Medicine* **2014**, *93*, e141. [CrossRef]
112. Elia, D.; Torre, O.; Cassandro, R.; Caminati, A.; Harari, S. Pulmonary Langerhans cell histiocytosis: A comprehensive analysis of 40 patients and literature review. *Eur. J. Intern. Med.* **2015**, *26*, 351–356. [CrossRef] [PubMed]
113. Mourah, S.; How-Kit, A.; Meignin, V.; Gossot, D.; Lorillon, G.; Bugnet, E.; Mauger, F.; Lebbe, C.; Chevret, S.; Tost, J.; et al. Recurrent NRAS mutations in pulmonary Langerhans cell histiocytosis. *Eur. Respir. J.* **2016**, *47*, 1785–1796. [CrossRef]
114. Tazi, A. Adult pulmonary Langerhans' cell histiocytosis. *Eur. Respir. J.* **2006**, *27*, 1272–1285. [CrossRef] [PubMed]
115. Harari, S.; Torre, O.; Cassandro, R.; Taveira-Dasilva, A.M.; Moss, J. Bronchoscopic diagnosis of Langerhans cell histiocytosis and lymphangioleiomyomatosis. *Respir. Med.* **2012**, *106*, 1286–1292. [CrossRef] [PubMed]
116. Lorillon, G.; Bergeron, A.; Detourmignies, L.; Jouneau, S.; Wallaert, B.; Frija, J.; Tazi, A. Cladribine is effective against cystic pulmonary Langerhans cell histiocytosis. *Am. J. Respir. Crit. Care Med.* **2012**, *186*, 930–932. [CrossRef]
117. Yusen, R.D.; Edwards, L.B.; Dipchand, A.I.; Goldfarb, S.B.; Kucheryavaya, A.Y.; Levvey, B.J.; Lund, L.H.; Meiser, B.; Rossano, J.W.; Stehlik, J. The Registry of the International Society for Heart and Lung Transplantation: Thirty-third Adult Lung and Heart–Lung Transplant Report—2016; Focus Theme: Primary Diagnostic Indications for Transplant. *J. Heart Lung Transplant.* **2016**, *35*, 1170–1184. [CrossRef]
118. Casal, A.; Suárez-Antelo, J.; Riveiro, V.; Ferreiro, L.; Rodríguez-Núñez, N.; Toubes, M.E.; Valdés, L. Smoking-related interstitial lung disease: A narrative review. *Chron. Respir. Dis.* **2024**, *21*, 14799731241291538. [CrossRef]
119. Zheng, M.; Marron, R.M.; Sehgal, S. Hard Metal Lung Disease: Update in Diagnosis and Management. *Curr. Pulmonol. Rep.* **2020**, *9*, 37–46. [CrossRef]
120. Lettieri, S.; Bonella, F.; Marando, V.A.; Franciosi, A.N.; Corsico, A.G.; Campo, I. Pathogenesis-driven treatment of primary pulmonary alveolar proteinosis. *Eur. Respir. Rev.* **2024**, *33*, 240064. [CrossRef] [PubMed]
121. Borie, R.; Danel, C.; Debray, M.P.; Taille, C.; Dombret, M.-C.; Aubier, M.; Epaud, R.; Crestani, B. Pulmonary alveolar proteinosis. *Eur. Respir. Rev.* **2011**, *20*, 98–107. [CrossRef] [PubMed]

122. Jehn, L.B.; Bonella, F. Pulmonary alveolar proteinosis—Current and future therapeutical strategies. *Curr. Opin. Pulm. Med.* **2023**, *29*, 465–474. [CrossRef] [PubMed]
123. Kitamura, T.; Tanaka, N.; Watanabe, J.; Uchida; Kanegasaki, S.; Yamada, Y.; Nakata, K. Idiopathic pulmonary alveolar proteinosis as an autoimmune disease with neutralizing antibody against granulocyte/macrophage colony-stimulating factor. *J. Exp. Med.* **1999**, *190*, 875–880. [CrossRef] [PubMed]
124. Kumar, A.; Abdelmalak, B.; Inoue, Y.; Culver, D.A. Pulmonary alveolar proteinosis in adults: Pathophysiology and clinical approach. *Lancet Respir. Med.* **2018**, *6*, 554–565. [CrossRef] [PubMed]
125. Divithotawela, C.; Apte, S.H.; Tan, M.E.; De Silva, T.A.; Chambers, D.C. Pulmonary alveolar proteinosis after lung transplantation. *Respirol. Case Rep.* **2020**, *8*, e00566. [CrossRef]
126. Yousem, S.A. Alveolar lipoproteinosis in lung allograft recipients. *Hum. Pathol.* **1997**, *28*, 1383–1386. [CrossRef]
127. Thachuthara-George, J.; Neeraj, S.; Buckner, B.; Mankidy, B.; Scheinin, S.; Kaleekal, T. Pulmonary Alveolar Proteinosis (PAP) After Lung Transplant. *Chest* **2015**, *148*, 380A. [CrossRef]
128. Du, E.Z.; Yung, G.L.; Le, D.T.; Masliah, E.; Yi, E.S.; Friedman, P.J. Severe alveolar proteinosis following chemotherapy for acute myeloid leukemia in a lung allograft recipient. *J. Thorac. Imaging* **2001**, *16*, 307–309. [CrossRef] [PubMed]
129. Khoor, A.; Roden, A.C.; Colby, T.V.; Roggli, V.L.; Elrefaei, M.; Alvarez, F.; Erasmus, D.B.; Mallea, J.M.; Murray, D.L.; Keller, C.A. Giant cell interstitial pneumonia in patients without hard metal exposure: Analysis of 3 cases and review of the literature. *Hum. Pathol.* **2016**, *50*, 176–182. [CrossRef] [PubMed]
130. Tanaka, J.; Moriyama, H.; Terada, M.; Takada, T.; Suzuki, E.; Narita, I.; Kawabata, Y.; Yamaguchi, T.; Hebisawa, A.; Sakai, F.; et al. An observational study of giant cell interstitial pneumonia and lung fibrosis in hard metal lung disease. *BMJ Open* **2014**, *4*, e004407. [CrossRef]
131. Nemery, B.; Verbeken, E.K.; Demedts, M. Giant cell interstitial pneumonia (hard metal lung disease, cobalt lung). *Semin. Respir. Crit. Care Med.* **2001**, *22*, 435–447. [CrossRef] [PubMed]
132. Ratto, D.; Balmes, J.; Boylen, T.; Sharma, O.P. Pregnancy in a woman with severe pulmonary fibrosis secondary to hard metal disease. *Chest* **1988**, *93*, 663–665. [CrossRef]
133. Nemery, B.; Nagels, J.; Verbeken, E.; Dinsdale, D.; Demedts, M. Rapidly fatal progression of cobalt lung in a diamond polisher. *Am. Rev. Respir. Dis.* **1990**, *141 Pt 1*, 1373–1378. [CrossRef]

Journal of
Clinical Medicine

MDPI

Article

Prognostic Role and Determinants of Ascending Aorta Dilatation in Non-Advanced Idiopathic Pulmonary Fibrosis: A Preliminary Observation from a Tertiary University Center

Andrea Sonaglioni [1,*], Antonella Caminati [2], Greta Behring [2], Gian Luigi Nicolosi [3], Gaetana Anna Rispoli [4], Maurizio Zompatori [5], Michele Lombardo [1] and Sergio Harari [2,6]

1 Division of Cardiology, MultiMedica IRCCS, 20123 Milan, Italy; michele.lombardo@multimedica.it
2 Semi-Intensive Care Unit, Division of Pneumology, MultiMedica IRCCS, 20123 Milan, Italy; antonella.caminati@multimedica.it (A.C.); greta.behring@unimi.it (G.B.); sergio.harari@unimi.it (S.H.)
3 Division of Cardiology, Policlinico San Giorgio, 33170 Pordenone, Italy; gianluigi.nicolosi@gmail.com
4 Division of Radiology, MultiMedica IRCCS, 20123 Milan, Italy; gaetanaanna.rispoli@multimedica.it
5 DIMES Department, University of Bologna, 40126 Bologna, Italy; maurizio.zompatori@unibo.it
6 Department of Clinical Sciences and Community Health, Università di Milano, 20122 Milan, Italy
* Correspondence: andrea.sonaglioni@multimedica.it; Tel.: +39-0285994276

Abstract: Background: Patients with idiopathic pulmonary fibrosis (IPF) have a high prevalence of cardiovascular (CV) risk factors and an increased CV disease burden. The aim of this study was to investigate the prognostic role of the ascending aorta (AA) diameter in patients with mild-to-moderate IPF and to identify the main determinants of AA dilatation. **Methods:** All IPF patients without severe pulmonary hypertension who underwent a multi-instrumental evaluation, comprehensive of high-resolution computed tomography (HRCT) and transthoracic echocardiography (TTE), between September 2017 and November 2023, were retrospectively analyzed. The primary endpoint was the composite of "all-cause mortality or re-hospitalization for all causes", over a medium-term follow-up. The secondary endpoint was to evaluate the independent predictors of AA dilatation. Additionally, Bland–Altman analysis was used to assess the accuracy and precision of echocardiography-derived AA diameters compared with non-ECG gated HRCT measurements. **Results:** A total of 105 IPF patients and 102 age-, sex-, and CV risk factor-matched controls without IPF were evaluated retrospectively. Over a follow-up of 3.9 ± 1.9 yrs, 31 patients died and 47 were re-hospitalized. AA/height (HR 1.15, 95% CI 1.06–1.25, $p < 0.001$) was independently associated with the primary endpoint, whereas unindexed AA (HR 1.01, 95% CI 0.96–1.06, $p = 0.83$) and AA/BSA (HR 1.00, 95% CI 0.89–1.11, $p = 0.39$) were not. An AA/height > 20 mm/m showed 100% sensitivity and 63% specificity (AUC = 0.78) for predicting the primary endpoint. C-reactive protein (OR 1.87; 95% CI 1.21–2.89, $p = 0.005$) and left ventricular mass index (OR 1.13, 95% CI 1.04–1.24, $p = 0.006$) were independently associated with an AA/height > 20 mm/m in the whole study group. The Bland–Altman analysis revealed a bias of +2.51 mm (with the 95% limits of agreement ranging from −3.62 to 8.65 mm) for AA estimation, suggesting a general overestimation of the AA diameter by TTE in comparison to HRCT. **Conclusions:** AA dilatation is predictive of poor outcomes in IPF patients without advanced lung disease over a mid-term follow-up. The AA/height assessment may improve the prognostic risk stratification of IPF patients.

Keywords: idiopathic pulmonary fibrosis; ascending aorta diameter; ascending aorta dilatation; mortality; outcome

1. Introduction

Idiopathic pulmonary fibrosis (IPF) is a chronic, progressive, fibrotic interstitial lung disease of unknown etiology, which occurs primarily in older adults [1]. The prognosis of IPF is poor, with an estimated median survival of 2–5 years from the time of diagnosis [2]. Several comorbidities, along with intrinsic and extrinsic risk factors, may contribute to the development of IPF [3–5].

The literature data indicate that IPF patients have a high prevalence of cardiovascular (CV) risk factors and increased CV disease burden, including coronary artery disease, heart failure, atrial fibrillation, and cerebrovascular disease [6–8]. Moreover, IPF may affect the vasculature beyond the lungs and, through an increased systemic inflammation, also accelerate atherosclerosis and degenerative processes of the arterial walls [9,10], thus potentially contributing to ascending aorta (AA) dilatation.

Recent population studies [11–16] have reported that an increased AA diameter is independently associated with a greater risk of CV events in large cohorts of individuals. As far as we know, no previous study was specifically focused on the prognostic role of AA diameters in IPF patients. Considering the high CV risk profile of IPF patients, we hypothesized that the AA diameter might be associated with poor outcome, over a mid-term follow-up period. Accordingly, the present study aimed at primarily investigating the prognostic role of the AA diameter in patients with mild-to-moderate IPF and determining the main parameters independently associated with AA dilatation in the same cohort of patients. The reproducibility of AA measurements by transthoracic echocardiography (TTE), in comparison to those derived from high-resolution computed tomography (HRCT) scans, will be discussed as well.

2. Materials and Methods

2.1. Study Population

The present study retrospectively analyzed all IPF patients without severe pulmonary hypertension (PH), followed up between September 2017 and November 2023 at the Division of Pneumology of our Institution. All patients with mild-to-moderate IPF who underwent a multi-instrumental evaluation, comprehensive of HRCT, spirometry and diffusing capacity of the lungs for carbon monoxide (DLCO), six-minute walking test (6MWT), electrocardiography (ECG), conventional TTE and carotid ultrasonography, were included. The same cohort of IPF patients was the object of previous investigations focusing on left atrial strain evaluation [17], sonographic examination of the carotid arteries [18], arterial elastance assessment [19], and finally on the prognostic role of the CHA_2DS_2-VASc score [20]. This retrospective cohort of IPF patients was compared with healthy individuals without IPF, matched by age, sex, and cardiovascular risk factors [21]. The control group was selected from the Outpatient Cardiology Division of our Institution.

IPF was defined according to the 2022 ATS/ERS/JRS/ALAT Clinical Practice Guidelines [1].

The inclusion criteria were: (1) mild-to-moderate IPF, defined by forced vital capacity (FVC) > 50%, DLCO > 35% and TTE-derived tricuspid regurgitation velocity (TRV) < 3.4 m/s [22]; (2) IPF diagnostic work-up comprehensive of blood tests, spirometry and DLCO, 6MWT, HRCT, ECG, TTE, and carotid ultrasonography; (3) hemodynamic stability.

The exclusion criteria were: (1) severe pulmonary hypertension [22] and/or congestive right heart failure at basal evaluation; (2) hemodynamic instability at basal evaluation; and (3) incomplete laboratory and instrumental data.

The following information was obtained from the patients' medical records: demographics and anthropometrics; prevalence of relevant cardiovascular risk factors; history of cardiovascular and/or cerebrovascular events; ECG data; main comorbidities; blood tests comprehensive of serum levels of C-reactive protein (CRP) and estimated glomerular filtration rate (eGFR) [23]; and finally, the medical treatment during the hospitalization.

Each IPF patient included in the study underwent anamnesis, objective examination, HRCT, spirometry and DLCO, 6MWT, ECG, TTE, and carotid ultrasonography, on the same day.

The study protocol was authorized by the Comitato Etico Territoriale Lombardia 5 (Committee's reference number 508/24, date of approval 22 October 2024).

2.2. High-Resolution Computed Tomography

A HRCT was obtained at the time of diagnosis in all IPF patients. Based on the HRCT characteristics, two expert radiologists (M.Z. and G.A.R.) classified each IPF patient into a definite usual interstitial pneumonia (UIP) pattern (subpleural and basal predominant honeycombing with or without traction bronchiectasis), a probable UIP pattern (subpleural and basal predominant reticular pattern with traction bronchiectasis or bronchiolectasis), or an indeterminate UIP pattern (peribronchovascular and subpleural ground-glass opacities, intermingled with fine reticulation but no honeycombing or traction bronchiectasis). The two radiologists also estimated the coronary artery calcification (CAC) score according to the Agatston method [24] by using semiautomatic software (CaScoring, Syngo.via VB30A, Siemens Healthineers). Coronary calcium was classified using a threshold of 130 Hounsfield units (HU) [25]. Internal diameters of the aortic root and AA were measured at end-expiration, without ECG-gating.

2.3. Conventional Transthoracic Echocardiography

All echocardiographic examinations were performed by using a Philips Sparq ultrasound machine (Philips, Andover, MA, USA) with a 2.5 MHz transducer.

The following M-mode and 2D echocardiographic parameters were recorded: relative wall thickness (RWT); left ventricular mass index (LVMi); left ventricular end-diastolic volume index, left ventricular end-systolic volume index, and left ventricular ejection fraction (LVEF), estimated with the biplane modified Simpson's method [26]; left atrial volume index; right ventricular inflow tract (RVIT), right ventricular (RV) to left ventricular (LV) basal diameter ratio, and tricuspid annular plane systolic excursion (TAPSE) from the apical four-chamber view; finally, the inferior vena cava (IVC) transverse diameter.

Doppler measurements included the E/A ratio and the average E/e' ratio, as indices of LV diastolic function and left ventricular filling pressures (LVFPs), respectively [27]. Systolic pulmonary artery pressure (sPAP) was derived by the modified Bernoulli equation [22]. The ratio between TAPSE and sPAP was measured as a noninvasive index of RV/pulmonary artery (PA) coupling [28].

The degree of valvulopathy was assessed according to the AHA/ACC recommendations [29].

Finally, aortic root and AA diameters were measured at end-diastole from the parasternal long-axis view, using the "leading edge-to-leading edge" convention, as recommended by the latest ESC guidelines [30]. The values of the aortic root and AA diameters were reported as unindexed and indexed to body surface area (BSA) and height.

2.4. Endpoint Definition

The primary endpoint of this study was to identify the independent predictors of the composite of "all-cause mortality or re-hospitalization for all causes" in a retrospective cohort of IPF patients without severe PH, over a medium-term follow-up.

The secondary endpoint was to evaluate the independent predictors of an increased AA diameter, whose cut-off value was statistically determined, in the same study group.

The causes of death and/or rehospitalizations were investigated, for each IPF patient, through the review of the medical records available in the hospital archive and/or telephone interviews.

2.5. Statistical Analysis

For statistical power calculation, we hypothesized that, by dividing IPF patients into two main categories (those with an AA diameter/BSA > 19 mm/m^2 and those with an AA diameter/BSA $\leq$ 19 mm/m^2), IPF patients with AA dilatation might have a significantly higher risk of "all-cause mortality or re-hospitalization for all causes" than those with normal AA size, over a mid-term follow-up period. Assuming that IPF patients with an AA diameter/BSA > 19 mm/m^2 and those with an AA diameter/BSA $\leq$ 19 mm/m^2 might have a 3-year "all-cause mortality or re-hospitalization for all causes" of 20% and 10%, respectively, a sample size of 105 IPF patients would reach a statistical power of 100% for determining a statistically significant difference in the rates of "all-cause mortality or re-hospitalization for all causes" between the two groups of individuals, using a two-tailed *t*-test with a type I error at 5%.

Given that all data were determined to be normally distributed, continuous data were summarized as mean $\pm$ standard deviation, while categorical data were presented as numbers (percentage). The difference between the means was estimated using the *t*-test, whereas categorical variables were compared using the Chi-square test.

Univariate and multivariate Cox regression analyses were performed to identify the independent predictors of the composite of "all-cause mortality or re-hospitalization for all causes" in IPF patients, over a medium-term follow-up. The following variables were included in the Cox regression analysis: age and male sex (as demographics), CRP (as a systemic marker of inflammation), FVC (as a measurement of pulmonary function), definite UIP pattern (as HRCT subtype of IPF), LVEF (as an index of LV systolic function), TAPSE/sPAP ratio (as an index of RV-PA coupling), unindexed and/or indexed AA diameters, CAC score (as an index of atherosclerotic burden), and, finally, beta-blocker treatment. For each variable investigated, correspondent hazard ratios with 95% confidence intervals (CIs) were calculated.

The receiver operating characteristics (ROC) curve analysis was performed to establish the sensitivity and specificity of the main statistically significant continuous variables for predicting the primary endpoint. The area under the curve (AUC) was estimated.

Kaplan–Meier survival curves were designed to measure the differences between the AA diameter categories in the rates of "all-cause mortality or rehospitalizations for all causes", over a mid-term follow-up, for the whole cohort of IPF patients. The survival curves were compared using the log-rank test.

Univariate and multivariate logistic regression analyses were performed for detecting the independent predictors of AA dilatation, whose optimal cut-off was determined using the Youden Index, in IPF patients.

Finally, Bland–Altman analysis [31] was used to assess the accuracy and precision of echocardiography-derived AA diameters compared with non-ECG gated HRCT measurements. The accuracy of echocardiography was assessed by estimating the mean difference between noninvasive and invasive measures of the AA diameters and their 95% confidence interval (CI). Precision was assessed by calculating the lower and upper limits of agreement between noninvasive and invasive measures of the AA diameters.

Statistical analysis was performed using SPSS software version 28 (SPSS Inc., Chicago, IL, USA).

3. Results

3.1. Clinical Findings

A total of 105 IPF patients and 102 age-, sex-, and cardiovascular risk factor-matched controls without IPF were evaluated retrospectively.

The two study groups showed a moderate-to-high prevalence of smoking history and a moderate prevalence of hypertension, type 2 diabetes mellitus, and dyslipidemia. Compared to controls, IPF patients had a significantly higher atherosclerotic burden, as expressed by the greater prevalence of ≥50% carotid artery stenosis, CAC on HRCT, lower extremity peripheral artery disease, and finally polidistrectual vasculopathy; however, IPF patients were not found to have a significantly increased prevalence of coronary artery disease and/or cerebrovascular events compared to controls. The two study groups showed a similar prevalence of non-cardiovascular comorbidities, such as cancers, chronic obstructive pulmonary disease (COPD), obstructive sleep apnea syndrome (OSAS), gastroesophageal reflux disease (GERD), hypothyroidism and mixed anxiety–depressive disorder. Analysis of blood tests revealed that serum levels of CRP were significantly increased in IFP patients compared to controls (1.7 ± 2.7 vs. 0.9 ± 2.1 mg/dL, p = 0.02), whereas no statistically significant differences were observed between the two groups of patients with regard to serum hemoglobin, eGFR glucose, N-terminal pro-B-type natriuretic peptide (NT-proBNP), and low-density lipoprotein (LDL) cholesterol. A cardioprotective treatment comprehensive of beta blockers and statins was more commonly prescribed to controls, whereas approximately half of the IPF patients were treated with oxygen therapy and anti-fibrotic agents (Table 1).

Table 1. Clinical characteristics of IPF patients and controls at basal evaluation.

Clinical Variables	IPF Patients (n = 105)	Controls (n = 102)	p-Value
Demographics and anthropometrics			
Age (yrs)	76.3 ± 6.8	76.4 ± 11.4	0.94
Male sex (%)	82 (78.1)	72 (70.6)	0.22
Height (cm)	166.0 ± 7.7	164.5 ± 9.3	0.21
Weight (Kg)	73.7 ± 13.3	70.7 ± 13.6	0.11
BSA (m^2)	1.86 ± 0.18	1.85 ± 0.21	0.71
BMI (Kg/m^2)	26.6 ± 3.5	26.3 ± 4.0	0.56
Yrs from IPF diagnosis	3.7 ± 1.9	/	
Cardiovascular risk factors			
Smoking history (%)	86 (81.9)	74 (72.5)	0.11
Hypertension (%)	55 (52.4)	60 (58.8)	0.35
Type 2 diabetes mellitus (%)	34 (32.4)	30 (29.4)	0.64
Dyslipidemia (%)	52 (49.5)	40 (39.2)	0.13
Atherosclerotic disease burden			
≥50% carotid artery stenosis (%)	34 (32.4)	19 (18.6)	**0.02**
Coronary artery calcification on HRCT (%)	41 (39.0)	25 (24.5)	**0.02**
Lower extremity peripheral artery disease (%)	12 (11.4)	4 (3.9)	**0.04**
Polidistrectual vasculopathy (%)	24 (22.8)	8 (7.8)	**0.003**

Table 1. *Cont.*

Clinical Variables	IPF Patients (n = 105)	Controls (n = 102)	*p*-Value
Cardiovascular disease burden			
History of CAD (previous PCI/CABG) (%)	23 (21.9)	17 (16.7)	0.34
Previous stroke/TIA (%)	7 (6.7)	12 (11.8)	0.20
Non-cardiovascular comorbidities			
Cancers (%)	19 (18.1)	13 (12.7)	0.29
COPD (%)	19 (18.1)	12 (11.8)	0.20
OSAS (%)	9 (8.6)	6 (5.9)	0.45
GERD (%)	24 (22.8)	15 (14.7)	0.13
Hypothyroidism (%)	11 (10.5)	6 (5.9)	0.23
Mixed anxiety–depressive disorder (%)	9 (8.6)	7 (6.9)	0.64
Blood tests			
Serum hemoglobin (g/dL)	14.0 ± 1.7	13.7 ± 1.9	0.23
eGFR (mL/min/m^2)	80.7 ± 17.0	78.0 ± 17.9	0.27
Serum glucose (mg/dL)	115.5 ± 20.6	110.4 ± 33.4	0.19
Serum NT-proBNP (pg/mL)	404.2 ± 1247.2	631.1 ± 1385.0	0.22
Serum CRP (mg/dL)	1.7 ± 2.7	0.9 ± 2.1	**0.02**
Serum LDL cholesterol (mg/dL)	115.1 ± 33.0	107.6 ± 36.4	0.12
Cardioprotective treatment			
Antiplatelets (%)	45 (42.8)	50 (49.0)	0.37
Anticoagulants (%)	12 (11.4)	10 (9.8)	0.70
ACEi-ARBs (%)	39 (37.1)	48 (47.0)	0.15
Calcium channel blockers (%)	21 (20.0)	30 (29.4)	0.12
Beta blockers (%)	25 (23.8)	42 (41.2)	**0.007**
Diuretics (%)	28 (26.7)	24 (23.5)	0.60
Statins (%)	22 (20.9)	35 (34.3)	**0.03**
Antidiabetic drugs (%)	28 (26.7)	25 (24.5)	0.72
Proton pump inhibitors (%)	22 (20.9)	13 (12.7)	0.11
Respiratory treatment			
Oxygen therapy (%)	55 (52.4)	/	
Oral corticosteroids (%)	38 (36.2)	/	
Inhalation therapy (%)	11 (10.5)	/	
Pirfenidone (%)	43 (40.9)	/	
Nintedanib (%)	55 (52.4)	/	

Data are expressed as mean ± SD or as number (percentage). Significant *p*-values are in bold. ACEIs, angiotensin-converting enzyme inhibitors; ARBs, angiotensin II receptor blockers; BMI, body mass index; BSA, body surface area; CAD, coronary artery disease; CABG, coronary artery bypass graft; COPD, chronic obstructive pulmonary disease; CRP, C-reactive protein; eGFR, estimated glomerular filtration rate; GERD, gastroesophageal reflux disease; HRCT, high resolution computed tomography; IPF, idiopathic pulmonary fibrosis; LDL, low-density lipoprotein; NT-proBNP, N-Terminal pro-B-Type Natriuretic Peptide; OSAS, Obstructive Sleep Apnea Syndrome; PCI, percutaneous coronary intervention; SD, standard deviation; TIA, transient ischemic attack.

3.2. Instrumental Findings

Table 2 summarizes all the relevant instrumental parameters measured in the two study groups.

Table 2. Baseline instrumental variables detected in the two study groups.

Instrumental Parameters	IPF Patients (n = 105)	Controls (n = 102)	*p*-Value
Radiological findings			
Definite UIP (%)	63 (60.0)	/	/
Probable UIP (%)	26 (24.8)	/	/
Indeterminate pattern (%)	16 (15.2)	/	/
CAC score (HU)	698.9 ± 879.8	/	/
Spirometry parameters			
FVC (L)	2.6 ± 0.6	/	/
FVC (%)	77.6 ± 16.7	/	/
FEV1 (L)	2.1 ± 0.5	/	/
FEV1 (%)	82.4 ± 16.1	/	/
FEV1/FVC ratio	0.8 ± 0.1	/	/
TLC (L)	4.8 ± 1.1	/	/
TLC (%)	76.4 ± 16.7	/	/
DLCO (mL/min/mmHg)	11.4 ± 4.0	/	/
DLCO (%)	47.9 ± 16.0	/	/
Restrictive pattern (%)	70 (66.7)	/	/
ΔSaO_2 (%)	6.6 ± 4.2	/	/
6MWT (m)	399.3 ± 110.6	/	/
ECG variables			
Heart rate (bpm)	74.9 ± 15.0	74.1 ± 12.2	0.67
AF (%)	12 (11.4)	10 (9.8)	0.70
Intraventricular delay (%)	21 (20.0)	25 (24.5)	0.43
EchoDoppler parameters			
LVEDD (mm)	46.5 ± 5.7	47.0 ± 6.2	0.55
RWT	0.43 ± 0.06	0.43 ± 0.07	>0.99
LVMi (g/m^2)	97.5 ± 23.3	102.6 ± 29.2	0.16
Normal LV geometric pattern (%)	36 (34.3)	30 (29.4)	0.45
LV concentric remodeling (%)	48 (45.7)	40 (39.2)	0.34
LV concentric hypertrophy (%)	10 (9.5)	16 (15.7)	0.18
LV eccentric hypertrophy (%)	11 (10.5)	16 (15.7)	0.26
LVEDVi (mL/m^2)	40.3 ± 11.8	38.7 ± 13.5	0.36
LVESVi (mL/m^2)	15.8 ± 8.2	14.7 ± 10.3	0.39
LVEF (%)	61.9 ± 9.1	63.8 ± 9.4	0.14
E/A ratio	0.78 ± 0.18	0.75 ± 0.44	0.52
E/average e′ ratio	14.0 ± 4.5	11.9 ± 4.9	**0.001**

Table 2. *Cont.*

Instrumental Parameters	IPF Patients (n = 105)	Controls (n = 102)	*p*-Value
LAVi (mL/m^2)	33.6 ± 10.9	34.1 ± 13.7	0.77
More than mild MR (%)	12 (11.4)	11 (10.8)	0.88
More than mild AR (%)	11 (10.5)	8 (7.8)	0.51
More than mild TR (%)	24 (22.8)	7 (6.9)	**0.001**
RVIT (mm)	33.1 ± 6.6	28.1 ± 4.3	**<0.001**
RV/LV basal diameter ratio	0.77 ± 0.23	0.70 ± 0.19	**0.02**
TAPSE (mm)	22.0 ± 4.7	22.9 ± 3.7	0.13
TRV (m/s)	3.3 ± 2.7	2.6 ± 0.3	**0.009**
IVC (mm)	19.7 ± 4.8	17.9 ± 3.8	**0.003**
sPAP (mmHg)	42.0 ± 13.3	27.7 ± 6.3	**<0.001**
TAPSE/sPAP (mm/mmHg)	0.57 ± 0.24	0.86 ± 0.22	**<0.001**
Unindexed aortic root (mm)	36.4 ± 3.8	34.9 ± 4.1	**0.007**
Aortic root indexed to BSA (mm/m^2)	19.6 ± 2.2	19.3 ± 2.4	0.35
Aortic root indexed to height (mm/m)	22.0 ± 2.3	21.2 ± 2.1	**0.009**
Unindexed ascending aorta (mm)	36.6 ± 4.9	35.0 ± 3.9	**0.01**
Ascending aorta indexed to BSA (mm/m^2)	19.8 ± 3.0	19.4 ± 2.7	0.31
Ascending aorta indexed to height (mm/m)	22.1 ± 2.9	21.3 ± 2.4	**0.03**

Data are expressed as mean ± SD or as number (percentage). Significant *p*-values are in bold. A 6MWT, six-minute walking test; ΔSaO2, absolute difference between peak exercise and rest oxygen saturation; AR, aortic regurgitation; BSA, body surface area; CAC, coronary artery calcification; DLCO, diffusing capacity of the lung for carbon monoxide; ECG, electrocardiogram; FEV1, forced expiratory volume in 1 s; FVC, forced vital capacity; HRCT, high resolution computed tomography; HU, Hounsfield unit; IPF, idiopathic pulmonary fibrosis; IVC, inferior vena cava; LAVi, left atrial volume index; LV, left ventricular; LVEDD, left ventricular end-diastolic diameter; LVEDVi, left ventricular end-diastolic volume index; LVEF, left ventricular ejection fraction; LVESVi, left ventricular end-systolic volume index; LVMi, left ventricular mass index; MR, mitral regurgitation; RV, right ventricular; RVIT, right ventricular inflow tract; RWT, relative wall thickness; SD, standard deviation; sPAP, systolic pulmonary artery pressure; TAPSE, tricuspid annular plane systolic excursion; TLC, total lung capacity; TR, tricuspid regurgitation; TRV, tricuspid regurgitation velocity; TTE, transthoracic echocardiography; UIP, usual interstitial pneumonia.

On HRCT, 60% of IPF patients were diagnosed with a "definite" UIP pattern, 24.8% with a "probable" UIP pattern, and the remaining 15.2% with an "indeterminate" pattern; moreover, an elevated CAC score (698.9 ± 879.8 HU) was obtained. Pulmonary function tests (PFTs) showed a mild reduction in FVC%, forced expiratory volume in 1 s (FEV1)%, and total lung capacity (TLC)%, whereas DLCO% was moderately impaired. The 6 min distance walked by IPF patients was slightly reduced in comparison to the normal range for healthy individuals (between 400 and 700 m) [32]. No statistically significant differences were observed between the two study groups in heart rate, atrial fibrillation prevalence, and intraventricular delay on resting ECG. On TTE, left-sided cardiac chamber cavity size did not differ between IPF patients and controls. The most common LV geometric pattern detected in both groups of patients was LV concentric remodeling with normal LV systolic function and first-degree diastolic dysfunction. However, LVFPs, as expressed by the E/average e' ratio (14.0 ± 4.5 vs. 11.9 ± 4.9, $p = 0.001$), were significantly higher in IPF patients than controls. No significant valvulopathy was reported in the two study groups. IPF patients were found with a mild degree of RV enlargement, as quantified by both RVIT diameter and RV/LV basal diameter ratio measured from the apical four-chamber view.

Nevertheless, RV systolic function, assessed by the M-mode derived TAPSE (22.0 ± 4.7 vs. 22.9 ± 3.7 mm, p = 0.13) was normal and similar in both groups of patients. The echocardiographic evaluation of pulmonary hemodynamics revealed significantly increased values of TRV, IVC diameter, and sPAP in IPF patients compared to controls, compatible with mild-to-moderate PH. A concomitant moderate impairment in TAPSE/sPAP ratio was observed in IPF patients in comparison to controls and to the accepted normal range, which is typically between 0.8 and 1.8 [28]. Concerning the assessment of the thoracic aorta, the aortic root and AA diameters indexed to BSA were similar in the two study groups. The majority of IPF patients (74.3% in total) were found with increased AA diameters indexed to BSA, in comparison to the accepted reference values [26]. Compared to controls, IPF patients were diagnosed with significantly larger unindexed aortic root and AA diameters and significantly larger aortic root and AA diameters indexed to height.

3.3. Survival Analysis

The mean follow-up time was 3.9 ± 1.9 yrs. During the follow-up period, 31 IPF patients died and 47 were re-hospitalized due to: (1) CV causes (21.3%): acute ischemic stroke/transient ischemic attack (6 patients) and acute coronary syndrome (4 patients); (2) cardiopulmonary causes (42.5%): right heart failure (12 patients) and acute pulmonary embolism (8 patients); (3) pulmonary causes (36.2%): acute respiratory failure secondary to IPF progression (7 patients), pneumonia (7 patients), pneumomediastinum (2 patients), and pneumothorax (1 patient). No case of acute aortic syndrome was recorded. The deaths recorded in IPF patients occurred within 4 years after hospital discharge in the great majority of cases.

On Cox regression analysis, CRP, FVC%, TAPSE/sPAP ratio, and AA indexed to height were independently associated with the primary endpoint (Table 3).

Table 3. Univariate and multivariate Cox regression analyses performed to identify the variables independently associated with the composite of "all-cause mortality plus re-hospitalization for all causes" in the whole cohort of IPF patients, over a medium-term follow-up.

	Univariate Cox Regression Analysis			Multivariate Cox Regression Analysis		
Variables	**HR**	**95% CI**	***p*-Value**	**HR**	**95% CI**	***p*-Value**
Age (yrs)	1.02	0.98–1.05	0.32			
Male sex	1.33	0.77–2.31	0.31			
Smoking	1.15	0.65–2.02	0.64			
CRP (mg/dL)	1.12	1.05–1.20	**<0.001**	1.09	1.01–1.18	**0.03**
FVC (%)	0.98	0.96–0.99	**0.002**	0.98	0.97–0.99	**0.02**
Definite UIP pattern	1.20	0.88–1.64	0.24			
LVEF (%)	0.97	0.94–0.99	**0.03**	0.98	0.95–1.00	0.11
TAPSE/sPAP ratio (mm/mmHg)	0.10	0.03–0.34	**<0.001**	0.23	0.07–0.76	**0.02**
Unindexed ascending aorta diameter	1.01	0.96–1.06	0.83			
Ascending aorta diameter indexed to BSA (mm/m^2)	1.00	0.89–1.11	0.39			
Ascending aorta diameter indexed to height (mm/m)	1.18	1.09–1.27	**<0.001**	1.15	1.06–1.25	**<0.001**
CAC score (HU)	1.00	0.97–1.03	0.98			
Beta blocker treatment	0.79	0.50–1.26	0.32			

Significant p-values are in bold. BSA, body surface area; CAC, coronary artery calcification; CRP, C-reactive protein; FVC, forced vital capacity; HU, Hounsfield unit; LVEF, left ventricular ejection fraction; sPAP, systolic pulmonary artery pressure; TAPSE, tricuspid annular plane systolic excursion; UIP, usual interstitial pneumonia.

ROC curve analysis revealed that a CRP > 0.37 mg/dL (72% sensitivity, 41% specificity, AUC = 0.54), a FVC < 73.5% (50% sensitivity, 37% specificity, AUC = 0.38), a TAPSE/sPAP ratio < 0.65 mm/mmHg (73% sensitivity, 63% specificity, AUC = 0.73), and an AA diameter indexed to height > 20 mm/m (100% sensitivity, 63% specificity, AUC = 0.78) showed the greatest sensitivity and specificity for predicting the composite endpoint in the whole study population.

Prognostic ROC curves and Kaplan–Meier survival curves were drawn to compare the rates of the composite of "all-cause mortality or re-hospitalization for all causes" over the follow-up period in IPF patients, categorized according to an AA diameter indexed to height ≤ 20 mm/m and >20 mm/m, as depicted in Figure 1A and Figure 1B, respectively.

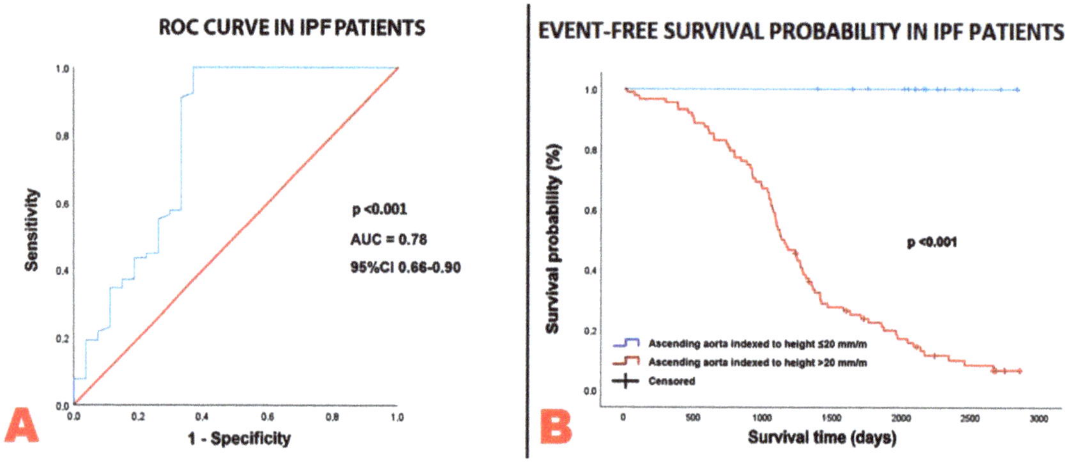

Figure 1. Prognostic ROC curve (**A**) and Kaplan–Meier survival curves (**B**) drawn to compare the rates of the endpoint "all-cause mortality or re-hospitalizations for all causes" in IPF patients, categorized according to ascending aorta indexed to height≤ and >20 mm/m, respectively. AUC, area under the curve; IPF, idiopathic pulmonary fibrosis; ROC, receiver operating characteristics.

In the multivariate logistic regression analysis performed to detect the variables independently associated with an AA indexed to height >20 mm/m in the entire cohort of IPF patients, only CRP and LVMi maintained statistical significance (Table 4).

Table 4. Univariate and multivariate logistic regression analyses performed to evaluate the parameters independently associated with an ascending aorta indexed to height > 20 mm/m in the entire cohort of IPF patients.

	Univariate Logistic Regression Analysis			Multivariate Logistic Regression Analysis		
Variables	**OR**	**95% CI**	***p*-Value**	**OR**	**95% CI**	***p*-Value**
Age (yrs)	1.03	0.95–1.11	0.43			
Male sex	1.62	0.51–5.19	0.42			
BSA (m^2)	1.66	0.10–30.5	0.73			
Hypertension	1.71	0.59–4.91	0.32			
Smoking	2.20	0.67–7.23	0.19			
CRP (mg/dL) x 0.1 U increase	2.00	1.30–3.06	**0.001**	1.87	1.21–2.89	**0.005**
FVC (%)	0.96	0.93–0.99	**0.03**	0.98	0.93–1.03	0.36

Table 4. *Cont.*

Variables	Univariate Logistic Regression Analysis			Multivariate Logistic Regression Analysis		
	OR	95% CI	*p*-Value	OR	95% CI	*p*-Value
Definite UIP pattern	1.05	0.52–2.13	0.88			
LVMi (g/m^2)	1.08	1.04–1.13	**<0.001**	1.13	1.04–1.24	**0.006**
CAC score (HU)	1.02	0.95–1.09	0.52			
Oral corticosteroids	1.77	0.53–5.89	0.35			

Significant *p*-values are in bold. BSA, body surface area; CAC, coronary artery calcification; CRP, C-reactive protein; FVC, forced vital capacity; HU, Hounsfield unit; LVMi, left ventricular mass index; UIP, usual interstitial pneumonia.

A CRP > 0.4 mg/dL (79% sensitivity, 99% specificity, AUC = 0.93) and an LVMi > 90 g/m^2 (72% sensitivity, 99% specificity, AUC = 0.83) were the best cut-off values for predicting the secondary endpoint.

3.4. Measurement Variability

The Bland–Altman analysis revealed a bias of +2.51 mm (with the 95% limits of agreement ranging from −3.62 to 8.65 mm) for AA estimation, suggesting a general overestimation of the AA diameter by TTE in comparison to non-ECG gated HRCT (Figure 2).

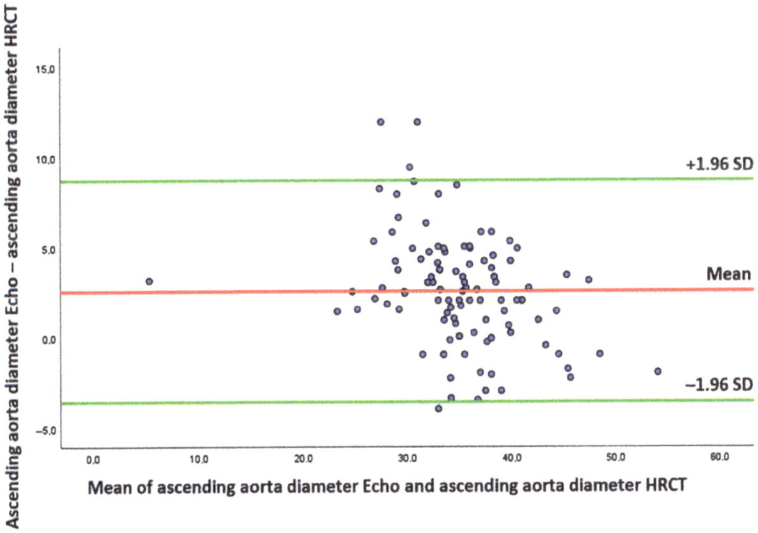

Figure 2. Bland–Altman analysis performed to assess the accuracy and precision of echocardiography-derived ascending aorta diameters compared with non-ECG gated HRCT measurements. ECG, electrocardiogram; HRCT, high-resolution computed tomography.

4. Discussion

4.1. Main Findings of the Study

The present study conducted on a retrospective series of IPF patients without advanced lung disease demonstrated that: (1) compared to matched controls, IPF patients had significantly larger unindexed aortic root and AA diameters and significantly larger aortic root and AA diameters indexed to a height; (2) the AA dilatation was independently associated with the occurrence of the composite of "all-cause mortality or re-hospitalization for all causes" over a mid-term follow-up; (3) the AA diameter indexed to height showed an incremental prognostic value over both the unindexed AA diameter and the AA diameter indexed to BSA; (4) serum levels of CRP and LVMi were independently correlated with AA dilatation in IPF patients; (5) TTE examination was associated with systematic overestimation of AA diameters in comparison to the measurements derived from non-ECG gated HRCT.

In our findings, an AA diameter indexed to height > 20 mm/m at basal evaluation was the best cut-off value for distinguishing between IPF patients with an increased probability of "all-cause mortality or re-hospitalization for all causes" from those with an increased probability of event-free survival, over the follow-up period. Serum CRP levels, FVC%, and the TTE-derived TAPSE/sPAP ratio were other independent prognostic indicators of an increased risk of mortality and adverse clinical events in IPF patients.

4.2. Prognostic Role of Ascending Aorta Dilatation

During the last two decades, a few studies have demonstrated the prognostic role of aortic root and AA size in various study populations. Gardin J.M. et al. [11], in a cohort of patients aged ≥ 65 years without clinical CV disease at baseline, found that aortic root dilatation was predictive of congestive heart failure, stroke, CV disease mortality, and all-cause mortality. Lai C.L. et al. [12], in the Chin-Shan Community Cardiovascular Cohort study, found a significant association between aortic root dimension and all-cause death in adults < 65 years. Cuspidi C. et al. [13], in the PAMELA study, demonstrated that the aortic root diameter indexed to height was predictive of nonfatal and fatal CV events among middle-aged individuals, showing an incremental prognostic value over the absolute aortic root diameter and the aortic root diameter indexed to BSA. Kamimura D. et al. [14], in the Jackson Heart Study, found that a greater proximal aortic diameter was associated with an increased risk of CV events in a community-based cohort of blacks. Canciello G. et al. [15] and Leone D. et al. [16] demonstrated that AA dilatation was associated with a greater risk of CV events in hypertensive patients, regardless of LV hypertrophy and other confounders.

Consistent with the PAMELA study's results, in our findings, the AA diameter indexed to height was the best indicator of poor outcomes in IPF patients. Our results are also in alignment with the recent evidence that indexing aortic dimensions to patient height may allow incremental prognostic information for evaluating the risk of natural complications in patients with AA dilatation [33]. Conversely, the weight might not contribute substantially to aortic size and growth.

The present study also confirmed the usefulness of the TAPSE/sPAP ratio for providing a prognostic risk stratification of IPF patients, as previously demonstrated by our study group [34]. This simple noninvasive index of the RV-PA coupling measures the relationship between RV contractility and RV afterload. The TAPSE/sPAP ratio impairment with consequent RV-PA uncoupling may be induced by a pre-capillary component, resulting from fibrotic destruction of lung parenchyma, leading to hypoxic vasoconstriction and a loss of vascular bed density, and a post-capillary component favored by increased arterial stiffness, moderate diastolic dysfunction, and left-sided heart chambers stiffness.

4.3. Pathophysiological Mechanisms of Ascending Aorta Dilatation in IPF Patients

A number of factors may synergically contribute to the AA dilatation in IPF patients (Figure 3).

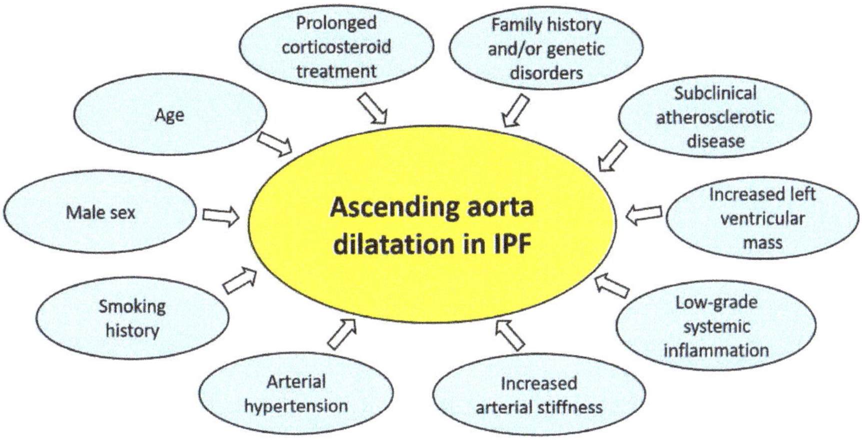

Figure 3. Main determinants of ascending aorta dilatation in IPF patients. IPF, idiopathic pulmonary fibrosis.

Firstly, it is important to consider that the profile of IPF patients is similar to the general profile of patients at higher risk for CV disease [35], due to the high prevalence of the most common CV risk factors, particularly older age, male sex, smoking history and hypertension, detected in these patients. AA dilatation is a common finding in arterial hypertension, affecting about 15% of hypertensive patients, and has been recently associated with a greater risk of CV events [16].

Secondly, it has been reported that there is an association between poorer pulmonary function and higher arterial stiffness, likely mediated by circulating inflammatory mediators, such as CRP and IL-6 [36]. Given the positive correlation between arterial stiffness and aortic size demonstrated in individuals without overt heart disease [37], in hypertensive patients [38], and in patients affected by type 2 diabetes [39], it is likely that an increased arterial stiffness, frequently observed in IPF patients [19], may have an important role in inducing the AA dilatation in IPF patients.

A low-grade systemic inflammation, which is commonly detected in IPF patients [18,40,41], might contribute to or trigger the process of remodeling within vascular walls of the aorta, with peculiar involvement of the media and adventitia, leading to media atrophy, thinning, and weakening of the aortic wall, and ultimately aortic dilatation [42].

Moreover, as observed in young individuals [43] and in patients with essential hypertension [44], the increase in aortic diameters detected in IPF patients may be related to the increased left ventricular mass. Indeed, LV remodeling is strongly associated with aortic wall remodeling: LV wall thickness, LVMi, and diastolic dysfunction may all contribute to an increase in aortic diameter.

Similarly to what is described in the general population [45], subclinical atherosclerotic disease, particularly CAC score, could be another possible determinant of increased AA diameter in IPF patients.

Aortic dilatation may also be promoted by prolonged corticosteroid treatment, which has been associated with aortic wall fragility due to its negative effect on collagen formation and connective tissue strength [46,47].

Finally, it is not possible to exclude that a number of cases of AA dilatation detected in IPF patients may be related to positive family history and/or genetic disorders, including Marfan syndrome, Ehlers–Danlos syndrome, Turner's syndrome, and bicuspid aortic valve [48].

In the present study, among the several parameters included in the logistic regression analysis performed to identify the independent predictors of AA dilatation in IPF patients (age, male sex, BSA, hypertension, smoking, CRP, FVC, LVMi, CAC score, and corticosteroid treatment), only serum CRP levels and LVMi showed an incremental prognostic value over the other variables. Our results would confirm that, in IPF patients, LV remodeling and aortic wall remodeling are strongly correlated and that a low-grade systemic inflammation might also affect the AA wall.

4.4. Implications for Clinical Practice

In light of our findings, the assessment of aortic diameters might help pulmonologists to optimize the prognostic risk stratification of IPF patients. Notably, IPF patients with AA diameter indexed to height > 20 mm/m at basal echocardiographic evaluation should be considered at high risk of major adverse CV events over a mid-term follow-up period. Due to their beneficial effect in attenuating AA dilation [49,50], the prescription of beta blockers and statins, commonly underutilized in IPF patients [51], should be implemented in clinical practice, especially for those patients with an AA diameter indexed to height > 20 mm/m. The initiation and/or up-titration of angiotensin-converting enzyme (ACE) inhibitors or angiotensin receptor blockers (ARBs) may also protect against further AA dilatation, thus preventing the occurrence of acute aortic syndromes. As observed in hypertensive patients, early cardioprotective treatment could induce a reduction in left ventricular mass [52], thus improving CV prognosis.

The present study also confirmed the accuracy and reliability of conventional TTE for measuring the AA diameters in IPF patients. By providing a systematic overestimation of the real aortic size, the "leading edge-to-leading edge" convention, strongly encouraged by international guidelines [26], is more effective than the "inner edge-to-inner edge" convention in identifying early those patients at increased risk of adverse CV events and/or life-threatening complications, such as aortic dissection.

4.5. Study Limitations

The main limitations of the present study were its monocentric design, its retrospective nature, and the limited number of IPF patients analyzed. However, the sample size calculation for survival analysis justified the total number of IPF patients included in the study. In addition, several traditional and innovative echocardiographic parameters, such as stroke volume, arterial elastance, and left atrial strain during the reservoir phase, were not included in our evaluation, as they were not measured in all patients at the basal echocardiographic examination. These parameters would have allowed us to obtain further information about the mechanisms underpinning AA dilatation in IPF patients. Finally, the aortic diameters were assessed by a non-ECG-gated HRCT, rather than computed tomography angiography; therefore, the aortic diameters, even if measured in all IPF patients, could not always be obtained at end-diastole in all cases.

5. Conclusions

AA dilatation is predictive of poor outcome in IPF patients without advanced lung disease, over a mid-term follow-up.

The AA diameter indexed to height might improve the prognostic risk stratification of IPF patients, and its dilatation may suggest the early initiation and/or up-titration of cardioprotective drugs.

Further multicentric prospective studies are needed to confirm our findings.

Author Contributions: Conceptualization, A.S. and A.C.; Methodology, A.S., G.A.R. and M.Z.; software, A.S.; Validation, A.C., M.L. and S.H.; Formal Analysis, A.S.; Investigation, A.S., A.C., G.B., G.A.R. and M.Z.; Resources, A.S. and S.H.; Data Curation, A.S., G.B., G.A.R. and M.Z.; Writing—Original Draft Preparation, A.S.; Writing—Review and Editing, G.L.N.; Visualization, G.L.N., M.L. and S.H.; Supervision, M.L. and S.H.; Project Administration, S.H.; Funding Acquisition, A.S. All authors have read and agreed to the published version of the manuscript.

Funding: This research was funded by the Italian Ministry of Health, Ricerca Corrente IRCCS MultiMedica.

Institutional Review Board Statement: The study was conducted in accordance with the Declaration of Helsinki and approved by the Comitato Etico Territoriale Lombardia 5 (Committee's reference number 508/24), date of approval 22 October 2024.

Informed Consent Statement: Informed consent was obtained from all individual participants included in the study.

Data Availability Statement: Data extracted from included studies will be publicly available on Zenodo (https://zenodo.orgaccessed on 31 October 2024).

Acknowledgments: The authors wish to thank Monica Fumagalli for her graphical support.

Conflicts of Interest: The authors declare no conflicts of interest.

References

1. Raghu, G.; Remy-Jardin, M.; Richeldi, L.; Thomson, C.C.; Inoue, Y.; Johkoh, T.; Kreuter, M.; Lynch, D.A.; Maher, T.M.; Martinez, F.J.; et al. Idiopathic Pulmonary Fibrosis (an Update) and Progressive Pulmonary Fibrosis in Adults: An Official ATS/ERS/JRS/ALAT Clinical Practice Guideline. *Am. J. Respir. Crit. Care Med.* **2022**, *205*, e18–e47. [CrossRef] [PubMed]
2. Nathan, S.D.; Shlobin, O.A.; Weir, N.; Ahmad, S.; Kaldjob, J.M.; Battle, E.; Sheridan, M.J.; du Bois, R.M. Long-term course and prognosis of idiopathic pulmonary fibrosis in the new millennium. *Chest* **2011**, *140*, 221–229. [CrossRef]
3. Conti, S.; Harari, S.; Caminati, A.; Zanobetti, A.; Schwartz, J.D.; Bertazzi, P.A.; Cesana, G.; Madotto, F. The association between air pollution and the incidence of idiopathic pulmonary fibrosis in Northern Italy. *Eur. Respir J.* **2018**, *51*, 1700397. [CrossRef]
4. Luppi, F.; Kalluri, M.; Faverio, P.; Kreuter, M.; Ferrara, G. Idiopathic pulmonary fibrosis beyond the lung: Understanding disease mechanisms to improve diagnosis and management. *Respir. Res.* **2021**, *22*, 109. [CrossRef] [PubMed]
5. Gandhi, S.; Tonelli, R.; Murray, M.; Samarelli, A.V.; Spagnolo, P. Environmental Causes of Idiopathic Pulmonary Fibrosis. *Int. J. Mol. Sci.* **2023**, *24*, 16481. [CrossRef]
6. Raghu, G.; Amatto, V.C.; Behr, J.; Stowasser, S. Comorbidities in idiopathic pulmonary fibrosis patients: A systematic literature review. *Eur. Respir. J.* **2015**, *46*, 1113–1130. [CrossRef]
7. Kärkkäinen, M.; Kettunen, H.P.; Nurmi, H.; Selander, T.; Purokivi, M.; Kaarteenaho, R. Effect of smoking and comorbidities on survival in idiopathic pulmonary fibrosis. *Respir. Res.* **2017**, *18*, 160. [CrossRef]
8. Caminati, A.; Lonati, C.; Cassandro, R.; Elia, D.; Pelosi, G.; Torre, O.; Zompatori, M.; Uslenghi, E.; Harari, S. Comorbidities in idiopathic pulmonary fibrosis: An underestimated issue. *Eur. Respir. Rev.* **2019**, *28*, 190044. [CrossRef] [PubMed]
9. Nathan, S.D.; Basavaraj, A.; Reichner, C.; Shlobin, O.A.; Ahmad, S.; Kiernan, J.; Burton, N.; Barnett, S.D. Prevalence and impact of coronary artery disease in idiopathic pulmonary fibrosis. *Respir. Med.* **2010**, *104*, 1035–1041. [CrossRef] [PubMed]
10. Kizer, J.R.; Zisman, D.A.; Blumenthal, N.P.; Kotloff, R.M.; Kimmel, S.E.; Strieter, R.M.; Arcasoy, S.M.; Ferrari, V.A.; Hansen-Flaschen, J. Association between pulmonary fibrosis and coronary artery disease. *Arch. Intern. Med.* **2004**, *164*, 551–556. [CrossRef]
11. Gardin, J.M.; Arnold, A.M.; Polak, J.; Jackson, S.; Smith, V.; Gottdiener, J. Usefulness of aortic root dimension in persons > or = 65 years of age in predicting heart failure, stroke, cardiovascular mortality, all-cause mortality and acute myocardial infarction (from the Cardiovascular Health Study). *Am. J. Cardiol.* **2006**, *97*, 270–275. [CrossRef]
12. Lai, C.L.; Chien, K.L.; Hsu, H.C.; Su, T.C.; Chen, M.F.; Lee, Y.T. Aortic root dimension as an independent predictor for all-cause death in adults < 65 years of age (from the Chin-Shan Community Cardiovascular Cohort Study). *Echocardiography* **2010**, *27*, 487–495. [PubMed]
13. Cuspidi, C.; Facchetti, R.; Bombelli, M.; Re, A.; Cairoa, M.; Sala, C.; Tadic, M.; Grassi, G.; Mancia, G. Aortic root diameter and risk of cardiovascular events in a general population: Data from the PAMELA study. *J. Hypertens.* **2014**, *32*, 1879–1887. [CrossRef]

14. Kamimura, D.; Suzuki, T.; Musani, S.K.; Hall, M.E.; Samdarshi, T.E.; Correa, A.; Fox, E.R. Increased Proximal Aortic Diameter is Associated with Risk of Cardiovascular Events and All-Cause Mortality in Blacks The Jackson Heart Study. *J. Am. Heart Assoc.* **2017**, *6*, e005005. [CrossRef]
15. Canciello, G.; Mancusi, C.; Losi, M.A.; Izzo, R.; Trimarco, B.; de Simone, G.; De Luca, N. Aortic Root Dilatation Is Associated with Incident Cardiovascular Events in a Population of Treated Hypertensive Patients: The Campania Salute Network. *Am. J. Hypertens.* **2018**, *31*, 1317–1323. [CrossRef] [PubMed]
16. Leone, D.; Airale, L.; Bernardi, S.; Mingrone, G.; Astarita, A.; Cesareo, M.; Sabia, L.; Avenatti, E.; Tosello, F.; Bruno, G.; et al. Prognostic role of the ascending aorta dilatation in patients with arterial hypertension. *J. Hypertens.* **2021**, *39*, 1163–1169. [CrossRef] [PubMed]
17. Sonaglioni, A.; Caminati, A.; Lipsi, R.; Nicolosi, G.L.; Lombardo, M.; Anzà, C.; Harari, S. Early left atrial dysfunction in idiopathic pulmonary fibrosis patients without chronic right heart failure. *Int. J. Cardiovasc. Imaging* **2020**, *36*, 1711–1723. [CrossRef]
18. Sonaglioni, A.; Caminati, A.; Lipsi, R.; Lombardo, M.; Harari, S. Association between C-reactive protein and carotid plaque in mild-to-moderate idiopathic pulmonary fibrosis. *Intern. Emerg. Med.* **2021**, *16*, 1529–1539. [CrossRef]
19. Sonaglioni, A.; Caminati, A.; Nicolosi, G.L.; Lombardo, M.; Harari, S. Incremental prognostic value of arterial elastance in mild-to-moderate idiopathic pulmonary fibrosis. *Int. J. Cardiovasc. Imaging* **2022**, *38*, 1473–1485. [CrossRef]
20. Sonaglioni, A.; Caminati, A.; Re, M.; Elia, D.; Trevisan, R.; Granato, A.; Zompatori, M.; Lombardo, M.; Harari, S. Prognostic role of CHA2DS2-VASc score for mortality risk assessment in non-advanced idiopathic pulmonary fibrosis: A preliminary observation. *Intern. Emerg. Med.* **2023**, *18*, 755–767. [CrossRef] [PubMed]
21. Piepoli, M.F.; Hoes, A.W.; Agewall, S.; Albus, C.; Brotons, C.; Catapano, A.L.; Cooney, M.T.; Corrà, U.; Cosyns, B.; Deaton, C.; et al. 2016 European Guidelines on cardiovascular disease prevention in clinical practice: The Sixth Joint Task Force of the European Society of Cardiology and Other Societies on Cardiovascular Disease Prevention in Clinical Practice (constituted by representatives of 10 societies and by invited experts)Developed with the special contribution of the European Association for Cardiovascular Prevention & Rehabilitation (EACPR). *Eur. Heart J.* **2016**, *37*, 2315–2381.
22. Humbert, M.; Kovacs, G.; Hoeper, M.M.; Badagliacca, R.; Berger, R.M.F.; Brida, M.; Carlsen, J.; Coats, A.J.S.; Escribano-Subias, P.; Ferrari, P.; et al. 2022 ESC/ERS Guidelines for the diagnosis and treatment of pulmonary hypertension. *Eur. Heart J.* **2022**, *43*, 3618–3731. [CrossRef] [PubMed]
23. Levey, A.S.; Bosch, J.P.; Lewis, J.B.; Greene, T.; Rogers, N.; Roth, D. A more accurate method to estimate glomerular filtration rate from serum creatinine: A new prediction equation. Modification of Diet in Renal Disease Study Group. *Ann. Intern Med.* **1999**, *130*, 461–470. [CrossRef]
24. Agatston, A.S.; Janowitz, W.R.; Hildner, F.J.; Zusmer, N.R.; Viamonte, M., Jr.; Detrano, R. Quantification of coronary artery calcium using ultrafast computed tomography. *J. Am. Coll. Cardiol.* **1990**, *15*, 827–832. [CrossRef] [PubMed]
25. Ohnesorge, B.; Flohr, T.; Fischbach, R.; Kopp, A.F.; Knez, A.; Schröder, S.; Schöpf, U.J.; Crispin, A.; Klotz, E.; Reiser, M.F.; et al. Reproducibility of coronary calcium quantification in repeat examinations with retrospectively ECG-gated multisection spiral CT. *Eur. Radiol.* **2002**, *12*, 1532–1540. [CrossRef] [PubMed]
26. Lang, R.M.; Badano, L.P.; Mor-Avi, V.; Afilalo, J.; Armstrong, A.; Ernande, L.; Flachskampf, F.A.; Foster, E.; Goldstein, S.A.; Kuznetsova, T.; et al. Recommendations for cardiac chamber quantification by echocardiography in adults: An update from the American Society of Echocardiography and the European Association of Cardiovascular Imaging. *J. Am. Soc. Echocardiogr.* **2015**, *28*, 1–39.e14. [CrossRef] [PubMed]
27. Nagueh, S.F.; Smiseth, O.A.; Appleton, C.P.; Byrd, B.F., 3rd; Dokainish, H.; Edvardsen, T.; Flachskampf, F.A.; Gillebert, T.C.; Klein, A.L.; Lancellotti, P.; et al. Recommendations for the Evaluation of Left Ventricular Diastolic Function by Echocardiography: An Update from the American Society of Echocardiography and the European Association of Cardiovascular Imaging. *J. Am. Soc. Echocardiogr.* **2016**, *29*, 277–314. [CrossRef] [PubMed]
28. Tello, K.; Wan, J.; Dalmer, A.; Vanderpool, R.; Ghofrani, H.A.; Naeije, R.; Roller, F.; Mohajerani, E.; Seeger, W.; Herberg, U.; et al. Validation of the Tricuspid Annular Plane Systolic Excursion/Systolic Pulmonary Artery Pressure Ratio for the Assessment of Right Ventricular-Arterial Coupling in Severe Pulmonary Hypertension. *Circ. Cardiovasc. Imaging* **2019**, *12*, e009047. [CrossRef]
29. Nishimura, R.A.; Otto, C.M.; Bonow, R.O.; Carabello, B.A.; Erwin, J.P., 3rd; Fleisher, L.A.; Jneid, H.; Mack, M.J.; McLeod, C.J.; O'Gara, P.T.; et al. 2017 AHA/ACC Focused Update of the 2014 AHA/ACC Guideline for the Management of Patients with Valvular Heart Disease: A Report of the American College of Cardiology/American Heart Association Task Force on Clinical Practice Guidelines. *Circulation* **2017**, *135*, e1159–e1195. [CrossRef]
30. Evangelista, A.; Sitges, M.; Jondeau, G.; Nijveldt, R.; Pepi, M.; Cuellar, H.; Pontone, G.; Bossone, E.; Groenink, M.; Dweck, M.R.; et al. Multimodality imaging in thoracic aortic diseases: A clinical consensus statement from the European Association of Cardiovascular Imaging and the European Society of Cardiology working group on aorta and peripheral vascular diseases. *Eur. Heart J. Cardiovasc. Imaging* **2023**, *24*, e65–e85. [CrossRef]
31. Bland, J.M.; Altman, D.G. Statistical methods for assessing agreement between two methods of clinical measurement. *Lancet* **1986**, *1*, 307–310. [CrossRef] [PubMed]

32. Enright, P.L.; Sherrill, D.L. Reference equations for the six-minute walk in healthy adults. *Am. J. Respir. Crit. Care Med.* **1998**, *158*, 1384–1387. [CrossRef]
33. Zafar, M.A.; Li, Y.; Rizzo, J.A.; Charilaou, P.; Saeyeldin, A.; Velasquez, C.A.; Mansour, A.M.; Bin Mahmood, S.U.; Ma, W.G.; Brownstein, A.J.; et al. Height alone, rather than body surface area, suffices for risk estimation in ascending aortic aneurysm. *J. Thorac. Cardiovasc. Surg.* **2018**, *155*, 1938–1950. [CrossRef] [PubMed]
34. Sonaglioni, A.; Caminati, A.; Grasso, E.; Colleoni, M.; Nicolosi, G.L.; Lombardo, M.; Harari, S. TAPSE/SPAP ratio stratifies mortality risk in mild-to-moderate idiopathic pulmonary fibrosis. *Int. J. Tuberc. Lung Dis.* **2024**, *28*, 183–188. [CrossRef] [PubMed]
35. Dalleywater, W.; Powell, H.A.; Hubbard, R.B.; Navaratnam, V. Risk factors for cardiovascular disease in people with idiopathic pulmonary fibrosis: A population-based study. *Chest* **2015**, *147*, 150–156. [CrossRef]
36. Okamoto, M.; Shipley, M.J.; Wilkinson, I.B.; McEniery, C.M.; Valencia-Hernández, C.A.; Singh-Manoux, A.; Kivimaki, M.; Brunner, E.J. Does Poorer Pulmonary Function Accelerate Arterial Stiffening?: A Cohort Study with Repeated Measurements of Carotid-Femoral Pulse Wave Velocity. *Hypertension* **2019**, *74*, 929–935. [CrossRef] [PubMed]
37. Vriz, O.; Driussi, C.; Bettio, M.; Ferrara, F.; D'Andrea, A.; Bossone, E. Aortic root dimensions and stiffness in healthy subjects. *Am. J. Cardiol.* **2013**, *112*, 1224–1229. [CrossRef]
38. Milan, A.; Tosello, F.; Caserta, M.; Naso, D.; Puglisi, E.; Magnino, C.; Comoglio, C.; Rabbia, F.; Mulatero, P.; Veglio, F. Aortic size index enlargement is associated with central hemodynamics in essential hypertension. *Hypertens. Res.* **2011**, *34*, 126–132. [CrossRef]
39. Li, L.; Xie, W.; Li, Q.; Hong, H. The positive correlation between brachial-ankle pulse wave velocity and aortic diameter in Chinese patients with diabetes. *J. Clin. Hypertens.* **2022**, *24*, 1059–1067. [CrossRef] [PubMed]
40. Zhang, K.; Li, A.; Zhou, J.; Zhang, C.; Chen, M. Genetic association of circulating C-reactive protein levels with idiopathic pulmonary fibrosis: A two-sample Mendelian randomization study. *Respir. Res.* **2023**, *24*, 7. [CrossRef] [PubMed]
41. Heukels, P.; Moor, C.C.; von der Thüsen, J.H.; Wijsenbeek, M.S.; Kool, M. Inflammation and immunity in IPF pathogenesis and treatment. *Respir. Med.* **2019**, *147*, 79–91. [CrossRef]
42. Syed, M.B.J.; Fletcher, A.J.; Dweck, M.R.; Forsythe, R.; Newby, D.E. Imaging aortic wall inflammation. *Trends Cardiovasc. Med.* **2019**, *29*, 440–448. [CrossRef] [PubMed]
43. Totaro, S.; Rabbia, F.; Milan, A.; Urbina, E.M.; Veglio, F. Aortic root dilatation in the children and young adults: Prevalence, determinants, and association with target organ damage. *J. Am. Soc. Hypertens.* **2016**, *10*, 782–789. [CrossRef]
44. Milan, A.; Tosello, F.; Naso, D.; Avenatti, E.; Leone, D.; Magnino, C.; Veglio, F. Ascending aortic dilatation, arterial stiffness and cardiac organ damage in essential hypertension. *J. Hypertens.* **2013**, *31*, 109–116. [CrossRef] [PubMed]
45. Ballegaard, C.R.; Pham, M.H.C.; Sigvardsen, P.E.; Kühl, J.T.; Sørgaard, M.; Taudorf, M.; Fuchs, A.; Nordestgaard, B.G.; Køber, L.V.; Kofoed, K.F. Aortic enlargement and coronary artery calcification in a general population cohort. *Eur. Heart J. Cardiovasc. Imaging* **2022**, *23*, 855–862. [CrossRef] [PubMed]
46. Kurata, A.; Kawakami, T.; Sato, J.; Sakamoto, A.; Muramatsu, T.; Nakabayashi, K. Aortic aneurysms in systemic lupus erythematosus: A meta-analysis of 35 cases in the literature and two different pathogeneses. *Cardiovasc. Pathol.* **2011**, *20*, e1–e7. [CrossRef]
47. Sato, O.; Takagi, A.; Miyata, T.; Takayama, Y. Aortic aneurysms in patients with autoimmune disorders treated with corticosteroids. *Eur. J. Vasc. Endovasc. Surg.* **1995**, *10*, 366–369. [CrossRef]
48. Chen, S.W.; Kuo, C.F.; Huang, Y.T.; Lin, W.T.; Chien-Chia Wu, V.; Chou, A.H.; Lin, P.J.; Chang, S.H.; Chu, P.H. Association of Family History with Incidence and Outcomes of Aortic Dissection. *J. Am. Coll. Cardiol.* **2020**, *76*, 1181–1192. [CrossRef] [PubMed]
49. Chen, S.W.; Chan, Y.H.; Lin, C.P.; Wu, V.C.; Cheng, Y.T.; Chen, D.Y.; Chang, S.H.; Hung, K.C.; Chu, P.H.; Chou, A.H. Association of Long-term Use of Antihypertensive Medications with Late Outcomes Among Patients with Aortic Dissection. *JAMA Netw. Open* **2021**, *4*, e210469. [CrossRef] [PubMed]
50. Pramana, K.A.A.P.; Pintaningrum, Y.; Rahmat, B. The effects of statin therapy on aneurysm size, growth rate, and matrix metalloproteinases-9 levels in patients with aortic aneurysm: A systematic review and meta-analysis. *Egypt. Heart J.* **2023**, *75*, 88. [CrossRef]
51. van Cleemput, J.; Sonaglioni, A.; Wuyts, W.A.; Bengus, M.; Stauffer, J.L.; Harari, S. Idiopathic Pulmonary Fibrosis for Cardiologists: Differential Diagnosis, Cardiovascular Comorbidities, and Patient Management. *Adv. Ther.* **2019**, *36*, 298–317. [CrossRef] [PubMed]
52. Salvetti, M.; Paini, A.; Bertacchini, F.; Stassaldi, D.; Aggiusti, C.; Agabiti Rosei, C.; Bassetti, D.; Agabiti-Rosei, E.; Muiesan, M.L. Changes in left ventricular geometry during antihypertensive treatment. *Pharmacol. Res.* **2018**, *134*, 193–199. [CrossRef]

Journal of
Clinical Medicine

MDPI

Review

Non-Pharmacological Management of Idiopathic Pulmonary Fibrosis

Jon B. Mullholand *, Catherine E. Grossman and Apostolos Perelas *

Division of Pulmonary Disease and Critical Care Medicine, Virginia Commonwealth University, Richmond, VA 23298, USA; catherine.grossman@vcuhealth.org
* Correspondence: jon.mullholand@vcuhealth.org (J.B.M.); apostolos.perelas@vcuhealth.org (A.P.)

Abstract: Idiopathic pulmonary fibrosis (IPF) is a relatively common progressive fibrotic interstitial lung disease associated with significant morbidity and mortality. The available medications for IPF only slow down the disease process, with lung transplantation the only option for a cure. Non-pharmacological therapies are significant adjuncts that can improve symptom burden and quality of life with minimal or no side effects. Supplemental oxygen can improve exercise capacity and the sensation of dyspnea in a significant portion of patients with resting or exertional hypoxemia and has been supported by several professional societies. Pulmonary rehabilitation is a comprehensive program that includes education and therapeutic exercises to improve patient stamina and strength. It is one of the few interventions that have been shown to produce a meaningful increase in a patient's exercise capacity, but its wide adoption is limited by availability, especially in rural areas. Sleep optimization with supplemental oxygen and positive airway pressure therapy should actively be investigated for all patients diagnosed with IPF. Although gastroesophageal reflux control with non-pharmacological means is still controversial as an intervention to reduce the rate of lung function decline, it can help control reflux symptoms and improve cough intensity. IPF patients should be educated on the importance of balanced nutrition and the potential benefits of screening for lung transplantation. Palliative medicine can help with symptom control and should be considered for all patients regardless severity, but especially in those in the later stages of disease.

Keywords: idiopathic pulmonary fibrosis (IPF); interstitial lung disease (ILD); supplemental oxygen; lung transplant; pulmonary rehabilitation; sleep; diet; palliative care; GERD; lung cancer

1. Introduction

Idiopathic pulmonary fibrosis (IPF) is a relatively common progressive fibrotic interstitial lung disease (ILD) associated with significant morbidity and mortality [1]. Despite the progress made in understanding its pathogenesis, the therapies available to date have only been shown to reduce the rate of disease progression without a major effect on symptom burden or quality of life [2,3]. Moreover, they are associated with a significant side effect risk and poor tolerance [4]. Consequently, lung transplantation remains the only definitive therapy for IPF, but it is plagued by high costs, limited donor availability, and suboptimal long-term outcomes [5]. This review will focus on non-pharmacological therapies for IPF; many of these interventions are directed towards symptoms and have been shown to improve quality of life with minimal or no side effects.

2. Supplemental Oxygen

IPF results in hypoxia through a variety of mechanisms; diffusion impairment, ventilation/perfusion mismatch, and pulmonary vasculopathy have all been demonstrated to be present and contribute to the phenomenon in varying degrees [6]. Hypoxia can initially be seen only during sleep or heavy exertion, but it eventually occurs at rest, and it has been associated with reduced exercise capacity, poor quality of life, and reduced survival [7,8]. It is thus not surprising that oxygen therapy is one of the key criteria for consideration for lung transplantation according to the latest guidelines [9]. Most patients with IPF will require supplemental oxygen at some time during their disease, and for most of them, it represents a major milestone in their life.

Despite its frequent use, there are surprisingly few quality data to guide strategies around oxygen supplementation in IPF, with most clinicians and even society guidelines relying on COPD data [10]. However, time after time, it has been shown that patients with IPF are different than those with COPD; in general, they tend to have a higher prevalence of hypoxemia, an increased degree of desaturation, and increased needs for supplemental oxygen to avoid exertional hypoxemia. The 2020 ATS guidelines, although succinct, were a very good initial step in bringing more attention to the practice of supplemental oxygen prescription for this population while raising awareness of the need for liquid oxygen [10].

Long-term oxygen therapy describes supplemental oxygen for at least 15 h a day. It has been advocated for patients with severe resting hypoxemia based on the most recent ATS guidelines [10] despite the lack of evidence supporting a mortality or quality of life benefit [11]. It has been recommended for patients with PaO2 of $\subseteq$ 55 mmHg or SpO2 of 88% or below at rest or in those with PaO2 55–59 mmHg or SpO2 89% with evidence of right ventricular dysfunction [10]. Ambulatory oxygen has been recommended in patients with severe hypoxemia while ambulating on room air [10]. The current evidence does not suggest a benefit in mortality, but supplemental oxygen has been shown to improve quality of life metrics, dyspnea, and exercise capacity among patients with IPF [12,13], although not in all patients [14].

High-flow oxygen has been examined in patients exercising, with promising results to date. Two trials have examined high-flow oxygen and compared it to the standard of care; Badenes-Bonet et al. demonstrated an increase in exercise tolerance during a CPET [15], whereas Harada et al. demonstrated increased ability to perform submaximal exercise with less desaturations and fatigue [16]. A meta-analysis showed that during exercise, high-flow oxygen systems had better outcomes than low-flow systems, and, among high-flow systems, nasal cannula outperformed venturi devices [17].

Traditionally, supplemental oxygen needs have been calculated with titration during a 6 min walk test. However, there are emerging data suggesting that this may underestimate the patient's real needs [18]. There are currently many commercially available wearable portable oximeters; however, so far, they have not been used to assist with accurate supplemental oxygen prescription. Continuous oxygen flow is preferred over pulse flow, especially for those with higher oxygen needs, and most patients will get the most benefit by using oxygen tanks despite their greater weight and reduced portability [10]. Liquid oxygen has been proposed for patients requiring >3 lt via NC through continuous flow; however, availability remains very limited, which is mostly driven by costs and poor reimbursement by insurance companies [10].

3. Pulmonary Rehabilitation

Pulmonary rehabilitation (PR) is "a comprehensive intervention based on a thorough patient assessment followed by patient-tailored therapies that include, but are not limited to, exercise training, education, and behavior change, designed to improve the physical and psychological condition of people with CRD and to promote the long-term adherence to health-enhancing behaviors" [19]. PR has been a staple of treatment for patients with advanced lung disease, including, in particular, individuals with COPD [20].

A recent meta-analysis of nine studies revealed a moderate increase in exercise capacity [estimated based on the 6 min walk distance (6 MWD)] and an improvement in dyspnea scores [21]. The improvement in the 6 MWD (37.25 m) reached the minimal clinically significant improvement for patients with fibrotic lung disease [22]. Additionally, there was a noted benefit in HRQoL (Health-Related Quality of Life), which was determined using the IPF-specific SGRQ-I (St. George Respiratory Questionnaire—Idiopathic Pulmonary Fibrosis) [21]. Unfortunately, neither of these benefits were sustained in the IPF-specific sub-group at the 6–12-month follow-up in contrast to the general ILD group. This led to an update in the ATS/ERS guidelines for a strong recommendation for the use of PR in ILD; however, no specific recommendations were made for IPF [20]. Moreover, a recommendation was made for repeating PR in regular intervals to sustain the benefits [23]. In practice, and given the limitations in the availability of PR, this is achieved with the help of maintenance programs, which the patients can join after completing PR.

Even though there are data for general use of PR in IPF, there are still many questions left as to the best model to provide PR. First is the role of supplemental oxygen during PR. Whereas most programs titrate supplemental oxygen based on a 6 min walk test to maintain SpO2 of 89% or above, there is evidence that high-flow oxygen may result in increased duration of exercise tolerance, along with less fatigue and less desaturations [16]. In a recent review of high-flow oxygen in the setting of PR, it was noted that these benefits are inconsistent across the board of ILD, most likely due to high heterogeneity when investigating the benefits [24]. There is an active multi-center trial in Canada studying the role of high-flow oxygen for pulmonary rehabilitation in individuals with clinically stable IPF (NCT02551068) [25]. Additionally, conflicting evidence exists on the types of training (high-intensity vs. traditional program). There is a large multi-center study in Australia currently in recruitment to assess high-intensity aerobic training compared to traditional PR (NCT03800914 http://clinicaltrials.gov/show/NCT03800914, accessed on 12 January 2024) [26].

The main barrier to the wide adoption of PR in patients with IPF is undeniably its limited availability; in the United States, easy access to PR is not guaranteed. There are generally not enough programs in rural areas with low population density, and in busy metropolitan areas there are also shortages of spots in PR programs [27]. The COVID-19 pandemic exacerbated these problems by increasing the number of patients needing PR while reducing class sizes to allow for social distancing and forcing shut downs of programs because of insufficient funding. Telehealth-based options were developed to address these deficiencies; the feasibility of this way of providing rehab services has been proven in multiple studies with COPD and post-inflammatory ILD. There have yet to be any data specifically for individuals with IPF [28,29].

4. Telehealth and Remote Monitoring

Remote monitoring has attracted interest for a variety of chronic conditions, including IPF. Telehealth programs have been shown to be feasible and attractive to both patients and providers; however, there are no high-quality data indicating whether they can replace routine in-office monitoring, increase medication adherence, or help detect acute exacerbations early [30–32]. Moreover, there are concerns around cost, availability, and usability among a population of mostly elderly patients who have traditionally had difficulties adjusting to newer technologies. Further studies are required to further define the type, setting, and population subgroup for which these technologies can provide the most benefit.

5. Sleep-Related Hypoxia

Sleep-related breathing disorders are found frequently in patients with IPF; obstructive sleep apnea (OSA) is reported at rates of up to 88% of IPF patients, central sleep apnea (CSA) prevalence rates are reported at 19–22%, and nocturnal hypoxemia (NH), also called sleep-sustained hypoxia (total sleep time with SpO2 under 88% > 5 min and AHI < 15/h), which is not related to obstructive central apnea, is reported in up to 12% of IPF patients [33,34]. The recognition and treatment of these disorders are important, as prolonged nocturnal hypoxia (regardless of etiology, i.e., obstructive vs. nonobstructive pathology) predicts higher mortality [35–37]. Treatment with positive pressure therapy and oxygen when indicated may improve mortality [35,37,38]. Many authors advocate for routine polysomnogram screening in all IPF patients given this evidence; furthermore, adherence to therapy with sleep-disordered breathing and nocturnal hypoxia is acceptable in patients with IPF (with varying rates of non-adherence reported in different articles) [34,39,40]. Serial polysomnography is advised over time, as several studies reveal that upon follow-up polysomnography, therapies may need to be added to prior nocturnal prescriptions (i.e., addition of oxygen to PAP or addition of PAP to oxygen therapy). However, the limited availability of sleep specialists makes the implementation of this recommendation challenging.

6. Gastroesophageal Reflux Control

Prior studies have demonstrated that up to 87–94% of patients with idiopathic pulmonary fibrosis (IPF) exhibit abnormal esophageal acid exposure, measured through ambulatory esophageal pH monitoring [41,42]. In 2015, guidelines recommended that all patients with IPF should receive pharmacologic GERD treatment, as at that time there was evidence supporting the improvement of respiratory outcomes [43]. However, more recent guidelines have rescinded this recommendation, as evidence for GERD treatment's effect on pulmonary function testing has not been robust and there have been some concerns about an increase in the risk of respiratory infections [44–46]. The association between GERD and IPF, including the role of GERD as a possible causative agent in IPF progression, is a complex and controversial topic. There appears to be an association between the two entities, but a causal relationship between the two has yet to be overtly established [47–49].

The initial recommendation for treatment of all patients with IPF with anti-reflux medications has been replaced with a more targeted approach towards patients with IPF and confirmed GERD, as further analyses failed to verify a benefit from global anti-reflux therapies [44,50]. An arsenal of approaches can be attempted, usually in combination, including medications, lifestyle and dietary modifications, and, in select cases, surgical intervention. Lifestyle and dietary modifications can be valuable adjuncts in managing GERD symptoms. Dietary recommendations emphasize educating patients on avoiding foods and beverages known to provoke reflux and encouraging cessation of eating at least 2–3 h before bedtime [51]. Sleep positioning is also essential; elevating the head of the bed and sleeping in a left lateral decubitus position can help prevent reflux by leveraging gravity to keep stomach contents from traveling up the esophagus. Additionally, smoking cessation and weight loss are recommended to further reduce reflux [52].

Surgical treatment, such as laparoscopic anti-reflux surgery, has not yet demonstrated a definitive impact on mortality or lung function in IPF patients with GERD [44]. Current American Thoracic Society (ATS) guidelines do not recommend anti-reflux surgery for the improvement of pulmonary outcomes in IPF, which were also summarized by the panel's meta-analysis [44,50]. However, surgery may be considered in cases of refractory GERD symptoms despite optimal medical management, as the WRAP-IPF trial found this approach to be safe and well-tolerated in this patient population [53].

7. Nutrition

Mounting evidence supports the interplay of nutrition with regard to age-related chronic diseases; observations of the interplay of aging and the development of pulmonary fibrosis have also spurned research into the role of diet and nutrition in the disease course of pulmonary fibrosis. Furthermore, patients with IPF commonly have comorbidities that often have nutritional counseling as part of their treatment strategies, such as cardiovascular disease, obesity, diabetes mellitus, and dyslipidemia [46,54,55]. In reference to IPF, the composition of the diet may be important in relation to disease development and progression. Two thought-provoking case-control studies in the Japanese population of IPF patients described diets higher in consumption of meat and saturated fats and lower in consumption of fruits and vegetables [56,57].

The effect of diet composition on lung inflammation has been further evaluated in mouse models; mice exposed to high-fat diets had higher amounts of age-related lung inflammation, mitochondrial deterioration, and decreased lung stem cell populations when compared to mice on calorie-restrictive or low-fat diets [58,59]. Furthermore, measured inflammation in the mice was able to be reduced once the animals' diets were switched to a low-fat diet [59]. There is not yet enough information on the use of antioxidant supplements in IPF; however, one study noted that combination therapy of vitamins D, C, and E showed improvement in FEV1 and TLC and reduction in systemic inflammation [60].

With respect to measurements of obesity, it has been shown that patients with a lower BMI (body mass index) have increased 3–5-year mortality [61–63]. However, data have shown that higher BMI is an independent risk factor for the development of IPF, although it may contribute to decreased mortality, the "obesity paradox" [62]. This paradox has been seen in other respiratory and non-respiratory diseases, such as COPD and heart failure. One of the current theories postulates that the protective factor associated with higher BMI is due to increased lean muscle density, which is not accurately assessed when using the BMI scale and thus is not an adequate prognostic measurement. Interestingly, when comparing the impact of cardio respiratory fitness (CRF) and obesity on mortality in heart failure and COPD, patients with good CRF had decreased mortality regardless of BMI status [64]. Future studies are needed to evaluate the role of body composition and outcomes in IPF as well as diet/nutrition as they relate to progression of disease. As of now, the interplay of nutrition and diet in patients with IPF is a recognized gap in the IPF research knowledge base.

8. Lung Cancer Screening

It is well-established that patients with idiopathic pulmonary fibrosis have a very significant risk of developing lung cancer, which is higher than that seen among patients with chronic obstructive pulmonary disease [65]. Moreover, patients with fibrotic ILD have a higher risk of complications, including radiation pneumonitis and chemotherapy-induced pneumonitis, and they are at a significant risk of developing IPF exacerbation after surgical resection [66,67].

Lung cancer screening has been proposed in patients with IPF to promote early detection and treatment [68]. Indeed, among suitable patients with IPF and early-stage lung cancer, surgical resection has been associated with acceptable long-term outcomes [69]. However, the value of early detection may be lower among patients who have more advanced disease and would not be a surgical candidate. In our practice, we perform yearly chest computed tomography among our patients with IPF, and we follow the Fleischner criteria to determine the need for follow-up vs. positron emission tomography or tissue sampling [70].

9. Symptom Control and Palliative Care

Palliative experts have described the progression of fibrotic lung diseases as comparable to the progression of malignancy due to the severity of the disease and the effect on QoL. Several studies have demonstrated that the inclusion of palliative care reduces symptom burden and improves quality of life [71]. Patients with IPF suffer not only from direct respiratory symptoms, profound breathlessness, and cough but also non-respiratory symptoms that can include fatigue, anorexia, anxiety, and depression [55]. The non-respiratory symptoms can significantly impact morbidity, with a reported difference in survival of 66 months (without non-respiratory comorbidities) compared to 35 months (with non-respiratory comorbidities) [46]. Unfortunately, non-respiratory symptoms are more difficult to control than direct respiratory symptoms.

To improve QoL, multiple studies, as well as a 2017 meta-analysis from Brighton et al., have shown that "breathlessness support services" and/or a multidisciplinary palliative team, including palliative physicians, respiratory therapists, and nurses, when working with severe fibrotic lung disease result in improvement of breathlessness as well as decreased overall distress related to the disease itself and associated symptoms [72–74]. Unfortunately, the impact of palliative multidisciplinary groups has not been as effective for all QoL metrics, including, most notably, anxiety and depression. Although the aforementioned studies saw some improvement in these outcomes, there have been several additional studies that have shown that involving palliative services did not change the individual's depression or anxiety and at times showed a trend towards worsening these comorbidities [75,76]. Given the variable progression of IPF, optimal timing when introducing palliative services is difficult to determine.

There is some concern that patients recognize the addition of palliative services as discontinuation of life-sustaining care or anti-fibrotic therapies, which is strongly discouraged by palliative groups [71]. This phenomenon has been seen in other chronic terminal diseases, with one study of individuals with malignancy showing that patients were more receptive to services offered through palliative care when the name was switched to supportive care [77]. Other patient barriers to palliative services are misconceptions about potential limitations of offered therapies (including limitations of transplant availability), cultural/religious practices, and misunderstanding of the goals of palliative care [71]. In addition to patient-related barriers, there are multiple health care system barriers that exist. Major deficiencies exist in the availability of palliative resources, which can be due to patients' geographic locations, adequate palliative care staffing, and, finally, limited expertise in providing palliative services to patients with non-oncologic-related terminal diseases [55,71,78]. While the benefits in terms of different measures are variable, benefits have been shown, and there is a lack of harm. ATS guidelines currently recommend palliative care consultation as an adjunct to other IPF treatments [44].

10. Conclusions

Non-pharmacological therapies are a significant part of the management of IPF. They work together with pharmacotherapy to help maintain patients' quality of life by improving symptom burden, exercise capacity, and the sensation of well-being (Table 1). Further research is needed to determine the nature and timing of the interventions that can provide the best benefit to the most suitable population.

Table 1. Summary of non-pharmacological interventions for the treatment of Idiopathic Pulmonary Fibrosis.

Non-Pharmacological Management of IPF					
Therapy	**Quality of Data**	**Benefits**	**Quality of Life**	**Guideline Recommendation Strength**	**Future Research**
Supplemental Oxygen	Low	Increased exercise capacity and improved levels of dyspnea	Improved	Strong	Investigations into needs for supplemental oxygen
Pulmonary Rehabilitation	Low	Increased exercise capacity and improved levels of dyspnea	Improved	Weak	Form of Pulmonary Rehabilitation Use of High-Flow oxygen devices during Pulmonary Rehabilitation Role of alternative models of Pulmonary Rehabilitation (Home or telehealth programs)
Telehealth/Remote Monitoring	Emerging	Potential role of improving medication compliance and early detection of exacerbation; Increased perceived support from patients	-	-	Identification of characteristics of patient's who would benefit from this intervention
Treatment of Sleep Related Hypoxia	High	Decreased nocturnal hypoxemia	-	-	Role of repeated polysomnography
GERD Management	Low	No improvement in pulmonary function If GERD is diagnosed improved GERD symptoms	No improvement in patients without symptoms of GERD	Conditional	Trials powered to evaluate pulmonary functionTrials investigating treatment in IPF population with and without GERD symptoms
Nutrition	Emerging	Negative correlation of BMI and mortality	-	-	Role of nutrition and registered dietician on disease progression
Lung Cancer Screening	High	Early detection of Lung cancer	-	Strong	-
Palliative Care	Low	Improvement in treatment related side effects and comorbid conditions Improved dyspnea Conflicting evidence of benefits of anxiety and depression	Improved	Recommended	Establishment of accepted triggers to initiate Palliative Care Consultation

GERD: Gastric Esophageal Reflux Disease.

Funding: This research received no external funding.

Conflicts of Interest: The authors declare no conflict of interest.

References

1. Richeldi, L.; Collard, H.R.; Jones, M.G. Idiopathic pulmonary fibrosis. *Lancet* **2017**, *389*, 1941–1952. [CrossRef] [PubMed]
2. King, T.E., Jr.; Bradford, W.Z.; Castro-Bernardini, S.; Fagan, E.A.; Glaspole, I.; Glassberg, M.K.; Gorina, E.; Hopkins, P.M.; Kardatzke, D.; Lancaster, L.; et al. A phase 3 trial of pirfenidone in patients with idiopathic pulmonary fibrosis. *N. Engl. J. Med.* **2014**, *370*, 2083–2092. [CrossRef]
3. Richeldi, L.; Du Bois, R.M.; Raghu, G.; Azuma, A.; Brown, K.K.; Costabel, U.; Cottin, V.; Flaherty, K.R.; Hansell, D.M.; Inoue, Y.; et al. Efficacy and safety of nintedanib in idiopathic pulmonary fibrosis. *N. Engl. J. Med.* **2014**, *370*, 2071–2082. [CrossRef] [PubMed]
4. Zhao, R.; Xie, B.; Wang, X.; Zhang, X.; Ren, Y.; Wang, C.; Dai, H. The tolerability and efficacy of antifibrotic therapy in patients with idiopathic pulmonary fibrosis: Results from a real-world study. *Pulm. Pharmacol. Ther.* **2024**, *84*, 102287. [CrossRef] [PubMed]
5. Brown, A.W.; Kaya, H.; Nathan, S.D. Lung transplantation in IIP: A review. *Respirology* **2016**, *21*, 1173–1184. [CrossRef] [PubMed]
6. Agusti, A.G.N.; Roca, J.; Gea, J.; Wagner, P.D.; Xaubet, A.; Rodriguez-Roisin, R. Mechanisms of gas-exchange impairment in idiopathic pulmonary fibrosis. *Am. Rev. Respir. Dis.* **1991**, *143*, 219–225. [CrossRef] [PubMed]
7. Kataoka, K.; Oda, K.; Takizawa, H.; Ogura, T.; Miyamoto, A.; Inoue, Y.; Akagawa, S.; Hashimoto, S.; Kishaba, T.; Sakamoto, K.; et al. Cohort study to evaluate prognostic factors in idiopathic pulmonary fibrosis patients introduced to oxygen therapy. *Sci Rep.* **2023**, *13*, 13664. [CrossRef] [PubMed]
8. Hook, J.L.; Arcasoy, S.M.; Zemmel, D.; Bartels, M.N.; Kawut, S.M.; Lederer, D.J. Titrated oxygen requirement and prognostication in idiopathic pulmonary fibrosis. *Eur. Respir. J.* **2012**, *39*, 359–365. [CrossRef]
9. Leard, L.E.; Holm, A.M.; Valapour, M.; Glanville, A.R.; Attawar, S.; Aversa, M.; Campos, S.V.; Christon, L.M.; Cypel, M.; Dellgren, G.; et al. Consensus document for the selection of lung transplant candidates: An update from the International Society for Heart and Lung Transplantation. *J. Heart Lung Transplant.* **2021**, *40*, 1349–1379. [CrossRef] [PubMed]
10. Jacobs, S.S.; Krishnan, J.A.; Lederer, D.J.; Ghazipura, M.; Hossain, T.; Tan, A.-Y.M.; Carlin, B.; Drummond, M.B.; Ekström, M.; Garvey, C.; et al. Home Oxygen Therapy for Adults with Chronic Lung Disease. An Official American Thoracic Society Clinical Practice Guideline. *Am. J. Respir. Crit. Care Med.* **2020**, *202*, E121–E141. [CrossRef]
11. Crockett, A.; Cranston, J.M.; Antic, N. Domiciliary oxygen for interstitial lung disease. *Cochrane Database Syst. Rev.* **2001**, *2001*, CD002883. [CrossRef]
12. Visca, D.; Mori, L.; Tsipouri, V.; Fleming, S.; Firouzi, A.; Bonini, M.; Pavitt, M.J.; Alfieri, V.; Canu, S.; Bonifazi, M.; et al. Effect of ambulatory oxygen on quality of life for patients with fibrotic lung disease (AmbOx): A prospective, open-label, mixed-method, crossover randomised controlled trial. *Lancet Respir. Med.* **2018**, *6*, 759–770. [CrossRef] [PubMed]
13. Arizono, S.; Furukawa, T.; Taniguchi, H.; Sakamoto, K.; Kimura, T.; Kataoka, K.; Ogawa, T.; Watanabe, F.; Kondoh, Y. Supplemental oxygen improves exercise capacity in IPF patients with exertional desaturation. *Respirology* **2020**, *25*, 1152–1159. [CrossRef] [PubMed]
14. Nishiyama, O.; Miyajima, H.; Fukai, Y.; Yamazaki, R.; Satoh, R.; Yamagata, T.; Sano, H.; Iwanaga, T.; Higashimoto, Y.; Nakajima, H.; et al. Effect of ambulatory oxygen on exertional dyspnea in IPF patients without resting hypoxemia. *Respir. Med.* **2013**, *107*, 1241–1246. [CrossRef]
15. Badenes-Bonet, D.; Cejudo, P.; Rodó-Pin, A.; Martín-Ontiyuelo, C.; Chalela, R.; Rodríguez-Portal, J.A.; Vázquez-Sánchez, R.; Gea, J.; Duran, X.; Caguana, O.A.; et al. Impact of high-flow oxygen therapy during exercise in idiopathic pulmonary fibrosis: A pilot crossover clinical trial. *BMC Pulm. Med.* **2021**, *21*, 355. [CrossRef] [PubMed]
16. Harada, J.; Nagata, K.; Morimoto, T.; Iwata, K.; Matsunashi, A.; Sato, Y.; Tachikawa, R.; Ishikawa, A.; Tomii, K. Effect of high-flow nasal cannula oxygen therapy on exercise tolerance in patients with idiopathic pulmonary fibrosis: A randomized crossover trial. *Respirology* **2022**, *27*, 144–151. [CrossRef] [PubMed]
17. Lin, L.Y.; Wu, Y.C.; Wu, J.S.; Tai, H.Y.; Huang, T.W.; Cheng, W.H. Oxygen therapy for exercise capacity in fibrotic interstitial lung disease: A systematic review and meta-analysis of randomised controlled trials. *Respir Med.* **2024**, *227*, 107657. [CrossRef] [PubMed]
18. Santos, C.D.; Santos, A.F.; das Neves, R.C.; Ribeiro, R.M.; Rodrigues, F.; Caneiras, C.; Spruit, M.A.; Bárbara, C. Telemonitoring of daily activities compared to the six-minute walk test further completes the puzzle of oximetry-guided interventions. *Sci. Rep.* **2021**, *11*, 16600. [CrossRef]
19. Spruit, M.A.; Singh, S.J.; Garvey, C.; ZuWallack, R.; Nici, L.; Rochester, C.; Hill, K.; Holland, A.E.; Lareau, S.C.; Man, W.D.-C.; et al. An official American Thoracic Society/European Respiratory Society statement: Key concepts and advances in pulmonary rehabilitation. *Am. J. Respir. Crit. Care Med.* **2013**, *188*, e13–e64. [CrossRef] [PubMed]
20. Rochester, C.L.; Alison, J.A.; Carlin, B.; Jenkins, A.R.; Cox, N.S.; Bauldoff, G.; Bhatt, S.P.; Bourbeau, J.; Burtin, C.; Camp, P.G.; et al. Pulmonary Rehabilitation for Adults with Chronic Respiratory Disease: An Official American Thoracic Society Clinical Practice Guideline. *Am. J. Respir. Crit. Care Med.* **2023**, *208*, e7–e26. [CrossRef] [PubMed]
21. Dowman, L.; Hill, C.J.; May, A.; Holland, A.E. Pulmonary rehabilitation for interstitial lung disease. *Cochrane Database Syst. Rev.* **2021**, *2*, CD006322. [CrossRef]

22. du Bois, R.M.; Weycker, D.; Albera, C.; Bradford, W.Z.; Costabel, U.; Kartashov, A.; Lancaster, L.; Noble, P.W.; Sahn, S.A.; Szwarcberg, J.; et al. Six-minute-walk test in idiopathic pulmonary fibrosis: Test validation and minimal clinically important difference. *Am. J. Respir. Crit. Care Med.* **2011**, *183*, 1231–1237. [CrossRef] [PubMed]
23. National Institute for Health and Care Excellence. *Idiopathic Pulmonary Fibrosis in Adults: Diagnosis and Management*; National Institute for Health and Care Excellence: London, UK, 2017.
24. Candia, C.; Lombardi, C.; Merola, C.; Ambrosino, P.; D'anna, S.E.; Vicario, A.; De Marco, S.; Molino, A.; Maniscalco, M. The Role of High-Flow Nasal Cannula Oxygen Therapy in Exercise Testing and Pulmonary Rehabilitation: A Review of the Current Literature. *J. Clin. Med.* **2023**, *13*, 232. [CrossRef]
25. Ryerson, C.J.; Camp, P.G.; Eves, N.D.; Schaeffer, M.; Syed, N.; Dhillon, S.; Jensen, D.; Maltais, F.; O'donnell, D.E.; Raghavan, N.; et al. High Oxygen Delivery to Preserve Exercise Capacity in Patients with Idiopathic Pulmonary Fibrosis Treated with Nintedanib. Methodology of the HOPE-IPF Study. *Ann. Am. Thorac. Soc.* **2016**, *13*, 1640–1647. [CrossRef]
26. Dowman, L.; McDonald, C.F.; Hill, C.J.; Lee, A.L.; Barker, K.; Boote, C.; Glaspole, I.; Goh, N.S.L.; Southcott, A.M.; Burge, A.T.; et al. The evidence of benefits of exercise training in interstitial lung disease: A randomised controlled trial. *Thorax* **2017**, *72*, 610–619. [CrossRef]
27. Rochester, C.L. Barriers to Pulmonary Rehabilitation. *Respir. Care* **2024**, *69*, 713–723. [CrossRef] [PubMed]
28. Cerdán de las Heras, J.; Hilberg, O.; Løkke, A.; Bendstrup, E. Tele-rehabilitation program in Idiopathic Pulmonary Fibrosis. In *M-Health/e-Health*; European Respiratory Society: Lausanne, Switzerland, 2019; p. PA2232. [CrossRef]
29. Rammaert, B.; Leroy, S.; Cavestri, B.; Wallaert, B.; Grosbois, J.M. Home-based pulmonary rehabilitation in idiopathic pulmonary fibrosis. *Rev. Mal. Respir.* **2009**, *26*, 275–282. [CrossRef]
30. Moor, C.C.; Mostard, R.L.M.; Grutters, J.C.; Bresser, P.; Aerts, J.G.J.V.; Chavannes, N.H.; Wijsenbeek, M.S. Home Monitoring in Patients with Idiopathic Pulmonary Fibrosis. A Randomized Controlled Trial. *Am. J. Respir. Crit. Care Med.* **2020**, *202*, 393–401. [CrossRef]
31. Wijsenbeek, M.S.; Moor, C.C.; A Johannson, K.; Jackson, P.D.; Khor, Y.H.; Kondoh, Y.; Rajan, S.K.; Tabaj, G.C.; E Varela, B.; van der Wal, P.; et al. Home monitoring in interstitial lung diseases. *Lancet Respir. Med.* **2023**, *11*, 97–110. [CrossRef] [PubMed]
32. Althobiani, M.A.; Evans, R.A.; Alqahtani, J.S.; Aldhahir, A.M.; Russell, A.-M.; Hurst, J.R.; Porter, J.C. Home monitoring of physiology and symptoms to detect interstitial lung disease exacerbations and progression: A systematic review. *ERJ Open Res.* **2021**, *7*, 441. [CrossRef] [PubMed]
33. Hagmeyer, L.; Herkenrath, S.D.; Treml, M.; Pietzke-Calcagnile, A.; Anduleit, N.; Randerath, W. Sleep-related breathing disorders in idiopathic pulmonary fibrosis are frequent and may be associated with pulmonary vascular involvement. *Sleep Breath.* **2023**, *27*, 961–971. [CrossRef]
34. Bordas-Martinez, J.; Salord, N.; Vicens-Zygmunt, V.; Pérez, S.; Prado, E.; Calvo, M.; Blavia, R.; Bermudo, G.; Montes-Worboys, A.; Santos, S.; et al. Characterization of Sleep-Disordered Breathing in Idiopathic Pulmonary Fibrosis. *Arch. Bronconeumol.* **2023**, *59*, 768–771. [CrossRef] [PubMed]
35. Myall, K.J.; West, A.G.; Martinovic, J.L.; Lam, J.L.; Roque, D.; Wu, Z.; Maher, T.M.; Molyneaux, P.L.; Suh, E.-S.; Kent, B.D. Nocturnal Hypoxemia Associates With Symptom Progression and Mortality in Patients With Progressive Fibrotic Interstitial Lung Disease. *Chest* **2023**, *164*, 1232–1242. [CrossRef] [PubMed]
36. Troy, L.K.; Young, I.H.; Lau, E.M.; Wong, K.K.; Yee, B.J.; Torzillo, P.J.; Corte, T.J. Nocturnal hypoxaemia is associated with adverse outcomes in interstitial lung disease. *Respirology* **2019**, *24*, 996–1004. [CrossRef] [PubMed]
37. Vozoris, N.T.; Wilton, A.S.; Austin, P.C.; Kendzerska, T.; Ryan, C.M.; Gershon, A.S. Morbidity and mortality reduction associated with polysomnography testing in idiopathic pulmonary fibrosis: A population-based cohort study. *BMC Pulm. Med.* **2021**, *21*, 185. [CrossRef]
38. Mermigkis, C.; Bouloukaki, I.; Schiza, S.E. Sleep as a New Target for Improving Outcomes in Idiopathic Pulmonary Fibrosis. *Chest* **2017**, *152*, 1327–1338. [CrossRef] [PubMed]
39. Papadogiannis, G.; Bouloukaki, I.; Mermigkis, C.; Michelakis, S.; Ermidou, C.; Mauroudi, E.; Moniaki, V.; Tzanakis, N.; Antoniou, K.M.; Schiza, S.E. Patients with idiopathic pulmonary fibrosis with and without obstructive sleep apnea: Differences in clinical characteristics, clinical outcomes, and the effect of PAP treatment. *J. Clin. Sleep Med.* **2021**, *17*, 533–544. [CrossRef]
40. Mermigkis, C.; Bouloukaki, I.; Antoniou, K.; Papadogiannis, G.; Giannarakis, I.; Varouchakis, G.; Siafakas, N.; Schiza, S.E. Obstructive sleep apnea should be treated in patients with idiopathic pulmonary fibrosis. *Sleep Breath.* **2015**, *19*, 385–391. [CrossRef]
41. Raghu, G.; Freudenberger, T.D.; Yang, S.; Curtis, J.R.; Spada, C.; Hayes, J.; Sillery, J.K.; Pope, C.E.; Pellegrini, C.A. High prevalence of abnormal acid gastro-oesophageal reflux in idiopathic pulmonary fibrosis. *Eur. Respir. J.* **2006**, *27*, 136–142. [CrossRef] [PubMed]
42. Tobin, R.W.; Pope, C.E.; Pellegrini, C.A.; Emond, M.J.; Sillery, J.; Raghu, G. Increased prevalence of gastroesophageal reflux in patients with idiopathic pulmonary fibrosis. *Am. J. Respir. Crit. Care Med.* **1998**, *158*, 1804–1808. [CrossRef]

43. Raghu, G.; Rochwerg, B.; Zhang, Y.; Cuello-Garcia, C.; Azuma, A.; Behr, J.; Brozek, J.L.; Collard, H.R.; Cunningham, W.; Homma, S.; et al. An Official ATS/ERS/JRS/ALAT Clinical Practice Guideline: Treatment of Idiopathic Pulmonary Fibrosis. An Update of the 2011 Clinical Practice Guideline. *Am. J. Respir. Crit. Care Med.* **2015**, *192*, e3–e19. [CrossRef] [PubMed]
44. Raghu, G.; Remy-Jardin, M.; Richeldi, L.; Thomson, C.C.; Inoue, Y.; Johkoh, T.; Kreuter, M.; Lynch, D.A.; Maher, T.M.; Martinez, F.J.; et al. Idiopathic Pulmonary Fibrosis (an Update) and Progressive Pulmonary Fibrosis in Adults: An Official ATS/ERS/JRS/ALAT Clinical Practice Guideline. *Am. J. Respir. Crit. Care Med.* **2022**, *205*, e18–e47. [CrossRef]
45. Yang, M.; Dong, J.; An, J.; Liu, L.; Chen, L. Effect of anti-reflux therapy on pulmonary function in idiopathic pulmonary fibrosis: A systematic review and meta-analysis. *J. Thorac. Dis.* **2021**, *13*, 5776–5787. [CrossRef] [PubMed]
46. Kreuter, M.; Ehlers-Tenenbaum, S.; Palmowski, K.; Bruhwyler, J.; Oltmanns, U.; Muley, T.; Heussel, C.P.; Warth, A.; Kolb, M.; Herth, F.J.F. Impact of Comorbidities on Mortality in Patients with Idiopathic Pulmonary Fibrosis. *PLoS ONE* **2016**, *11*, e0151425. [CrossRef] [PubMed]
47. Bédard Méthot, D.; Leblanc, É.; Lacasse, Y. Meta-analysis of Gastroesophageal Reflux Disease and Idiopathic Pulmonary Fibrosis. *Chest* **2019**, *155*, 33–43. [CrossRef] [PubMed]
48. Molina-Molina, M. The relationship between gastro-oesophageal reflux and pulmonary fibrosis: A never-ending story. *Eur. Respir. J.* **2023**, *61*, 2300566. [CrossRef]
49. Raghu, G.; Morrow, E.; Collins, B.F.; Ho, L.A.; Hinojosa, M.W.; Hayes, J.M.; Spada, C.A.; Oelschlager, B.; Li, C.; Yow, E.; et al. Laparoscopic anti-reflux surgery for idiopathic pulmonary fibrosis at a single centre. *Eur. Respir. J.* **2016**, *48*, 826–832. [CrossRef]
50. Khor, Y.H.; Bissell, B.; Ghazipura, M.; Herman, D.; Hon, S.M.; Hossain, T.; Kheir, F.; Knight, S.L.; Kreuter, M.; Macrea, M.; et al. Antacid Medication and Antireflux Surgery in Patients with Idiopathic Pulmonary Fibrosis: A Systematic Review and Meta-Analysis. *Ann. Am. Thorac. Soc.* **2022**, *19*, 833–844. [CrossRef]
51. Chen, J.W.; Vela, M.F.; Peterson, K.A.; Carlson, D.A. AGA Clinical Practice Update on the Diagnosis and Management of Extraesophageal Gastroesophageal Reflux Disease: Expert Review. *Clin. Gastroenterol. Hepatol.* **2023**, *21*, 1414–1421.e3. [CrossRef] [PubMed]
52. Ness-Jensen, E.; Hveem, K.; El-Serag, H.; Lagergren, J. Lifestyle Intervention in Gastroesophageal Reflux Disease. *Clin. Gastroenterol. Hepatol.* **2016**, *14*, e1–e3. [CrossRef] [PubMed]
53. Raghu, G.; Remy-Jardin, M.; Myers, J.L.; Richeldi, L.; Ryerson, C.J.; Lederer, D.J.; Behr, J.; Cottin, V.; Danoff, S.K.; Morell, F.; et al. Diagnosis of Idiopathic Pulmonary Fibrosis. An Official ATS/ERS/JRS/ALAT Clinical Practice Guideline. *Am. J. Respir. Crit. Care Med.* **2018**, *198*, e44–e68. [CrossRef] [PubMed]
54. Mercader-Barceló, J.; Truyols-Vives, J.; Río, C.; López-Safont, N.; Sala-Llinàs, E.; Chaplin, A. Insights into the Role of Bioactive Food Ingredients and the Microbiome in Idiopathic Pulmonary Fibrosis. *Int. J. Mol. Sci.* **2020**, *21*, 6051. [CrossRef] [PubMed]
55. Micco, A.; Carpentieri, E.; Di Sorbo, A.; Chetta, A.; Del Donno, M. Palliative care and end of life management in patients with idiopathic pulmonary fibrosis. *Multidiscip. Respir. Med.* **2023**, *18*, 896. [CrossRef]
56. Miyake, Y.; Sasaki, S.; Yokoyama, T.; Chida, K.; Azuma, A.; Suda, T.; Kudoh, S.; Sakamoto, N.; Okamoto, K.; Kobashi, G.; et al. Vegetable, Fruit, and Cereal Intake and Risk of Idiopathic Pulmonary Fibrosis in Japan. *Ann. Nutr. Metab.* **2004**, *48*, 390–397. [CrossRef]
57. Miyake, Y.; Sasaki, S.; Yokoyama, T.; Chida, K.; Azuma, A.; Suda, T.; Kudoh, S.; Sakamoto, N.; Okamoto, K.; Kobashi, G.; et al. Dietary fat and meat intake and idiopathic pulmonary fibrosis: A case-control study in Japan. *Int. J. Tuberc. Lung Dis.* **2006**, *10*, 333–339. [PubMed]
58. Della Vedova, M.C.; Garcia, F.M.S.; Muñoz, M.D.; Fornes, M.W.; Mejiba, S.E.G.; Gómez, N.N.; Ramirez, D.C. Diet-Induced Pulmonary Inflammation and Incipient Fibrosis in Mice: A Possible Role of Neutrophilic Inflammation. *Inflammation* **2019**, *42*, 1886–1900. [CrossRef] [PubMed]
59. Hegab, A.E.; Ozaki, M.; Meligy, F.Y.; Kagawa, S.; Ishii, M.; Betsuyaku, T. High fat diet activates adult mouse lung stem cells and accelerates several aging-induced effects. *Stem. Cell Res.* **2018**, *33*, 25–35. [CrossRef] [PubMed]
60. Yavari, M.; Mousavi, S.A.J.; Janani, L.; Feizy, Z.; Vafa, M. Effects of supplementation of vitamins D, C and E on Idiopathic Pulmonary Fibrosis (IPF): A clinical trial. *Clin. Nutr. ESPEN* **2022**, *49*, 295–300. [CrossRef]
61. Pan, D.; Wang, Q.; Yan, B.; Su, X. Higher body mass index was associated with a lower mortality of idiopathic pulmonary fibrosis: A meta-analysis. *J. Health Popul. Nutr.* **2024**, *43*, 124. [CrossRef]
62. He, X.; Ji, J.; Liu, C.; Luo, Z.; Tang, J.; Yan, H.; Guo, L. Body mass index and weight loss as risk factors for poor outcomes in patients with idiopathic pulmonary fibrosis: A systematic review and meta-analysis. *Ann. Med.* **2024**, *56*, 2311845. [CrossRef]
63. Faverio, P.; Bocchino, M.; Caminati, A.; Fumagalli, A.; Gasbarra, M.; Iovino, P.; Petruzzi, A.; Scalfi, L.; Sebastiani, A.; Stanziola, A.A.; et al. Nutrition in Patients with Idiopathic Pulmonary Fibrosis: Critical Issues Analysis and Future Research Directions. *Nutrients.* **2020**, *12*, 1131. [CrossRef] [PubMed]
64. Ravindran, S.G.; Saha, D.; Iqbal, I.; Jhaveri, S.; Avanthika, C.; Naagendran, M.S.; Bethineedi, L.D.; Santhosh, T. The Obesity Paradox in Chronic Heart Disease and Chronic Obstructive Pulmonary Disease. *Cureus* **2022**, *14*, e25674. [CrossRef]

65. Jung, H.I.; Park, J.S.; Lee, M.-Y.; Park, B.M.; Kim, H.J.; Park, S.H.; Choi, W.-I.; Lee, C.W. Prevalence of lung cancer in patients with interstitial lung disease is higher than in those with chronic obstructive pulmonary disease. *Medicine* **2018**, *97*, e0071. [CrossRef]
66. Sato, S.; Koike, T.; Hashimoto, T.; Ishikawa, H.; Okada, A.; Watanabe, T.; Tsuchida, M. Surgical Outcomes of Lung Cancer Patients with Combined Pulmonary Fibrosis and Emphysema and Those with Idiopathic Pulmonary Fibrosis without Emphysema. *Ann. Thorac. Cardiovasc. Surg.* **2016**, *22*, 216–223. [CrossRef]
67. Abu Qubo, A.; Numan, J.; Snijder, J.; Padilla, M.; Austin, J.H.; Capaccione, K.M.; Pernia, M.; Bustamante, J.; O'Connor, T.; Salvatore, M.M. Idiopathic pulmonary fibrosis and lung cancer: Future directions and challenges. *Breathe* **2022**, *18*, 220147. [CrossRef] [PubMed]
68. Tzouvelekis, A.; Spagnolo, P.; Bonella, F.; Vancheri, C.; Tzilas, V.; Crestani, B.; Kreuter, M.; Bouros, D. Patients with IPF and lung cancer: Diagnosis and management. *Lancet Respir. Med.* **2018**, *6*, 86–88. [CrossRef] [PubMed]
69. Saito, Y.; Kawai, Y.; Takahashi, N.; Ikeya, T.; Murai, K.; Kawabata, Y.; Hoshi, E. Survival after surgery for pathologic stage IA non-small cell lung cancer associated with idiopathic pulmonary fibrosis. *Ann. Thorac. Surg.* **2011**, *92*, 1812–1817. [CrossRef]
70. MacMahon, H.; Naidich, D.P.; Goo, J.M.; Lee, K.S.; Leung, A.N.C.; Mayo, J.R.; Mehta, A.C.; Ohno, Y.; Powell, C.A.; Prokop, M.; et al. Guidelines for Management of Incidental Pulmonary Nodules Detected on CT Images: From the Fleischner Society 2017. *Radiology* **2017**, *284*, 228–243. [CrossRef]
71. Kreuter, M.; Bendstrup, E.; Russell, A.-M.; Bajwah, S.; Lindell, K.; Adir, Y.; E Brown, C.; Calligaro, G.; Cassidy, N.; Corte, T.J.; et al. Palliative care in interstitial lung disease: Living well. *Lancet Respir. Med.* **2017**, *5*, 968–980. [CrossRef] [PubMed]
72. Bassi, I.; Guerrieri, A.; Carpano, M.; Gardini, A.; Prediletto, I.; Polastri, M.; Curtis, J.R.; Nava, S. Feasibility and efficacy of a multidisciplinary palliative approach in patients with advanced interstitial lung disease. A pilot randomised controlled trial. *Pulmonology* **2023**, *29*, S54–S62. [CrossRef] [PubMed]
73. Brighton, L.J.; Miller, S.; Farquhar, M.; Booth, S.; Yi, D.; Gao, W.; Bajwah, S.; Man, W.D.-C.; Higginson, I.J.; Maddocks, M. Holistic services for people with advanced disease and chronic breathlessness: A systematic review and meta-analysis. *Thorax* **2019**, *74*, 270–281. [CrossRef] [PubMed]
74. Higginson, I.J.; Bausewein, C.; Reilly, C.C.; Gao, W.; Gysels, M.; Dzingina, M.; McCrone, P.; Booth, S.; Jolley, C.J.; Moxham, J. An integrated palliative and respiratory care service for patients with advanced disease and refractory breathlessness: A randomised controlled trial. *Lancet Respir. Med.* **2014**, *2*, 979–987. [CrossRef] [PubMed]
75. Janssen, K.; Rosielle, D.; Wang, Q.; Kim, H.J. The impact of palliative care on quality of life, anxiety, and depression in idiopathic pulmonary fibrosis: A randomized controlled pilot study. *Respir. Res.* **2020**, *21*, 2. [CrossRef]
76. Lindell, K.O.; Klein, S.J.; Veatch, M.S.; Gibson, K.F.; Kass, D.J.; Nouraie, M.; Rosenzweig, M.Q. Nurse-Led Palliative Care Clinical Trial Improves Knowledge and Preparedness in Caregivers of Patients with Idiopathic Pulmonary Fibrosis. *Ann. Am. Thorac. Soc.* **2021**, *18*, 1811–1821. [CrossRef] [PubMed]
77. Dalal, S.; Palla, S.; Hui, D.; Nguyen, L.; Chacko, R.; Li, Z.; Fadul, N.; Scott, C.; Thornton, V.; Coldman, B.; et al. Association between a name change from palliative to supportive care and the timing of patient referrals at a comprehensive cancer center. *Oncologist* **2011**, *16*, 105–111. [CrossRef] [PubMed]
78. Quinn, K.L.; Wegier, P.; Stukel, T.A.; Huang, A.; Bell, C.M.; Tanuseputro, P. Comparison of Palliative Care Delivery in the Last Year of Life Between Adults With Terminal Noncancer Illness or Cancer. *JAMA Netw. Open* **2021**, *4*, e210677. [CrossRef] [PubMed]

Journal of
Clinical Medicine

MDPI

Review

Telomeropathies in Interstitial Lung Disease and Lung Transplant Recipients

Brian D. Southern * and Shruti K. Gadre

Integrated Hospital-Care Institute, Department of Pulmonary Medicine, Cleveland Clinic, Cleveland, OH 44195, USA; gadres@ccf.org
* Correspondence: southeb@ccf.org

Abstract: Telomeropathies, or telomere biology disorders (TBDs), are syndromes that can cause a number of medical conditions, including interstitial lung disease (ILD), bone marrow failure, liver fibrosis, and other diseases. They occur due to genetic mutations to the telomerase complex enzymes that result in premature shortening of telomeres, the caps on the ends of cellular DNA that protect chromosome length during cell division, leading to early cell senescence and death. Idiopathic pulmonary fibrosis (IPF) is the most common manifestation of the telomere biology disorders, although it has been described in other interstitial lung diseases as well, such as rheumatoid arthritis-associated ILD and chronic hypersensitivity pneumonitis. Telomere-related mutations can be inherited or can occur sporadically. Identifying these patients and offering genetic counseling is important because telomerapathies have been associated with poorer outcomes including death, lung transplantation, hospitalization, and FVC decline. Additionally, treatment with immunosuppressants has been shown to be associated with worse outcomes. Currently, there is no specific treatment for TBD except to transplant the organ that is failing, although there are a number of promising treatment strategies currently under investigation. Shortened telomere length is routinely discovered in patients undergoing lung transplantation for IPF. Testing to detect early TBD in patients with suggestive signs or symptoms can allow for more comprehensive treatment and multidisciplinary care pre- and post-transplant. Patients with TBD undergoing lung transplantation have been reported to have both pulmonary and extrapulmonary complications at a higher frequency than other lung transplant recipients, such as graft-specific complications, increased infections, and complications related to immunosuppressive therapy.

Keywords: telomere biology disorders; telomeropathies

1. Telomere Biology Disorders

Telomeres are regions of non-coding tandem repeat DNA sequences that are added to the end of all chromosomes to hinder progressive chromosomal shortening during replication of the cell. This prevents the chromosomes from becoming so short that they are no longer able to divide, which would result in cell death [1]. With aging, DNA replication does not always copy to the telomere end, so telomeres gradually become shorter, eventually causing senescence and cell death. Thus, in most somatic cells, telomere shortening is a consequence of aging. Not long after the discovery of telomeres, the existence of an enzyme with specific telomere terminal transferase-like properties that added repeat units to telomeric DNA to compensate for incomplete terminal replication was discovered [2]. Carol Greider, Elizabeth Blackburn, and Jack Szostak were awarded the 2009 Nobel prize in physiology or medicine for their work identifying the telomerase protein [3]. An oncologist and pediatrician in Dr. Grieder's laboratory, Mary Armanios, was studying a population of mice that had been genetically modified to lack telomerase. Serendipitously, she was introduced by a colleague to a patient with aplastic anemia who was discovered to have a mutation in a gene called human telomerase reverse transcriptase, or hTERT, which provides critical instructions for making a component of telomerase. She discovered that, like her mice, this patient seemed to be becoming old "before his time". She contacted his family members and collected blood for analysis. Three months later, the patient's father died of liver disease and bone marrow failure at age 49. She discovered an aunt and uncle who both suffered from pulmonary fibrosis and would die in their 50s. All of these family members had the same abnormality in the TERT gene and suffered from a rare inherited disease called dyskeratosis congenita (DC) [4]. She went on to identify additional families who suffered from DC who had mutations in the gene DKC1, which also encodes for a component of telomerase, and who later developed idiopathic pulmonary fibrosis (IPF) [5].

It is now known that telomerase is composed of two key components, hTERT, the reverse transcriptase component of telomerase, and hTR (or TERC), the RNA portion that serves as the template for nucleotide addition by hTERT (Figure 1). Mutations in these genes result in short telomeres associated with aplastic anemia and pulmonary fibrosis, which can lead to premature death [6]. Other genes important in telomerase biology include TINF2 and other members of the shelterin complex, which caps, protects, and regulates telomeres [7]. The dyskerin complex is essential for regulating the accumulation of hTR and is therefore important in maintaining proper telomerase activity [8]. RTEL1 (DNA helicase in telomerase maintenance) regulates telomere elongation [9], and PARN (poly(A)-specific ribonuclease) is involved in 3′-end maturation of the telomerase RNA [10]. Mutations in any of these components can lead to shortened telomeres, causing IPF and other disorders [11–14] (Table 1).

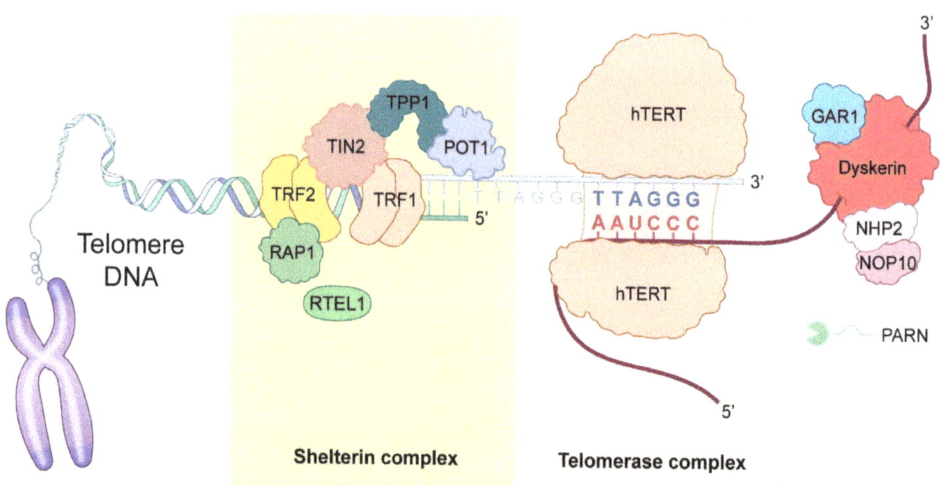

Figure 1. Telomerase and telomerase-associated proteins that are affected in telomeropathies associated with IPF and other ILDs.

Table 1. Known mutations in telomerase and shelterin complex subunits.

Gene	Chromosome	Inheritance	Effect of Mutation on Telomerase Complex	Refs.
DKC1	Xq28	XLR	Decreases TERT/TERC expression, suppresses telomerase activity	[15,16]
TERC	3q26.3	AD	Slows or stops cell proliferation independent of telomerase activity, accelerates shortening of longer telomeres, increases oxidative DNA damage at telomeres	[17–19]
TERT	5p15.53	AD, AR	Loss of function of the telomerase complex	[11,20]
NOP10	15q14-q15	AR	Diminishes telomerase activity via TERC downregulation	[21]
NHP2	5q35.5	AR	Diminishes telomerase activity via TERC downregulation	[22]
TINF2	14q11.2	AD	Lack of stabilization of TRF1 on telomeres; loss of protection of telomere and genome stability	[23,24]
RTEL	20q13.33	AR	Lack of disassembly of DNA loops for proper access to the telomere; lack of telomere stability	[25–27]
PARN	16p13.12	AD, AR, XLR	Does not allow for removal of poly(A) tails from hTR, causing lack of maturation of telomerase	[28,29]

XLR = X-linked recessive, AD = autosomal dominant, AR = autosomal recessive.

In addition to IPF, shortened telomeres have been associated with bone marrow failure syndromes [30], emphysema [31], cryptogenic liver cirrhosis [32], premature hair graying [33], avascular necrosis of the hips and shoulders [34], periodontal disease [35], and increased predisposition to various types of myelodysplasia/malignancies [36]. Patients with any of these manifestations may be said to have a TBD, short telomere syndrome (STS), or a telomeropathy. All modes of genetic inheritance can be seen in the TBDs. DKC1 is the only X-linked telomere-related gene that can result in X-linked recessive disease. Four TBD-causing genes have been shown to have an autosomal recessive mode of inheritance, and carriers are asymptomatic, although they may manifest TBD-related disorders as adults. TINF2 variants are strictly autosomal dominant. The remaining eleven known TBD-related genes can be autosomal dominant or recessive and can be represented by early manifestation of disease [37]. Genetic anticipation can occur in TBD with individuals who carry autosomal dominant variants and pass the mutation, along with shortened telomeres, to their children [38]. This can result in an earlier onset of disease with each successive generation. This has been observed in families with pulmonary fibrosis carrying monoallelic variants of TERC, TERT, or other genes, resulting in early-onset pulmonary fibrosis and other disorders, such as bone marrow failure [39]. In addition, the phenomenon of phenocopy can occur, as shown in a systematic study of 99 families with familial pulmonary fibrosis, where five individuals lacked the TBD gene mutation but had shortened telomeres and developed pulmonary fibrosis [40]. The primary determinant of whether or not a TBD will develop is the presence of shortened telomeres, as the absence of telomerase by itself may not be sufficient to cause disease [41]. In mouse models with telomerase deletion, no phenotypic changes are observed, but phenotypic changes related to aging can be seen after several generations [42]. The true prevalence of TBDs is unknown, largely due to the incomplete penetration of disease features in many carriers. Patients with IPF, aplastic anemia, or cryptogenic cirrhosis may have a subtle clinical phenotype and may not be tested for telomeropathies.

Several methods have been developed to measure telomere length, and telomere restriction fragment length analysis is the gold standard. However, its utilization is limited as large amounts of DNA are needed for analysis [43]. Flow-FISH (fluorescence in situ hybridization) of blood involves the use of a fluorescent probe that labels telomeres and uses flow cytometry to analyze the telomere length in specific cell types, most commonly granulocytes and leukocytes. Flow-FISH takes into account the age-related telomere length, which is necessary because telomere attrition is a normal process in aging. The presence of a telomere length at or below the lowest 10th percentile of normal length is diagnostic for short telomere syndrome [44].

2. Telomere Disorders in IPF

IPF is the most prevalent interstitial lung disease (ILD), with an annual incidence rate of approximately 10 cases per 100,000 people in Europe and North America [45]. IPF is the most frequent manifestation of TBD in adults [6]. Mutations related to telomeres have been reported in approximately 25% of familial instances and 1–3% of sporadic IPF instances, a percentage that is greater than that of patients exhibiting hematologic phenotypes [46]. Genetic studies in IPF have revealed that around 40% of familial IPF cases and 25% of sporadic IPF cases exhibit shortened telomeres, suggesting hence-undiscovered gene mutations in IPF [47,48]. Importantly, there is evidence to support the notion that short telomere syndrome plays a greater role in sporadic IPF. First, it has been shown that patients with IPF, irrespective of whether there is a telomere mutation, have short telomeres compared to the population, with approximately half having a leukocyte telomere length (LTL) below the 10th age-adjusted percentile [49]. In fact, the severity of telomere shortening in sporadic IPF is like that seen in telomerase mutation carriers. Second, in a Mendelian randomization study that compared 82 other adult-onset diseases, pulmonary fibrosis had the strongest association with telomere length, with an estimated effect size of 10-fold [50]. Finally, it is clearly observed that patients with sporadic IPF and shortened telomeres can have the same extrapulmonary manifestations seen in those with familial IPF [48]. These lines of evidence support the premise that shortened telomeres are common in sporadic IPF, and telomere length, not necessarily the underlying mutation, has the greatest impact on the development of sporadic IPF. Thus, telomere shortening alone, without a mutation in a telomere-related gene, is a heritable trait that can occur and result in IPF. The most common pattern seen radiographically or histologically in patients with IPF and with or without shortened telomeres is the usual interstitial pneumonia pattern (UIP). However, it has been well established that patients with inheritable forms of IPF can present with "atypical" findings on imaging or pathology, and affected members with the same germline mutation may have discordant diagnoses. In an analysis of 15 families where at least two members were diagnosed with ILD through a multidisciplinary approach, it was found that 12 families (80%) had differing diagnoses, while only 3 families (20%) had a consistent diagnosis of IPF [51]. For example, in one family harboring the same TERC mutation, individual family members had histologic diagnoses that were consistent with UIP, chronic hypersensitivity pneumonitis, desquamative interstitial pneumonia, and pleuroparenchymal fibroelastosis [51].

There are currently no guidelines informing clinicians on how to proceed if genetic IPF is suspected. Offering genetic counseling and screening to all patients with IPF could be useful in counseling family members with shortened telomeres to avoid substances that are harmful to the lung, such as those associated with smoking or other inhaled exposures [52]. The average age of patients carrying a telomerase mutation is younger than that of those without mutations [53], and individuals with shorter telomeres have been found to experience faster disease progression and reduced survival rates without a transplant [51]; identifying these patients earlier could lead to closer monitoring and more aggressive treatment. Moreover, a subsequent analysis of patients from the PANTHER-IPF trial revealed that administering prednisone, N-aceylcysteine, and azathioprine to patients with a leukocyte telomere length below the 10% percentile of normal correlated with a higher combined outcome of death, lung transplantation, hospitalization, or a decrease in FVC [54]. These findings were replicated in additional cohorts. Avoidance of immunosuppressant therapy in patients with shortened telomeres could lead to improved outcomes. These examples demonstrate how a precision medicine approach using telomere length analysis could lead to changes in treatment strategies and patient care.

3. Telomere Disorders in Other ILDs

Over the past decade, telomere-related mutations and short telomeres have been implicated in various forms of non-IPF ILD. Examples include non-specific interstitial pneumonia (NSIP), pleuroparenchymal fibroelastosis (PPFE), hypersensitivity pneumonitis, and combined pulmonary fibrosis and emphysema [55]. Using whole-exome sequencing, it was demonstrated that TERT, RTEL1, and PARN mutations occur in patients with rheumatoid arthritis-associated ILD at a 3-fold higher odds ratio than they do in a control population. Furthermore, LTLs in patients with RA-ILD and TERT, RTEL1, or PARN mutations were shorter compared to those in control patients [56]. These data support the contribution of shortened telomeres to the risk of developing RA-ILD. In a prospective cohort study comparing chronic hypersensitivity pneumonitis patients on mycophenolate with shortened peripheral blood LTL and those with normal telomere length, every quartile reduction in LTL was linked to a similar decrease in survival without a transplant [57]. In patients with chronic hypersensitivity pneumonitis, an observational study of two independent cohorts showed an association between the extent of radiographic fibrosis and short telomere length and, similarly to previous studies in IPF, reduced survival in the short telomere population [58]. In a different study that contrasted patients with UIP against those with interstitial pneumonia with autoimmune features (IPAF) and connective tissue disease-associated interstitial lung disease (CTD-ILD), it was found that telomere length was greater in patients with idiopathic pneumonia with autoimmune features and CTD-ILD compared to those with UIP [59]. Among the IPAF patient group, those with LTL less than the 10th percentile had a more rapid decline in lung function and poorer transplant-free survival compared to those with LTL greater than the 10th percentile. RA-ILD patients had shorter LTLs than non-RA CT-ILD patients, but this was not associated with any differences in transplant-free survival. Telomere length in unclassifiable ILD was linked to transplant-free survival, even when potential confounding factors were taken into account. Patients whose telomere length was in the lowest quartile had almost the same transplant-free survival rate as IPF patients [60]. As seen in these various studies and others, a shortened LTL is usually associated with worse outcomes regardless of the ILD phenotype, perhaps more associated with the histological pattern than the clinical diagnosis.

4. Treatment of Telomere Biology Disorders in ILD

Currently, there is no available treatment for TBDs other than transplanting the organ that is failing. Based on a theory that there is an estrogen-responsive element in the TERT gene, the NIH conducted a phase 1–2 study where the synthetic sex hormone danazol was administered to patients with various manifestations of TBD, with the primary outcome being a 20% decrease in the annual rate of telomere attrition at 24 months [61]. The study was halted prematurely as 12 of the patients met the primary endpoint. In almost all of these patients (11/12), there was an increase in telomere length at 24 months compared to the baseline length, and there was an improvement in blood counts. Based on this work, danazol was administered to 50 patients with IPF after they showed progressive disease with either of the two approved therapies for IPF, pirfenidone or nintedanib, with the primary outcome being a change in forced vital capacity (FVC) over 12 months of treatment [62]. After one year, only 22% (11 patients) continued the danazol treatment, while 39 patients had ceased therapy, predominantly due to side effects (56%) or death (33%). The lung function of all patients significantly deteriorated, with an average FVC reduction of 485 mL observed in the year following the commencement of treatment. Despite this negative study, other studies utilizing danazol are currently ongoing. High-throughput screening has identified an inhibitor of PAPD5 (a non-canonical polymerase that oligoadenylates and destabilizes TERC) called BCH001 that restores telomere length in induced pluripotent stem cells from patients with DC [63]. Imetelstat, a lipid-conjugated oligonucleotide that competitively blocks telomerase, was examined in a preliminary myelofibrosis study, and 21% of the participants achieved either partial or full remission [64]. A separate trial involving imetelstat in patients with advanced non-small cell lung cancer and shortened telomeres indicated a potential trend of improvement in both progression-free and overall survival [65]. The progression of fibrosis in a mouse model with short telomeres exposed to bleomycin was halted by activating telomerase using an adenovirus-associated vector (AAV) [66]. These investigators went on to show that physiologic aging leads to short telomeres and fibrosis in the lung of mice, and that administration of their AAV gene therapy prevented the onset of fibrosis [67]. These and other exciting strategies to reverse telomere shortening are novel and may be potential future therapeutic options for patients with TBD.

There are currently two approved therapies for IPF (pirfenidone, nintedanib) [68,69] and one approved therapy for progressive pulmonary fibrosis (nintedanib) [70]. There have been studies demonstrating that the use of these anti-fibrotic therapies in patients with telomerase gene mutations is safe and efficacious in slowing FVC decline [71]. A post hoc analysis of the pirfenidone trials CAPACITY and ASCEND revealed a significant treatment advantage for patients with telomere lengths both above and below the median. Nevertheless, individuals with telomere mutations underwent a more rapid decrease in FVC compared to those without mutations [53]. A retrospective analysis showed that both pirfenidone and nintedanib were linked to a slower rate of FVC decline compared to the rate prior to treatment [72]. These studies support the safety of using anti-fibrotics in progressive fibrosis regardless of telomere length.

5. Telomere Biology Disorders and Lung Transplantation

The only intervention that can extend the life of patients with end-stage pulmonary fibrosis is lung transplantation. Among patients with ILD who are referred for lung transplantation, it has been discovered that up to 25% possess a genetic variant associated with TBDs [73]. This percentage is believed to be higher due to the typically earlier onset and increased severity of ILD associated with TBD. The prevalence of TBDs is reported to be two times higher in IPF patients who receive a lung transplant compared to those with IPF who do not have a transplant [73]. In a particular group, it was found that 32% of IPF lung transplant recipients had a telomere length that was less than the 10th percentile [74].

Patients with TBD undergoing lung transplantation have been reported to have both pulmonary and extrapulmonary complications at a higher frequency than other lung transplant recipients. These include airway complications such as anastomotic dehiscence or bronchial stenosis [75], chronic allograft dysfunction [75], and severe infectious, hematological, hepatic, renal, and gastrointestinal complications [75–78]. The identification of telomere biology disorders may allow for strategies to prevent complications of short telomere syndrome in lung transplant recipients. It should be noted that the presence of a telomere biology disorder by itself is not considered to be a contraindication to lung transplantation.

Standard post-lung-transplant immunosuppressive protocols include a combination of calcineurin inhibitors (tacrolimus/cyclosporine), targeting varying trough levels, steroids (prednisone/dexamethasone), and antimetabolites (mycophenolate mofetil/azathioprine). Standard infection prophylaxis protocols include lifelong pneumocystis jirovecii pneumonia (PJP) prophylaxis (trimethoprim–sulfamethoxazole/pentamidine/dapsone) and varying durations of cytomegalovirus (CMV) (valganciclovir) and fungal (posaconazole/itraconazole/voriconazole) prophylaxis depending on the transplant center. These protocols often need to be modified in TBD patients to improve medication tolerance and mitigate potential adverse outcomes.

6. Graft-Specific Complications

Research comparing lung transplant recipients with telomere biology disorders to recipients with normal telomere length has produced inconsistent results regarding survival and graft outcomes such as Primary Graft Dysfunction (PGD), acute cellular rejection (ACR), and Chronic Lung Allograft Dysfunction (CLAD). In a single-center observational cohort of 82 patients with IPF, Newton and colleagues reported that short telomere length was associated with increased rates of PGD and CLAD [74]. There was nearly an 11-fold increased risk of death in the short telomere cohort compared to recipients with normal telomere length. Courtwright et al. reported that a shorter telomere length was linked to reduced CLAD-free survival [79]. In contrast, a more recent study by Alder et al. showed that post-transplant survival and CLAD-free survival did not differ with the telomere length within IPF lung transplant recipients [73]. This inconsistency in results could potentially be due to the fact that the definition of short telomeres was not uniform across different studies.

Acute cellular rejection is a less frequent occurrence in lung transplant recipients with TBD compared to recipients with normal telomere length. This is predominantly attributed to T-cell immunosenescence in patients with TBD. In Snyder et al.'s research, it was discovered that IPF lung transplant recipients with short telomeres experienced premature "aging" in their circulating T-cell compartment and a significant age-related decrease in early ACR burden [80]. While lung transplant recipients with telomere biology disorders may exhibit lower rates of acute graft rejection, they remain susceptible to chronic rejection.

7. Wound Healing and Airway Issues

The literature on wound healing and airway issues in lung transplant recipients with shortened telomeres is sparse. In a retrospective multicenter study of 63 lung transplant recipients with a telomere length in the <10th percentile, increased rates of dehiscence or stenosis in the large airway were reported in the short telomere group compared to a Scientific Registry of Transplant Recipients (SRTR) control group [81]. Individuals who have received a lung transplant and have TBD are more susceptible to complications in healing their airways. This is due to the premature aging of various cells such as fibroblasts, immune cells, endothelial cells, and epithelial cells. Infectious complications further complicate airway healing issues. The procedure of direct bronchial artery revascularization (BAR) during lung transplant surgery has been reported to lessen airway ischemia and enhance the healing of the airway in the early postoperative phase [82,83]. The feasibility of BAR at the time of transplant surgery should be considered in potential lung transplant recipients with TBD at the time of listing. Expert opinion also suggests that lung transplant recipients with TBD are at increased risk for sternal and chest wall wound dehiscence at a higher rate compared to recipients with normal telomere length, although the published literature is lacking.

8. Hematological Complications

Patients with TBD are more likely to develop a reduction in blood cells when given medications that suppress bone marrow, which are usually well tolerated in individuals without short telomeres. Silhan et al. compiled an international series of individuals carrying telomerase mutations who underwent lung transplantation in the USA, Australia, and Sweden [78]. Seven recipients were included in the study, with a median follow-up of 1.9 years. The predominant complications in this group were of a hematological nature, with 88% of recipients needing platelet transfusion assistance. All recipients required an adjustment in their immunosuppressive medications. Most patients were able to tolerate only two drug immunosuppressive regimens. The platelet counts increased after the immunosuppressive drugs were modified; however, they stayed below the levels before the transplant.

Short telomere length is a risk factor for clinically significant leucopenia as well [78]. In another study involving IPF lung transplant recipients with TBD, it was more common for patients with short telomeres to have their immunosuppression medications stopped due to cytopenias, compared to recipients without IPF. Bone marrow dysfunction requiring a bone marrow biopsy and increased requirements for transfusions and growth factor support were also noted among short telomere patients [84]. These studies emphasize the delicate state of the bone marrow reserve in patients with short telomeres and lung disease, which may become apparent after a transplant.

Strategies to prevent bone marrow suppression involve modifying the dosage of standard immunosuppression treatments by either pausing or reducing the amount of antimetabolite therapy, altering CMV prophylaxis, or using dapsone in place of trimethoprim/sulphamethoxazole for PJP prophylaxis [78]. The additional treatment for post-transplant cytopenias is mostly supportive. The use of blood or platelet transfusions and granulocyte colony-stimulating factor for neutropenia has been implemented. Danazol is typically not used in this patient group due to insufficient evidence and the potential danger of developing myelodysplastic syndrome (MDS) and acute myeloid leukemia (AML) [85]. In some instances, due to the heightened risk of MDS and AML, a bone marrow biopsy may be required to investigate cytopenias [84]. It is beneficial to include hematologists in the multidisciplinary team caring for lung transplant recipients with TBD.

9. Immunity and Infectious Complications

The decrease in T-cell numbers and function with age is referred to as T-cell immunosenescence. In patients with TBD, T cells show premature aging phenotypes compared to those in patients with normal telomere length. Short telomere syndromes in children and adults, caused by apoptosis induced by short telomeres and secondary depletion of T-cell precursors, result in low T-cell counts. These syndromes also lead to significant functional impairments, such as depleted pools of naïve T cells and a limited T-cell repertoire [79]. In a study group of 26 patients with TBD at Johns Hopkins, all of whom were under 60 years old, 32% (or 9 individuals) developed opportunistic infections linked to T-cell immunodeficiency. The infections were mainly related to herpes viruses (cytomegalovirus and varicella zoster virus), accounting for 66% of the infections. When CMV led to end-organ disease, such as encephalitis or pneumonitis, the infection resulted in death. Interestingly, adults can develop immunodeficiency without bone marrow failure, which can make them susceptible to life-threatening opportunistic infections.

An increased risk for other infectious complications is seen in lung transplant recipients with TBD as well. In an international case series of lung transplant recipients with TBD, 85% of the patients developed infectious complications with the first 2 years after transplantation [78]. The primary infections reported were Gram-negative pneumonia/sepsis and opportunistic infections, like pulmonary aspergillosis and cytomegalovirus pneumonitis.

Similarly, lung transplant recipients with TBD remain at higher risk for herpes viridae infections due to T-cell immunodeficiency [86]. Recipients of lung transplants with IPF and TBD have a risk that is up to five times higher for recurring CMV viremia [77]. These patients are also at higher risk of CMV end-organ disease compared to age-matched controls with and without IPF [77]. Simultaneously, multiple factors can make the treatment of CMV viremia more complex in this group. Lung transplant recipients with TBD are prone to CMV drug resistance and may experience bone marrow suppression as a side effect of antiviral drugs such as ganciclovir and valganciclovir. The use of alternative treatments such as foscarnet or cidofovir can be restricted in some circumstances due to their side effects like kidney and bone marrow suppression and poor tolerance. Letermovir, a new anti-CMV medication, targets the viral terminase complex, which is involved in the latter stages of the viral replication process. It has received approval for preventing CMV infection in allogenic stem cell transplants. Letermovir was examined for off-label use in preventing CMV in thoracic transplant patients, including 37 individuals who had lung transplants, and it was found to be both safe and successful [87]. Letermovir was used as primary prophylaxis in 62% and secondary prophylaxis in 38% of the patients due to myelosuppression or prior CMV resistance. Adverse effects such as myelosuppression, nausea, and lightheadedness required the cessation of letermovir in 12% of the patients. There were 12 episodes of low-level CMV DNAemia that did not require letermovir cessation and only 1 episode of clinically significant breakthrough CMV infection [87]. Additional research is needed to ascertain whether letermovir could be effective for CMV prevention, particularly in lung transplant recipients with TBD.

Iasella et al. found that lung transplant recipients with IPF were at a higher risk of developing post-transplant lymphoproliferative disorder associated with the Epstein–Barr virus (EBV), which they hypothesized was due to immune dysfunction related to short telomeres [88].

When designing care protocols to manage lung transplant recipients with TBD, consultation with transplant infectious disease physicians to consider alternative agents to prevent and manage infections is imperative. Lifelong CMV/HSV and antifungal prophylaxis and prolonged durations of antimicrobial therapy for other infections may be considered.

10. Liver Disease and Cirrhosis

Approximately 10% of patients with short telomeres have been reported to have liver abnormalities. Severe short telomere syndrome is typically associated with a classic triad of IPF, liver disease, and bone marrow failure [88]. Several case studies have reported successful early outcomes for patients with TBD who have undergone combined liver and lung transplants due to end-stage IPF and cirrhosis [89,90]. It is advised to conduct early screening for liver dysfunction in patients identified with short telomere length before the transplant period. Continued surveillance for liver disease with appropriate laboratory evaluation, imaging, and hepatology evaluation should be carried out in the post-transplant period.

11. Other Complications

Lung transplant recipients with TBD have been described to have a higher incidence of renal dysfunction after transplantation. Tokman et al. described outcomes in 14 lung transplant recipients with telomerase mutations, of which more than half developed acute renal failure, and 83% of the recipients developed chronic renal insufficiency during 3 years of follow-up [75]. Kidney biopsies from patients needing extended dialysis revealed tubular abnormalities and epithelial cell vacuolization, which are strongly indicative of toxicity from calcineurin inhibitors [78]. These findings suggest that lung transplant recipients with TBD may be more susceptible to the nephrotoxic effects of calcineurin inhibitors. It is plausible that patients with subclinical liver disease are prone to reduced clearance, as calcineurin inhibitors are metabolized by the hepatic p450 enzyme.

Gastrointestinal bleeding requiring blood transfusions was reported in more than one-third of lung transplant recipients with TBD in the cohort described by Silhan and colleagues [78]. Interestingly, in one of the patients, the bleeding was secondary to ischemic colitis with histopathologic findings documented in telomere-related enteropathy [78].

12. Comprehensive Care of Lung Transplant Recipients with Telomere Biology Disorders

Before transplantation, it might be justified to establish a diagnosis of underlying TBD due to the frequency of TBD in lung transplant recipients, potential post-transplant complications, and the need to alter post-transplant protocols. Recognizing short telomeres may enable the development of methods to avoid permanent complications of short telomere syndrome in patients who have undergone lung transplants. Tables 2 and 3 provide a suggested multidisciplinary team evaluation of STS in the pre- and post-transplant period. A multidisciplinary approach will help facilitate early diagnosis with screening protocols, early genetic counselling, and risk stratification and mitigation strategies such as induction protocols, modified immunosuppression protocols, and assessments for dual organ transplantation.

Table 2. Comprehensive pre-transplant care of lung transplant recipients with telomere biology disorders.

Consult to hematology to evaluate cytopenias and need for bone marrow biopsy
Consult to genetic counselling for assessment of familial risk of telomere biology disorder
Consult to hepatology for evaluation of liver dysfunction, appropriate imaging, and need for liver transplantation
Consult to infectious disease for counselling regarding infectious risks and to determine perioperative antibiotic choice and duration
Determine surgical feasibility of bronchial artery revascularization at time of lung transplant surgery to decrease risk of airway complications
If lung transplant candidate with telomere biology disorder is CMV IgG negative and stable, it would be ideal to consider CMV-negative donor, if possible

Table 3. Comprehensive post-transplant care of lung transplant recipients with telomere biology disorders.

Immunosuppression modification: avoid antimetabolite use, early reduction in steroid dose
Early initiation of antifungal and antiviral prophylaxis
Seek advice from infectious disease specialist for handling antimicrobial and antiviral prophylaxis in context of cytopenias
Consult to hematology to evaluate cytopenias and need for bone marrow biopsy
Consult to interventional bronchoscopy for expeditious management of airway complications
Consult to hepatology for continued surveillance of liver dysfunction
Age-appropriate cancer screening and yearly dermatology evaluation for skin cancer assessment

13. Conclusions

Telomeres and their associated proteins are essential for maintaining the telomere length in dividing cells, preventing cellular senescence and cell death. A number of mutations in the components of the telomerase complex, the shelterin complex, and other associated proteins have been implicated in the development of IPF and other ILDs. Approximately 25% of familial cases and 1–3% of sporadic IPF cases have been found to have telomere-related mutations. They have also been described in cases of ILD, such as in rheumatoid arthritis and hypersensitivity pneumonitis. Currently there is no available treatment for TBDs other than transplanting the affected organ, although studies are ongoing using molecules that lengthen the telomere or enhance telomerase activity. There has been an increasing interest in the impact of telomere length in lung transplant recipients. Telomere length could potentially be used as a pre-transplant biomarker to evaluate the risk of outcomes after transplantation. Nonetheless, one should be cautious when interpreting the limited and inconsistent evidence from a series of studies conducted at a single center. It is not adequate to disqualify lung transplant recipients from listing solely based on the length of their telomeres. There remain significant unknowns regarding standardizing the approach to care in this patient population. It is clear, however, that the complexity of these patients necessitates a comprehensive multidisciplinary approach to the pre- and post-lung-transplant care of this patient population.

Funding: This research received no external funding.

Conflicts of Interest: The authors declare no conflict of interest.

References

1. Turner, K.J.; Vasu, V.; Griffin, D.K. Telomere Biology and Human Phenotype. *Cells* **2019**, *8*, 73. [CrossRef] [PubMed]
2. Murray, A.W.; Szostak, J.W. Construction of artificial chromosomes in yeast. *Nature* **1983**, *305*, 189–193. [CrossRef] [PubMed]
3. Greider, C.W.; Blackburn, E.H. Identification of a specific telomere terminal transferase activity in Tetrahymena extracts. *Cell* **1985**, *43*, 405–413. [CrossRef] [PubMed]
4. Walter, J.E.; Armanios, M.; Shah, U.; Friedmann, A.M.; Spitzer, T.; Sharatz, S.M.; Hagen, C. CASE RECORDS of the MASSACHUSETTS GENERAL HOSPITAL. Case 41-2015. A 14-Year-Old Boy with Immune and Liver Abnormalities. *N. Engl. J. Med.* **2015**, *373*, 2664–2676. [CrossRef]
5. Gaysinskaya, V.; Stanley, S.E.; Adam, S.; Armanios, M. Synonymous Mutation in DKC1 Causes Telomerase RNA Insufficiency Manifesting as Familial Pulmonary Fibrosis. *Chest* **2020**, *158*, 2449–2457. [CrossRef] [PubMed]
6. Armanios, M.Y.; Chen, J.J.; Cogan, J.D.; Alder, J.K.; Ingersoll, R.G.; Markin, C.; Lawson, W.E.; Xie, M.; Vulto, I.; Phillips, J.A., 3rd; et al. Telomerase mutations in families with idiopathic pulmonary fibrosis. *N. Engl. J. Med.* **2007**, *356*, 1317–1326. [CrossRef]
7. Mir, S.M.; Samavarchi Tehrani, S.; Goodarzi, G.; Jamalpoor, Z.; Asadi, J.; Khelghati, N.; Qujeq, D.; Maniati, M. Shelterin Complex at Telomeres: Implications in Ageing. *Clin. Interv. Aging* **2020**, *15*, 827–839. [CrossRef] [PubMed]
8. Garus, A.; Autexier, C. Dyskerin: An essential pseudouridine synthase with multifaceted roles in ribosome biogenesis, splicing, and telomere maintenance. *RNA* **2021**, *27*, 1441–1458. [CrossRef]
9. Hourvitz, N.; Awad, A.; Tzfati, Y. The many faces of the helicase RTEL1 at telomeres and beyond. *Trends Cell Biol.* **2024**, *34*, 109–121. [CrossRef]
10. Moon, D.H.; Segal, M.; Boyraz, B.; Guinan, E.; Hofmann, I.; Cahan, P.; Tai, A.K.; Agarwal, S. Poly(A)-specific ribonuclease (PARN) mediates 3′-end maturation of the telomerase RNA component. *Nat. Genet.* **2015**, *47*, 1482–1488. [CrossRef] [PubMed]
11. Tsakiri, K.D.; Cronkhite, J.T.; Kuan, P.J.; Xing, C.; Raghu, G.; Weissler, J.C.; Rosenblatt, R.L.; Shay, J.W.; Garcia, C.K. Adult-onset pulmonary fibrosis caused by mutations in telomerase. *Proc. Natl. Acad. Sci. USA* **2007**, *104*, 7552–7557. [CrossRef] [PubMed]
12. Alder, J.K.; Stanley, S.E.; Wagner, C.L.; Hamilton, M.; Hanumanthu, V.S.; Armanios, M. Exome sequencing identifies mutant TINF2 in a family with pulmonary fibrosis. *Chest* **2015**, *147*, 1361–1368. [CrossRef] [PubMed]
13. Kannengiesser, C.; Borie, R.; Ménard, C.; Réocreux, M.; Nitschké, P.; Gazal, S.; Mal, H.; Taillé, C.; Cadranel, J.; Nunes, H.; et al. Heterozygous RTEL1 mutations are associated with familial pulmonary fibrosis. *Eur. Respir. J.* **2015**, *46*, 474–485. [CrossRef] [PubMed]
14. Stuart, B.D.; Choi, J.; Zaidi, S.; Xing, C.; Holohan, B.; Chen, R.; Choi, M.; Dharwadkar, P.; Torres, F.; Girod, C.E.; et al. Exome sequencing links mutations in PARN and RTEL1 with familial pulmonary fibrosis and telomere shortening. *Nat. Genet.* **2015**, *47*, 512–517. [CrossRef] [PubMed]
15. Richards, L.A.; Kumari, A.; Knezevic, K.; Thoms, J.A.; von Jonquieres, G.; Napier, C.E.; Ali, Z.; O'Brien, R.; Marks-Bluth, J.; Maritz, M.F.; et al. DKC1 is a transcriptional target of GATA1 and drives upregulation of telomerase activity in normal human erythroblasts. *Haematologica* **2020**, *105*, 1517–1526. [CrossRef]

16. Kan, G.; Wang, Z.; Sheng, C.; Yao, C.; Mao, Y.; Chen, S. Inhibition of DKC1 induces telomere-related senescence and apoptosis in lung adenocarcinoma. *J. Transl. Med.* **2021**, *19*, 161. [CrossRef] [PubMed]
17. Wu, S.; Ge, Y.; Lin, K.; Liu, Q.; Zhou, H.; Hu, Q.; Zhao, Y.; He, W.; Ju, Z. Telomerase RNA TERC and the PI3K-AKT pathway form a positive feedback loop to regulate cell proliferation independent of telomerase activity. *Nucleic Acids Res.* **2022**, *50*, 3764–3776. [CrossRef]
18. Goldman, F.; Bouarich, R.; Kulkarni, S.; Freeman, S.; Du, H.Y.; Harrington, L.; Mason, P.J.; Londoño-Vallejo, A.; Bessler, M. The effect of TERC haploinsufficiency on the inheritance of telomere length. *Proc. Natl. Acad. Sci. USA* **2005**, *102*, 17119–17124. [CrossRef]
19. Fernández-Varas, B.; Manguan-García, C.; Rodriguez-Centeno, J.; Mendoza-Lupiáñez, L.; Calatayud, J.; Perona, R.; Martín-Martínez, M.; Gutierrez-Rodriguez, M.; Benítez-Buelga, C.; Sastre, L. Clinical mutations in the TERT and TERC genes coding for telomerase components induced oxidative stress, DNA damage at telomeres and cell apoptosis besides decreased telomerase activity. *Human. Mol. Genet.* **2024**, *33*, 818–834. [CrossRef]
20. Min, J.; Shay, J.W. TERT Promoter Mutations Enhance Telomerase Activation by Long-Range Chromatin Interactions. *Cancer Discov.* **2016**, *6*, 1212–1214. [CrossRef] [PubMed]
21. Ibáñez-Cabellos, J.S.; Pérez-Machado, G.; Seco-Cervera, M.; Berenguer-Pascual, E.; García-Giménez, J.L.; Pallardó, F.V. Acute telomerase components depletion triggers oxidative stress as an early event previous to telomeric shortening. *Redox Biol.* **2018**, *14*, 398–408. [CrossRef] [PubMed]
22. Vulliamy, T.; Beswick, R.; Kirwan, M.; Marrone, A.; Digweed, M.; Walne, A.; Dokal, I. Mutations in the telomerase component NHP2 cause the premature ageing syndrome dyskeratosis congenita. *Proc. Natl. Acad. Sci. USA* **2008**, *105*, 8073–8078. [CrossRef]
23. Schmutz, I.; Mensenkamp, A.R.; Takai, K.K.; Haadsma, M.; Spruijt, L.; de Voer, R.M.; Choo, S.S.; Lorbeer, F.K.; van Grinsven, E.J.; Hockemeyer, D.; et al. TINF2 is a haploinsufficient tumor suppressor that limits telomere length. *eLife* **2020**, *9*, e61235. [CrossRef]
24. Choo, S.; Lorbeer, F.K.; Regalado, S.G.; Short, S.B.; Wu, S.; Rieser, G.; Bertuch, A.A.; Hockemeyer, D. Editing TINF2 as a potential therapeutic approach to restore telomere length in dyskeratosis congenita. *Blood* **2022**, *140*, 608–618. [CrossRef] [PubMed]
25. Ding, H.; Schertzer, M.; Wu, X.; Gertsenstein, M.; Selig, S.; Kammori, M.; Pourvali, R.; Poon, S.; Vulto, I.; Chavez, E.; et al. Regulation of Murine Telomere Length by Rtel: An Essential Gene Encoding a Helicase-like Protein. *Cell* **2004**, *117*, 873–886. [CrossRef]
26. Vannier, J.-B.; Pavicic-Kaltenbrunner, V.; Petalcorin, M.I.R.; Ding, H.; Boulton, S.J. RTEL1 Dismantles T Loops and Counteracts Telomeric G4-DNA to Maintain Telomere Integrity. *Cell* **2012**, *149*, 795–806. [CrossRef] [PubMed]
27. Hassani, M.A.; Murid, J.; Yan, J. Regulator of telomere elongation helicase 1 gene and its association with malignancy. *Cancer Rep. (Hoboken)* **2023**, *6*, e1735. [CrossRef] [PubMed]
28. Benyelles, M.; Episkopou, H.; O'Donohue, M.F.; Kermasson, L.; Frange, P.; Poulain, F.; Burcu Belen, F.; Polat, M.; Bole-Feysot, C.; Langa-Vives, F.; et al. Impaired telomere integrity and rRNA biogenesis in PARN-deficient patients and knock-out models. *EMBO Mol. Med.* **2019**, *11*, e10201. [CrossRef] [PubMed]
29. Corbett, A.H.; Fasken, M.B. A-Tail of Telomerase RNA Maturation. *Mol. Cell* **2019**, *74*, 635–636. [CrossRef] [PubMed]
30. Townsley, D.M.; Dumitriu, B.; Young, N.S. Bone marrow failure and the telomeropathies. *Blood* **2014**, *124*, 2775–2783. [CrossRef]
31. Stanley, S.E.; Merck, S.J.; Armanios, M. Telomerase and the Genetics of Emphysema Susceptibility. Implications for Pathogenesis Paradigms and Patient Care. *Ann. Am. Thorac. Soc.* **2016**, *13* (Suppl. S5), S447–S451. [CrossRef]
32. Nault, J.-C.; Ningarhari, M.; Rebouissou, S.; Zucman-Rossi, J. The role of telomeres and telomerase in cirrhosis and liver cancer. *Nat. Rev. Gastroenterol. Hepatol.* **2019**, *16*, 544–558. [CrossRef] [PubMed]
33. Wang, C.; Bi, L.; Du, Y.; Lu, C.; Zhao, M.; Lin, X.; Ding, Y.; Fan, W. The role of telomerase in hair growth and relevant disorders: A review. *J. Cosmet. Dermatol.* **2023**, *22*, 2925–2929. [CrossRef]
34. Niknafs, A.M.; Savage, S.A.; Niewisch, M.R.; Giri, N. Avascular Necrosis and Minimal Trauma Bone Fractures in Patients with Dyskeratosis Congenita. *Blood* **2022**, *140*, 2947–2948. [CrossRef]
35. Song, W.; Yang, J.; Niu, Z. Association of periodontitis with leukocyte telomere length in US adults: A cross-sectional analysis of NHANES 1999 to 2002. *J. Periodontol.* **2021**, *92*, 833–843. [CrossRef] [PubMed]
36. Maciejowski, J.; de Lange, T. Telomeres in cancer: Tumour suppression and genome instability. *Nat. Rev. Mol. Cell Biol.* **2017**, *18*, 175–186. [CrossRef]
37. Revy, P.; Kannengiesser, C.; Bertuch, A.A. Genetics of human telomere biology disorders. *Nat. Rev. Genet.* **2023**, *24*, 86–108. [CrossRef]
38. Vulliamy, T.; Marrone, A.; Szydlo, R.; Walne, A.; Mason, P.J.; Dokal, I. Disease anticipation is associated with progressive telomere shortening in families with dyskeratosis congenita due to mutations in TERC. *Nat. Genet.* **2004**, *36*, 447–449. [CrossRef]
39. Alder, J.K.; Cogan, J.D.; Brown, A.F.; Anderson, C.J.; Lawson, W.E.; Lansdorp, P.M.; Phillips, J.A., 3rd; Loyd, J.E.; Chen, J.J.; Armanios, M. Ancestral mutation in telomerase causes defects in repeat addition processivity and manifests as familial pulmonary fibrosis. *PLoS Genet.* **2011**, *7*, e1001352. [CrossRef] [PubMed]

40. van der Vis, J.J.; van der Smagt, J.J.; van Batenburg, A.A.; Goldschmeding, R.; van Es, H.W.; Grutters, J.C.; van Moorsel, C.H.M. Pulmonary fibrosis in non-mutation carriers of families with short telomere syndrome gene mutations. *Respirology* **2021**, *26*, 1160–1170. [CrossRef]
41. Blasco, M.A.; Lee, H.W.; Hande, M.P.; Samper, E.; Lansdorp, P.M.; DePinho, R.A.; Greider, C.W. Telomere shortening and tumor formation by mouse cells lacking telomerase RNA. *Cell* **1997**, *91*, 25–34. [CrossRef] [PubMed]
42. Strong, M.A.; Vidal-Cardenas, S.L.; Karim, B.; Yu, H.; Guo, N.; Greider, C.W. Phenotypes in mTERT$^{+}/^{-}$ and mTERT$^{-}/^{-}$ mice are due to short telomeres, not telomere-independent functions of telomerase reverse transcriptase. *Mol. Cell. Biol.* **2011**, *31*, 2369–2379. [CrossRef]
43. Mangaonkar, A.A.; Patnaik, M.M. Short Telomere Syndromes in Clinical Practice: Bridging Bench and Bedside. *Mayo Clin. Proc.* **2018**, *93*, 904–916. [CrossRef]
44. Baerlocher, G.M.; Vulto, I.; de Jong, G.; Lansdorp, P.M. Flow cytometry and FISH to measure the average length of telomeres (flow FISH). *Nat. Protoc.* **2006**, *1*, 2365–2376. [CrossRef] [PubMed]
45. Hutchinson, J.; Fogarty, A.; Hubbard, R.; McKeever, T. Global incidence and mortality of idiopathic pulmonary fibrosis: A systematic review. *Eur. Respir. J.* **2015**, *46*, 795–806. [CrossRef]
46. Dokal, I. Dyskeratosis congenita in all its forms. *Br. J. Haematol.* **2000**, *110*, 768–779. [CrossRef]
47. Molina-Molina, M.; Borie, R. Clinical implications of telomere dysfunction in lung fibrosis. *Curr. Opin. Pulm. Med.* **2018**, *24*, 440–444. [CrossRef] [PubMed]
48. Cronkhite, J.T.; Xing, C.; Raghu, G.; Chin, K.M.; Torres, F.; Rosenblatt, R.L.; Garcia, C.K. Telomere shortening in familial and sporadic pulmonary fibrosis. *Am. J. Respir. Crit. Care Med.* **2008**, *178*, 729–737. [CrossRef] [PubMed]
49. Alder, J.K.; Chen, J.J.; Lancaster, L.; Danoff, S.; Su, S.C.; Cogan, J.D.; Vulto, I.; Xie, M.; Qi, X.; Tuder, R.M.; et al. Short telomeres are a risk factor for idiopathic pulmonary fibrosis. *Proc. Natl. Acad. Sci. USA* **2008**, *105*, 13051–13056. [CrossRef] [PubMed]
50. Haycock, P.C.; Burgess, S.; Nounu, A.; Zheng, J.; Okoli, G.N.; Bowden, J.; Wade, K.H.; Timpson, N.J.; Evans, D.M.; Willeit, P.; et al. Association Between Telomere Length and Risk of Cancer and Non-Neoplastic Diseases: A Mendelian Randomization Study. *JAMA Oncol.* **2017**, *3*, 636–651. [CrossRef]
51. Newton, C.A.; Batra, K.; Torrealba, J.; Kozlitina, J.; Glazer, C.S.; Aravena, C.; Meyer, K.; Raghu, G.; Collard, H.R.; Garcia, C.K. Telomere-related lung fibrosis is diagnostically heterogeneous but uniformly progressive. *Eur. Respir. J.* **2016**, *48*, 1710–1720. [CrossRef] [PubMed]
52. Šelb, J.; Osolnik, K.; Kern, I.; Korošec, P.; Rijavec, M. Utility of Telomerase Gene Mutation Testing in Patients with Idiopathic Pulmonary Fibrosis in Routine Practice. *Cells* **2022**, *11*, 372. [CrossRef]
53. Dressen, A.; Abbas, A.R.; Cabanski, C.; Reeder, J.; Ramalingam, T.R.; Neighbors, M.; Bhangale, T.R.; Brauer, M.J.; Hunkapiller, J.; Reeder, J.; et al. Analysis of protein-altering variants in telomerase genes and their association with MUC5B common variant status in patients with idiopathic pulmonary fibrosis: A candidate gene sequencing study. *Lancet Respir. Med.* **2018**, *6*, 603–614. [CrossRef] [PubMed]
54. Newton, C.A.; Zhang, D.; Oldham, J.M.; Kozlitina, J.; Ma, S.F.; Martinez, F.J.; Raghu, G.; Noth, I.; Garcia, C.K. Telomere Length and Use of Immunosuppressive Medications in Idiopathic Pulmonary Fibrosis. *Am. J. Respir. Crit. Care Med.* **2019**, *200*, 336–347. [CrossRef]
55. Courtwright, A.M.; El-Chemaly, S. Telomeres in Interstitial Lung Disease: The Short and the Long of It. *Ann. Am. Thorac. Soc.* **2019**, *16*, 175–181. [CrossRef] [PubMed]
56. Juge, P.A.; Borie, R.; Kannengiesser, C.; Gazal, S.; Revy, P.; Wemeau-Stervinou, L.; Debray, M.P.; Ottaviani, S.; Marchand-Adam, S.; Nathan, N.; et al. Shared genetic predisposition in rheumatoid arthritis-interstitial lung disease and familial pulmonary fibrosis. *Eur. Respir. J.* **2017**, *49*, 1602314. [CrossRef] [PubMed]
57. Adegunsoye, A.; Morisset, J.; Newton, C.A.; Oldham, J.M.; Vittinghoff, E.; Linderholm, A.L.; Strek, M.E.; Noth, I.; Garcia, C.K.; Wolters, P.J.; et al. Leukocyte telomere length and mycophenolate therapy in chronic hypersensitivity pneumonitis. *Eur. Respir. J.* **2021**, *57*, 2002872. [CrossRef]
58. Ley, B.; Newton, C.A.; Arnould, I.; Elicker, B.M.; Henry, T.S.; Vittinghoff, E.; Golden, J.A.; Jones, K.D.; Batra, K.; Torrealba, J.; et al. The MUC5B promoter polymorphism and telomere length in patients with chronic hypersensitivity pneumonitis: An observational cohort-control study. *Lancet Respir. Med.* **2017**, *5*, 639–647. [CrossRef] [PubMed]
59. Newton, C.A.; Oldham, J.M.; Ley, B.; Anand, V.; Adegunsoye, A.; Liu, G.; Batra, K.; Torrealba, J.; Kozlitina, J.; Glazer, C.; et al. Telomere length and genetic variant associations with interstitial lung disease progression and survival. *Eur. Respir. J.* **2019**, *53*, 1801641. [CrossRef]
60. Ley, B.; Liu, S.; Elicker, B.M.; Henry, T.S.; Vittinghoff, E.; Golden, J.A.; Jones, K.D.; Wolters, P.J. Telomere length in patients with unclassifiable interstitial lung disease: A cohort study. *Eur. Respir. J.* **2020**, *56*, 2000268. [CrossRef] [PubMed]
61. Townsley, D.M.; Dumitriu, B.; Liu, D.; Biancotto, A.; Weinstein, B.; Chen, C.; Hardy, N.; Mihalek, A.D.; Lingala, S.; Kim, Y.J.; et al. Danazol Treatment for Telomere Diseases. *N. Engl. J. Med.* **2016**, *374*, 1922–1931. [CrossRef]

62. Hoffman, T.W.; van Moorsel, C.H.M.; van der Vis, J.J.; Biesma, D.H.; Grutters, J.C. No effect of danazol treatment in patients with advanced idiopathic pulmonary fibrosis. *ERJ Open Res.* **2023**, *9*, 00131–02023. [CrossRef] [PubMed]
63. Nagpal, N.; Wang, J.; Zeng, J.; Lo, E.; Moon, D.H.; Luk, K.; Braun, R.O.; Burroughs, L.M.; Keel, S.B.; Reilly, C.; et al. Small-Molecule PAPD5 Inhibitors Restore Telomerase Activity in Patient Stem Cells. *Cell Stem Cell* **2020**, *26*, 896–909.e8. [CrossRef] [PubMed]
64. Tefferi, A.; Lasho, T.L.; Begna, K.H.; Patnaik, M.M.; Zblewski, D.L.; Finke, C.M.; Laborde, R.R.; Wassie, E.; Schimek, L.; Hanson, C.A.; et al. A Pilot Study of the Telomerase Inhibitor Imetelstat for Myelofibrosis. *N. Engl. J. Med.* **2015**, *373*, 908–919. [CrossRef] [PubMed]
65. Chiappori, A.A.; Kolevska, T.; Spigel, D.R.; Hager, S.; Rarick, M.; Gadgeel, S.; Blais, N.; Von Pawel, J.; Hart, L.; Reck, M.; et al. A randomized phase II study of the telomerase inhibitor imetelstat as maintenance therapy for advanced non-small-cell lung cancer. *Ann. Oncol.* **2015**, *26*, 354–362. [CrossRef]
66. Povedano, J.M.; Martinez, P.; Serrano, R.; Tejera, Á.; Gómez-López, G.; Bobadilla, M.; Flores, J.M.; Bosch, F.; Blasco, M.A. Therapeutic effects of telomerase in mice with pulmonary fibrosis induced by damage to the lungs and short telomeres. *eLife* **2018**, *7*, e31299. [CrossRef]
67. Piñeiro-Hermida, S.; Autilio, C.; Martínez, P.; Bosch, F.; Pérez-Gil, J.; Blasco, M.A. Telomerase treatment prevents lung profibrotic pathologies associated with physiological aging. *J. Cell Biol.* **2020**, *219*, e202002120. [CrossRef]
68. King, T.E., Jr.; Bradford, W.Z.; Castro-Bernardini, S.; Fagan, E.A.; Glaspole, I.; Glassberg, M.K.; Gorina, E.; Hopkins, P.M.; Kardatzke, D.; Lancaster, L.; et al. A phase 3 trial of pirfenidone in patients with idiopathic pulmonary fibrosis. *N. Engl. J. Med.* **2014**, *370*, 2083–2092. [CrossRef] [PubMed]
69. Richeldi, L.; du Bois, R.M.; Raghu, G.; Azuma, A.; Brown, K.K.; Costabel, U.; Cottin, V.; Flaherty, K.R.; Hansell, D.M.; Inoue, Y.; et al. Efficacy and safety of nintedanib in idiopathic pulmonary fibrosis. *N. Engl. J. Med.* **2014**, *370*, 2071–2082. [CrossRef] [PubMed]
70. Flaherty, K.R.; Wells, A.U.; Cottin, V.; Devaraj, A.; Walsh, S.L.F.; Inoue, Y.; Richeldi, L.; Kolb, M.; Tetzlaff, K.; Stowasser, S.; et al. Nintedanib in Progressive Fibrosing Interstitial Lung Diseases. *N. Engl. J. Med.* **2019**, *381*, 1718–1727. [CrossRef] [PubMed]
71. Justet, A.; Klay, D.; Porcher, R.; Cottin, V.; Ahmad, K.; Molina Molina, M.; Nunes, H.; Reynaud-Gaubert, M.; Naccache, J.M.; Manali, E.; et al. Safety and efficacy of pirfenidone and nintedanib in patients with idiopathic pulmonary fibrosis and carrying a telomere-related gene mutation. *Eur. Respir. J.* **2021**, *57*, 2003198. [CrossRef]
72. Justet, A.; Thabut, G.; Manali, E.; Molina Molina, M.; Kannengiesser, C.; Cadranel, J.; Cottin, V.; Gondouin, A.; Nunes, H.; Magois, E.; et al. Safety and efficacy of pirfenidone in patients carrying telomerase complex mutation. *Eur. Respir. J.* **2018**, *51*, 1701875. [CrossRef] [PubMed]
73. Alder, J.K.; Sutton, R.M.; Iasella, C.J.; Nouraie, M.; Koshy, R.; Hannan, S.J.; Chan, E.G.; Chen, X.; Zhang, Y.; Brown, M.; et al. Lung transplantation for idiopathic pulmonary fibrosis enriches for individuals with telomere-mediated disease. *J. Heart Lung Transplant.* **2022**, *41*, 654–663. [CrossRef] [PubMed]
74. Newton, C.A.; Kozlitina, J.; Lines, J.R.; Kaza, V.; Torres, F.; Garcia, C.K. Telomere length in patients with pulmonary fibrosis associated with chronic lung allograft dysfunction and post-lung transplantation survival. *J. Heart Lung Transplant.* **2017**, *36*, 845–853. [CrossRef]
75. Tokman, S.; Singer, J.P.; Devine, M.S.; Westall, G.P.; Aubert, J.D.; Tamm, M.; Snell, G.I.; Lee, J.S.; Goldberg, H.J.; Kukreja, J.; et al. Clinical outcomes of lung transplant recipients with telomerase mutations. *J. Heart Lung Transplant.* **2015**, *34*, 1318–1324. [CrossRef] [PubMed]
76. Borie, R.; Kannengiesser, C.; Hirschi, S.; Le Pavec, J.; Mal, H.; Bergot, E.; Jouneau, S.; Naccache, J.M.; Revy, P.; Boutboul, D.; et al. Severe hematologic complications after lung transplantation in patients with telomerase complex mutations. *J. Heart Lung Transplant.* **2015**, *34*, 538–546. [CrossRef] [PubMed]
77. Popescu, I.; Mannem, H.; Winters, S.A.; Hoji, A.; Silveira, F.; McNally, E.; Pipeling, M.R.; Lendermon, E.A.; Morrell, M.R.; Pilewski, J.M.; et al. Impaired Cytomegalovirus Immunity in Idiopathic Pulmonary Fibrosis Lung Transplant Recipients with Short Telomeres. *Am. J. Respir. Crit. Care Med.* **2019**, *199*, 362–376. [CrossRef]
78. Silhan, L.L.; Shah, P.D.; Chambers, D.C.; Snyder, L.D.; Riise, G.C.; Wagner, C.L.; Hellström-Lindberg, E.; Orens, J.B.; Mewton, J.F.; Danoff, S.K.; et al. Lung transplantation in telomerase mutation carriers with pulmonary fibrosis. *Eur. Respir. J.* **2014**, *44*, 178–187. [CrossRef] [PubMed]
79. Courtwright, A.M.; Lamattina, A.M.; Takahashi, M.; Trindade, A.J.; Hunninghake, G.M.; Rosas, I.O.; Agarwal, S.; Raby, B.A.; Goldberg, H.J.; El-Chemaly, S. Shorter telomere length following lung transplantation is associated with clinically significant leukopenia and decreased chronic lung allograft dysfunction-free survival. *ERJ Open Res.* **2020**, *6*. [CrossRef] [PubMed]
80. Snyder, M.E.; Anderson, M.R.; Benvenuto, L.J.; Sutton, R.M.; Bondonese, A.; Koshy, R.; Burke, R.; Clifford, S.; Craig, A.; Iasella, C.J.; et al. Impact of age and telomere length on circulating T cells and rejection risk after lung transplantation for idiopathic pulmonary fibrosis. *J. Heart Lung Transplant.* **2023**, *42*, 1666–1677. [CrossRef] [PubMed]

81. Choi, B.; Messika, J.; Courtwright, A.; Mornex, J.F.; Hirschi, S.; Roux, A.; Le Pavec, J.; Quêtant, S.; Froidure, A.; Lazor, R.; et al. Airway complications in lung transplant recipients with telomere-related interstitial lung disease. *Clin. Transplant.* **2022**, *36*, e14552. [CrossRef] [PubMed]
82. Pettersson, G.B.; Karam, K.; Thuita, L.; Johnston, D.R.; McCurry, K.R.; Kapadia, S.R.; Budev, M.M.; Avery, R.K.; Mason, D.P.; Murthy, S.C.; et al. Comparative study of bronchial artery revascularization in lung transplantation. *J. Thorac. Cardiovasc. Surg.* **2013**, *146*, 894–900.e893. [CrossRef] [PubMed]
83. Yun, J.J.; Unai, S.; Pettersson, G. Lung transplant with bronchial arterial revascularization: Review of surgical technique and clinical outcomes. *J. Thorac. Dis.* **2019**, *11*, S1821–S1828. [CrossRef]
84. Hannan, S.J.; Iasella, C.J.; Sutton, R.M.; Popescu, I.D.; Koshy, R.; Burke, R.; Chen, X.; Zhang, Y.; Pilewski, J.M.; Hage, C.A.; et al. Lung transplant recipients with telomere-mediated pulmonary fibrosis have increased risk for hematologic complications. *Am. J. Transplant.* **2023**, *23*, 1590–1602. [CrossRef] [PubMed]
85. Schratz, K.E. Extrahematopoietic manifestations of the short telomere syndromes. *Hematol. Am. Soc. Hematol. Educ. Program.* **2020**, *2020*, 115–122. [CrossRef] [PubMed]
86. Kapse, B.; Budev, M.M.; Singer, J.P.; Greenland, J.R. Immune aging: Biological mechanisms, clinical symptoms, and management in lung transplant recipients. *Front. Transplant.* **2024**, *3*, 1356948. [CrossRef] [PubMed]
87. Saullo, J.L.; Baker, A.W.; Snyder, L.D.; Reynolds, J.M.; Zaffiri, L.; Eichenberger, E.M.; Ferrari, A.; Steinbrink, J.M.; Maziarz, E.K.; Bacchus, M.; et al. Cytomegalovirus prevention in thoracic organ transplantation: A single-center evaluation of letermovir prophylaxis. *J. Heart Lung Transplant.* **2022**, *41*, 508–515. [CrossRef] [PubMed]
88. Iasella, C.J.; Winters, S.A.; Kois, A.; Cho, J.; Hannan, S.J.; Koshy, R.; Moore, C.A.; Ensor, C.R.; Lendermon, E.A.; Morrell, M.R.; et al. Idiopathic pulmonary fibrosis lung transplant recipients are at increased risk for EBV-associated posttransplant lymphoproliferative disorder and worse survival. *Am. J. Transplant.* **2020**, *20*, 1439–1446. [CrossRef] [PubMed]
89. Lebeer, M.; Wuyts, W.A.; Cassiman, D.; Laleman, W.; Nevens, F.; Pirenne, J.; Monbaliu, D.; Roskams, T.; Verbeken, E.K.; Neyrinck, A.P.; et al. Multiple Solid Organ Transplantation in Telomeropathy: Case Series and Literature Review. *Transplantation* **2018**, *102*, 1747–1755. [CrossRef]
90. Moschouri, E.; Vionnet, J.; Giostra, E.; Daccord, C.; Lazor, R.; Sciarra, A.; Letovanec, I.; Sempoux, C.; Gonzalez, M.; Unger, S.; et al. Combined Lung and Liver Transplantation for Short Telomere Syndrome. *Liver Transpl.* **2020**, *26*, 840–844. [CrossRef]

Journal of
Clinical Medicine

MDPI

Brief Report

Improved Survival in Patients with Idiopathic Pulmonary Fibrosis Hospitalized for Acute Exacerbation

Federico Lionello, Giovanna Arcaro, Leonardo Bertagna De Marchi, Fausto Braccioni, Alessia Achille, Sara Lococo, Michele Ciresi, Gabriella Guarnieri and Andrea Vianello *

Department of Cardiac, Thoracic, Vascular Sciences and Public Health, University of Padova, via Giustiniani 2, 35128 Padova, Italy; federico.lionello@aopd.veneto.it (F.L.); giovanna.arcaro@aopd.veneto.it (G.A.); leonardo.bertagnademarchi@aopd.veneto.it (L.B.D.M.); fausto.braccioni@aopd.veneto.it (F.B.); alessia.achille@aopd.veneto.it (A.A.); sara.lococo@aopd.veneto.it (S.L.); michele.ciresi@aopd.veneto.it (M.C.); gabriella.guarnieri@unipd.it (G.G.)
* Correspondence: andrea.vianello@aopd.veneto.it; Tel.: +39-049-8218587; Fax: +39-049-8218590

Abstract: Background: Patients suffering from idiopathic pulmonary fibrosis (IPF) may experience acute exacerbation (AE-IPF), which frequently results in acute respiratory failure (ARF) requiring hospitalization. **Objective**: This study aims to determine if survival has improved over the last decade in patients hospitalized for ARF consequent to AE-IPF, in view of the progress recently made in pharmacological and supportive treatment strategies. **Methods**: This was an observational retrospective single-center study. The data of 14 patients admitted to an Intermediate Respiratory Care Unit (IRCU) between 1 January 2004 and 31 December 2013 (group A) were compared with those of 26 patients admitted between 1 January 2014 and 31 December 2023 (group B). This study's primary endpoint was survival following IRCU admission. **Results**: Survival time was significantly longer in the second group of patients compared to the first one [median survival time: 134 (31–257) vs. 25.5 (20–50) days; $p < 0.001$]. Group B patients also had a lower IRCU mortality rate (6/26 vs. 10/14; $p = 0.003$) and a significantly shorter stay in the IRCU [6 (1–60) vs. 14 (1–43) days; $p = 0.039$]. **Conclusions**: Innovative pharmacologic treatments and supportive therapeutic strategies are able to prolong survival and reduce the risk of in-hospital mortality in patients with AE-IPF hospitalized for ARF.

Keywords: idiopathic pulmonary fibrosis; acute exacerbation; nintedanib; pirfenidone; high-flow nasal oxygen; acute respiratory failure

1. Introduction

A rare disease of unknown etiology, idiopathic pulmonary fibrosis (IPF) is characterized by progressive, irreversible scarring of the lung interstitium, leading to respiratory function decline and early mortality [1]. During the course of the disease, patients suffering from IPF may experience acute exacerbation (AE-IPF), which often results in acute respiratory failure (ARF), requiring hospitalization [2]. Crucially, approximately one-half of patients hospitalized with AE-IPF do not survive [3], and those admitted to Intensive Care Units (ICUs) have a nearly 90% mortality rate [4]. Worth mentioning, survivors have a life-expectancy significantly shorter compared to patients with IPF who do not experience an AE, ranging between 15.5 and 36 months [2,5,6].

Although progress over the past twenty years in the development of pharmacologic and supportive treatments for IPF has not always been linear, growing evidence has been underlining an improved survival rate in patients experiencing acute exacerbation

(AE). Pirfenidone and nintedanib, respectively, approved for the treatment of IPF by the European Medicines Agency (EMA) in February 2011 and January 2015, have been associated with a decrease in in-hospital mortality [5–7]. Patients receiving pirfenidone were found, in fact, to have better three-month survival rate (55% vs. 34%) and a longer survival time (137.0 versus 16.0 days) compared to controls [7,8]. Moreover, subjects treated with nintedanib showed an in-hospital mortality rate significantly lower with respect to their counterparts (13.7% vs. 6.0%; OR: 0.43) [9].

The utilization of a corticosteroid and immunomodulator combination therapy was instead found to be associated with a worse prognosis during hospitalization [10] and discontinued after the ATS/ERS/JRS/ALAT released a consensus statement recommendation against its use in 2011 [5]. Several innovative supportive measures such as high-flow nasal oxygen (HFNO) therapy, extracorporeal membrane oxygenation (ECMO), and extracorporeal CO_2 removal ($ECCO_2R$), which were developed to improve oxygenation and reverse CO_2 retention in the event of ARF, have been linked to promising results [4,11,12]. In view of these considerations, the current study aimed to determine if survival has improved over the last decade in patients admitted to an Intermediate Respiratory Care Unit (IRCU) for ARF due to AE-IPF.

2. Methods

This observational retrospective single-center study was conducted in a tertiary teaching hospital located in Northeast Italy. At admission, all the study participants were asked to sign informed consent forms agreeing to the use of their de-identified clinical data for research, analysis, and reporting purposes. Ethical approval was waived by the facility's Institutional Review Committee in view of the fact that the study was retrospective in nature, and all the interventions prescribed were part of the hospital's internal protocols (No.: 2772-30 December 2022). This study was carried out in accordance with the Declaration of Helsinki of 1975.

2.1. Patients

All the patients with IPF and AE who were admitted to the IRCU of the University of Padua Medical Center between 1 January 2004 and 31 December 2023 for ARF were considered eligible for our study. The criteria for the patients' admission to our IRCU was failure of conventional O_2-therapy (COT) to maintain $SaO_2 \geq 92\%$. The patients' diagnoses of IPF formulated in accord with the criteria proposed by the ATS/ERS/JRS/ALAT consensus statement [5] and later updates [13] were confirmed. The patients' diagnoses of AE were confirmed in accordance with the recommendations of an international working group [14]. Patients who underwent lung transplant (LT) at a later date were excluded from this study.

The patients' medical records, including their medical histories, demographic and clinical characteristics, and laboratory and pulmonary function data, were retrieved, reviewed, and analyzed. Pulmonary function data were obtained from pulmonary function testing (PFT) carried out in the six months prior to IRCU admission. The patients were divided into 2 groups depending on the decade during which they were admitted to the IRCU [i.e., 1 January 2004–31 December 2013 = group A or 1 January 2014–31 December 2023 = group B]. Their outcomes, calculated on the basis of their clinical status parameters at the time they were discharged from the IRCU and at the end of the follow-up period, as well as the number of days they remained in the IRCU, were analyzed.

2.2. Interventions

Between 2004 and 2013, patients with IPF attending our Medical Center were generally prescribed immunosuppressive therapy in the absence of contraindications. The therapy was no longer utilized after the ATS/ERS/JRS/ALAT consensus guideline recommendations [5] were released in 2011. Pirfenidone and nintedanib, which were, respectively, approved for the treatment of IPF by the Italian Medicines Agency (AIFA) in June 2013 and April 2016, were accordingly routinely prescribed to our patients with IPF but always following a frank discussion regarding the drugs' potential side effects. High-dose corticosteroid therapy (prednisolone: 1 mg/kg/die) and broad-spectrum antibiotic regimens were administered to all the patients admitted to the IRCU over the entire study period.

COT, which was provided through standard non-rebreathing face masks, was the first-line supportive treatment that was utilized throughout the first decade of this study. In accordance with the center's standard protocol, non-invasive ventilation (NIV) was provided to patients with exacerbated IPF showing signs of respiratory muscle fatigue or severe hypoxemia [15]. In the presence of contraindications to a prolonged use of NIV, they were shifted to invasive mechanical ventilation (IMV) by endotracheal intubation (ETI) unless they had already expressed the decision not to be intubated. A step-by-step protocol including the use of high-flow nasal oxygen (HFNO) as a second-line therapy in hypoxemic patients not responding to COT has been followed in our center since May 2013 [12]. Elective intubation and IMV following HFNO failure were not situations that were considered by the current treatment algorithm. Only patients on a waiting list for lung transplant (LT) were eligible for extracorporeal membrane oxygenation (ECMO). The strategies utilized as supportive treatments over the two decades analyzed by this study are outlined in Table 1.

Table 1. Supportive treatments available to treat the patients admitted to the Respiratory Intermediate Care Unit during the two decades studied. ECMO was considered only for those patients on a waiting list for lung transplant. (COT = conventional oxygen therapy released through non-rebreathing face masks; $ECCO_2R$ = extracorporeal CO_2 removal; ECMO = extracorporeal membrane oxygenation; ETI = endotracheal intubation; HFNO = high-flow nasal oxygen; IMV = invasive mechanical ventilation; NIV = non-invasive ventilation; and RMF = respiratory muscle fatigue).

	Group A (Admission: 2004-13)	Group B (Admission: 2014-23)
First-line treatment	COT	COT
Refractory hypoxemia	NIV	HFNO
Hypercapnia, signs of RMF	NIV	NIV
NIV failure	IMV via ETI	$ECCO_2R$
HFNO failure	-	ECMO

2.3. *Study Endpoints and Statistical Analysis*

Survival following IRCU admission was considered the primary study endpoint. The mortality rate during the stay in the IRCU and the number of days in the IRCU were the secondary endpoints. The results were expressed, as appropriate, as mean values, ranges, and percentages. The continuous variables were compared, depending on the normality of the distributions, using Student's t test or the Mann–Whitney U test. The categorical variables were compared, as appropriate, using the Chi-squared test or Fisher's exact test. Survival from the time the patient was admitted to the IRCU was calculated using the Kaplan–Meier method; the log-rank test was used to compare the survival curves of the two groups. A bilateral p value < 0.05 was considered statistically significant for all the comparisons. All the statistical calculations were carried out using the Jamovy, Version 2.3, 2022 software.

3. Results

All forty-eight patients who were admitted to our IRCU with a diagnosis of AE-IPF during the study period (1 January 2004 to 31 December 2023) were considered eligible to participate in our retrospective study. The data of the eight patients who underwent LT at a later date were not included in the analysis. The age range of the patients included in the study was 44–83 years. Fourteen patients (group A) were admitted during the earlier decade and twenty-six (group B) during the later one. No group B patients had received immunosuppressive therapy before admission; meanwhile, six patients in group A had been administered azathioprine in combination with low-dose corticosteroids. Group B patients also showed better respiratory function (in particular, higher DLCO % values) (Table 2).

Table 2. Patients' baseline demographic, clinical, and pulmonary–cardiac function characteristics and laboratory data at the time of their admission to our Intermediate Respiratory Care Unit and their outcomes. (ACCI = Age-Adjusted Charlson Comorbidity Index; APACHE = Acute Physiology and Chronic Health Evaluation; BMI = body mass index; BNP = B-type natriuretic peptide; CRP = C-reactive protein; DLCO = diffusing capacity for carbon monoxide; FVC = forced vital capacity; FEV_1 = forced expiratory volume in the first second; GCS = Glasgow Coma Scale; IRCU = Intermediate Respiratory Care Unit; OCSs = oral corticosteroids; PaO_2/FiO_2 = ratio of arterial oxygen tension to inspired oxygen fraction; PCT = procalcitonin; and PH = pulmonary hypertension).

	Group A (Admission: 2004-13) (n = 14)	Group B (Admission: 2014-23) (n = 26)	*p* Value
Baseline demographic and clinical data			
Age (years), mean (range)	71.6 (10.8)	68.3 (10)	0.33
Gender (male/female)	7/7	21/5	0.55
BMI (kg/m^2), mean (range)	24.3 (3.2)	24.7 (3.1)	0.75
Smokers, n (%)	10 (71.4)	21 (80.8)	0.69
Length of time from diagnosis to IRCU admission (yrs), mean (range)	2.0 (0.2–6.0)	2.2 (0.0–9.0)	0.95
Pts with comorbidities, n (%)	11 (78.6)	24 (92.3)	0.32
ACCI score, median (range)	5 (1–6)	4 (2–12)	0.38
Pts with cancer disease, n (%)	2 (14.3)	2 (7.7)	0.50
Pts administered immunosuppressive therapy, n (%)	6 (42.8)	0 (0)	<0.001
Pts administered OCS therapy, n (%)	6 (42.8)	0 (0)	<0.001
Pts administered antifibrotic therapy, n (%)			
- Pirfenidone	0 (0)	11 (42.3)	<0.001
- Nintedanib	0 (0)	15 (57.7)	
Pts receiving home oxygen therapy, n (%)	7 (50)	14 (53.8)	0.71
FVC, L mean (range)	1.41 (0.73–2.94)	1.82 (0.95–2.75)	0.37
FVC, % mean (range)	51 (21–107)	55 (36–101)	0.99
FEV_1, L mean (range)	1.25 (0.72–2.70)	1.70 (0.91–2.66)	0.25
FEV_1, % mean (range)	63 (24–113)	68 (41–120)	0.92
DLCO, mL/min/mmHg, mean (range)	3.42 (1.04–13.00)	5.95 (2.33–8.38)	0.10
DLCO, % mean (range)	15 (5–51)	28 (11–49)	0.050
Pts with PH, n (%)	2 (14.3)	10 (38.5)	0.11
GAP Index, mean (range)	4 (2–7)	5 (1–7)	0.38
Clinical, laboratory, and blood gas data at the time of IRCU admission			
Respiratory rate (breaths/min), median (range)	32 (22–47)	25 (25–47)	0.003
Heart rate (beats/min), mean (range)	104 (86–170)	99 (58–130)	0.097
GCS media (range)	15 (12–15)	15 (12–15)	0.21

Table 2. *Cont.*

	Group A (Admission: 2004-13) (n = 14)	Group B (Admission: 2014-23) (n = 26)	*p* Value
Pts with fever (temperature > 38 °C), n (%)	6 (42.9)	5 (19.2)	0.11
Pts with leukocytosis (WBC > 12,000 × 10^6/L), n (%)	10 (71.4)	12 (46.2)	0.12
PaO_2 * (mmHg), mean (range)	64.8 (34.0–97.5)	80.0 (39.0–317)	0.051
$PaCO_2$ (mmHg), mean (range)	46.9 (25.3–90.0)	39.4 (27.5–82.3)	0.13
Arterial pH, mean (range)	7.40 (7.25–7.49)	7.42 (7.26–7.51)	0.56
PaO_2/FiO_2 (mmHg), median (range)	100 (35–268)	173 (46–421)	0.002
Pts with abnormal BNP level, n (%)	8 (57.1)	8 (30.8)	0.011
CRP (μg/mL), mean (range)	86.3 (2.9–181.0)	38.0 (2.1–395.0)	0.55
Pts with CRP level > 100 μg/mL, n (%)	4 (28.6)	1 (3.8)	0.042
Pts with PCT level > 0.5 μg/L, n (%)	1 (7.1)	4 (15.4)	0.92
APACHE score, median (range)	21 (14–26)	13 (5–33)	0.032
Clinical outcomes			
Patients who died during IRCU stay, n (%)	10 (71.4%)	6 (23.1)	0.003
Length of IRCU stay, days	14 (1–43)	6 (1–60)	0.039

* during supplemental O_2-therapy

In group B, 11 patients were receiving pirfenidone at the recommended full dosage, i.e., three times daily at oral doses of 801 mg, while 15 were administered nintedanib at the twice-daily oral dose of 150 mg, prior to being hospitalized, and that dosage was continued throughout the time they were hospitalized. Survivors continued to receive the treatment after discharge from the hospital. When they were admitted to the IRCU, group B patients had significantly lower respiratory rates (RRs) and APACHE II score values and significantly higher PaO_2/FiO_2 values compared to their counterparts. Moreover, there were significantly fewer group B patients with plasma BNP levels above the reference range and CRP level > 100 μg/mL (Table 2). All patients received the appropriate supportive and pharmacologic interventions for ARF during their stay in the IRCU according to current internal protocols [12,15].

The stratified log-rank test uncovered that group B patients survived for a significantly longer time compared to their counterparts [median survival time: 134 (31–257) vs. 25.5 (20–50) days; $p < 0.001$] (Figure 1); their hazard ratio for death was 0.27 (95% CI, 0.12 to 0.62, $p = 0.002$). Group 2 patients also had a lower IRCU mortality rate compared to their counterparts (6/26 vs. 10/14; $p = 0.003$). Finally, they spent significantly fewer days in the IRCU (Table 2).

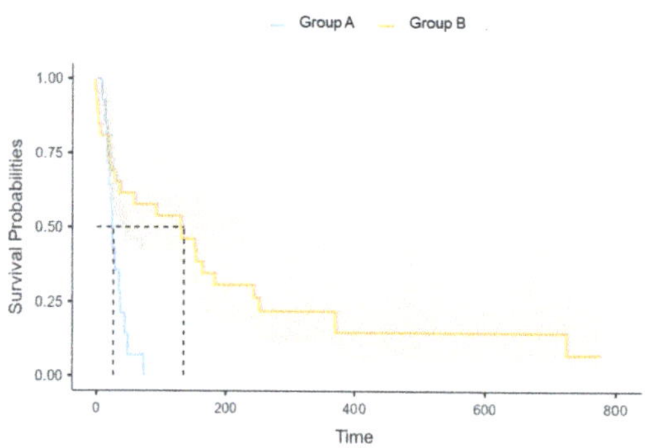

Figure 1. Kaplan–Maier estimates of survival function after Intermediate Respiratory Care Unit admission, stratified according to the group of origin. Dashed lines indicate median survival time.

4. Discussion

Although important advancements in the pharmacologic and supportive therapies used to treat patients with IPF and AE have been made over the past two decades, it is unclear if the outcomes of these patients have likewise improved. This study examined the question retrospectively by analyzing the survival of patients with exacerbated IPF admitted to our IRCU for ARF over the past two decades. Data analysis uncovered that the group of patients hospitalized more recently (after 2013) showed a significant improvement in survival times compared to those hospitalized during the previous decade. Indeed, their survival times had increased fivefold, and their IRCU mortality rate was also significantly reduced. Although it is difficult to pinpoint how the different interventions impacted the patients' outcomes, several important considerations can be made.

(A) Impact of Antifibrotic Therapy

At the time of their IRCU admission, the patients belonging to group B (more recent) tended to have better lung diffusing capacity values compared to their counterparts. This finding led us to assume that their improved survival was linked, at least in part, to the fact that they had better preserved pulmonary function than their counterparts. Other studies have reported that AE is more severe when respiratory function declines [16]. Better respiratory function in group B patients could be explained by the impact of antifibrotic treatment on lung function. Indeed, it has been demonstrated that both pirfenidone and nintedanib effectively delay lung function deterioration in patients with IPF [17,18]. Group B patients also showed higher levels of PaO_2/FiO_2 at the time they were admitted to the IRCU. Hypothetically, a smaller decrease in PaO_2/FiO_2 values could reflect limited pulmonary parenchyma damage and less-severe AE-IPF [19]; for this reason, the better survival rates could be partially explained by reduced lung inflammation during the acute disease phase. In accordance with data from experimental models of lung fibrosis, nintedanib could inhibit the progression of lung inflammation [20,21]. In line with this hypothesis, a recent study by Urushiyama et al. showed that initiating nintedanib within 14 days of being admitted to a hospital for AE was significantly associated with a lower risk of in-hospital death in patients with fibrosing interstitial lung disease (ILD) [9]. Moreover, pirfenidone was found to suppress inflammatory cytokines such as TGF-b and basic fibroblast growth factor (b-FGF), which are related to lung inflammation during an acute phase and subsequent fibrosis progression [7]. Interestingly, there was a significantly lower number of patients with a CRP level consistent with severe inflammation (>100 μg/mL) [22] in group B patients.

(B) Avoidance of Immunosuppressive Medication

At the time of IRCU admission, no group B patient was receiving steroid and/or immunosuppressive medication compared to 6 out of the 14 patients in group A. Considering that a history of immunosuppression before AE-IPF may adversely influence patients' survival [10,23], avoiding immunosuppressive therapy could have contributed to improved prognosis in patients hospitalized after 2013.

(C) Impact of Novel Supports for Oxygenation and CO_2 Removal

A significant percentage of group B patients who were unable to achieve sufficient oxygenation using standard non-rebreathing face masks had a satisfactory response to HFNO, which was prescribed in accordance with an internal protocol [12]. As refractory hypoxemia due to marked ventilation/perfusion (V/Q) mismatch and impairment in lung diffusing capacity is a predictor of poor outcome in patients with exacerbated IPF [24], the patients' satisfactory response to HFNO may have contributed to improving their survival. Indeed, the IRCU mortality rate was lower than 50% in the patients with AE-IPF who developed hypoxemia refractory to COT and showed a satisfactory response to HFNO [12]. A small single-center retrospective observational study likewise reported potential survival benefits in a cohort of 32 patients with ARF secondary to ILD treated with HFNO. That study found that the 30-day mortality was 23% as opposed to 63% in the patients receiving NIV [25]. We recently reported that a limited number of patients admitted to our IRCU over the past decade with severe CO_2 retention refractory to NIV were successfully treated with $ECCO_2R$ as an alternative to IMV [26]. Since transitioning patients with AE-IPF to IMV is associated with a mortality rate of approximately 90% [27], $ECCO_2R$ may have also contributed to improving the patients' survival.

This study has important limitations given its single-center, retrospective, and observational nature. Its population was also quite small, which is generally the case for clinical studies focusing on rare diseases and/or conditions. Its most important strength was that both IPF and AE-IPF were diagnosed following standard internationally accepted recommendations.

5. Conclusions

Despite its limitations, the preliminary results reported here corroborate the hypothesis that innovative pharmacologic and supportive treatments may prolong survival in patients with IPF hospitalized for AE. This strongly calls for collaborations between IPF specialists to develop novel clinical guidelines recommending the optimal management of this deadly complication.

Author Contributions: F.L.: conceptualization, methodology, and review and editing. G.A.: investigation, and review and editing. L.B.D.M.: data curation, formal analysis, and review and editing. F.B.: investigation and review and editing. A.A.: investigation and review and editing. S.L.: investigation and review and editing. M.C.: investigation and review and editing. G.G.: investigation, original draft preparation, and review and editing. A.V.: conceptualization, writing, and review and editing. All authors have read and agreed to the published version of the manuscript.

Funding: This research received no external funding.

Institutional Review Board Statement: This observational retrospective single-center study was conducted in a tertiary teaching hospital located in Northeast Italy. Ethical approval was waived by the facility's Institutional Review Committee in view of the fact that the study was retrospective in nature, and all the interventions prescribed were part of the hospital's internal protocols (No.: 2772; 30 December 2022). This study was carried out in accordance with the Declaration of Helsinki of 1975.

Informed Consent Statement: At admission, all the study participants were asked to sign informed consent forms agreeing to the use of their de-identified clinical data for research, analysis, and reporting purposes.

Data Availability Statement: The data presented in this study are available upon request from the corresponding author. The data are not publicly available due to privacy restrictions.

Conflicts of Interest: All the authors declare that they do not have any potential or actual conflicts of interest, including financial or personal relationships with persons or organizations which could have inappropriately influenced (biased) this study. No study sponsor was involved in designing or conceptualizing this study, collecting and analyzing/interpreting the data, drafting the manuscript, or the decision to submit the manuscript for publication.

References

1. Margaritopoulos, G.A.; Romagnoli, M.; Poletti, V.; Siafakas, N.M.; Wells, A.U.; Antoniou, K.M. Recent advances in the pathogenesis and clinical evaluation of pulmonary fibrosis. *Eur. Respir. Rev.* **2012**, *21*, 48–56. [CrossRef]
2. Song, J.W.; Hong, S.B.; Lim, C.M.; Koh, Y.; Kim, D.S. Acute exacerbation of idiopathic pulmonary fibrosis: Incidence, risk factors and outcome. *Eur. Respir. J.* **2011**, *37*, 356–363. [CrossRef]
3. Kreuter, M.; Polke, M.; Walsh, S.L.F.; Krisam, J.; Collard, H.R.; Chaudhuri, N.; Avdeev, S.; Behr, J.; Calligaro, G.; Corte, T.; et al. Acute exacerbation of idiopathic pulmonary fibrosis: International survey and call for harmonization. *Eur. Respir. J.* **2020**, *55*, 1901760. [CrossRef]
4. Faverio, P.; De Giacomi, F.; Sardella, L.; Fiorentino, G.; Carone, M.; Salerno, F.; Ora, J.; Rogliani, P.; Pellegrino, G.; Papa, G.F.S.; et al. Management of acute respiratory failure in interstitial lung diseases: Overview and clinical insights. *BMC Pulm. Med.* **2018**, *18*, 70. [CrossRef]
5. Raghu, G.; Collard, H.R.; Egan, J.J.; Martinez, F.J.; Behr, J.; Brown, K.K.; Colby, T.V.; Cordier, J.-F.; Flaherty, K.R.; Lasky, J.A.; et al. ATS/ERS/JRS/ALAT Committee on Idiopathic Pulmonary Fibrosis. An official ATS/ERS/JRS/ALAT statement: Idiopathic pulmonary fibrosis: Evidence-based guidelines for diagnosis and management. *Am. J. Respir. Crit. Care Med.* **2011**, *183*, 788–824. [CrossRef]
6. Yamazaki, R.; Nishiyama, O.; Yoshikawa, K.; Saeki, S.; Sano, H.; Iwanaga, T.; Tohda, Y. Clinical course and prognosis in survivors of acute exacerbations of idiopathic pulmonary fibrosis. *Respir. Investig.* **2021**, *59*, 408–413. [CrossRef]
7. Furuya, K.; Sakamoto, S.; Shimizu, H.; Sekiya, M.; Kinoshita, A.; Isshiki, T.; Sugino, K.; Matsumoto, K.; Homma, S. Pirfenidone for acute exacerbation of idiopathic pulmonary fibrosis: A retrospective study. *Respir. Med.* **2017**, *126*, 93–99. [CrossRef]
8. Vianello, A.; Molena, B.; Turato, C.; Braccioni, F.; Arcaro, G.; Paladini, L.; Andretta, M.; Saetta, M. Pirfenidone improves the survival of patients with idiopathic pulmonary fibrosis hospitalized for acute exacerbation. *Curr. Med. Res. Opin.* **2019**, *35*, 1187–1190. [CrossRef]
9. Urushiyama, H.; Jo, T.; Hasegawa, W.; Yokoyama, A.; Ando, T.; Sakamoto, Y.; Kumazawa, R.; Uda, K.; Michihata, N.; Awano, N.; et al. Effect of nintedanib on acute exacerbations of fibrosing interstitial lung diseases: A national database study in Japan. *ERJ Open Res.* **2022**, *8*, 00209–02022. [CrossRef]
10. Idiopathic Pulmonary Fibrosis Clinical Research Network; Raghu, G.; Anstrom, K.J.; King, T.E., Jr.; Lasky, J.A.; Martinez, F.J. Prednisone, Azathioprine, and *N*-Acetylcysteine for Pulmonary Fibrosis. *N. Engl. J. Med.* **2012**, *366*, 1968–1977. [CrossRef]
11. Trudzinski, F.C.; Kaestner, F.; Schäfers, H.J.; Fähndrich, S.; Seiler, F.; Böhmer, P.; Linn, O.; Kaiser, R.; Haake, H.; Langer, F.; et al. Outcome of patients with interstitial lung disease treated with extracorporeal membrane oxygenation for acute respiratory failure. *Am. J. Respir. Crit. Care Med.* **2016**, *193*, 527–533. [CrossRef]
12. Vianello, A.; Arcaro, G.; Molena, B.; Turato, C.; Braccioni, F.; Paladini, L.; Vio, S.; Ferrarese, S.; Peditto, P.; Gallan, F.; et al. High-flow nasal cannula oxygen therapy to treat acute respiratory failure in patients with acute exacerbation of idiopathic pulmonary fibrosis. *Ther. Adv. Respir. Dis.* **2019**, *13*, 1753466619847130. [CrossRef]
13. Raghu, G.; Remy-Jardin, M.; Richeldi, L.; Thomson, C.C.; Inoue, Y.; Johkoh, T.; Kreuter, M.; Lynch, D.A.; Maher, T.M.; Martinez, F.J.; et al. Idiopathic pulmonary fibrosis (an update) and progressive pulmonary fibrosis in adults: An official ATS/ERS/JRS/ALAT clinical practice guideline. *Am. J. Respir. Crit. Care Med.* **2022**, *205*, e18–e47. [CrossRef]
14. Collard, H.R.; Ryerson, C.J.; Corte, T.J.; Jenkins, G.; Kondoh, Y.; Lederer, D.J.; Lee, J.S.; Maher, T.M.; Wells, A.U.; Antoniou, K.M.; et al. Acute Exacerbation of Idiopathic Pulmonary Fibrosis. An International Working Group Report. *Am. J. Respir. Crit. Care Med.* **2016**, *194*, 265–275. [CrossRef]
15. Vianello, A.; Arcaro, G.; Battistella, L.; Pipitone, E.; Vio, S.; Concas, A.; Paladini, L.; Gallan, F.; Marchi, M.R.; Tona, F.; et al. Noninvasive ventilation in the event of acute respiratory failure in patients with idiopathic pulmonary fibrosis. *J. Crit. Care* **2014**, *29*, 562–567. [CrossRef]
16. Johannson, K.; Collard, H.R. Acute Exacerbation of Idiopathic Pulmonary Fibrosis: A Proposal. *Curr. Respir. Care Rep.* **2013**, *2*, 233–240. [CrossRef]
17. Noble, P.W.; Albera, C.; Bradford, W.Z.; Costabel, U.; Glassberg, M.K.; Kardatzke, D.; King, T.E., Jr.; Lancaster, L.; Sahn, S.A.; Szwarcberg, J.; et al. CAPACITY Study Group. Pirfenidone in patients with idiopathic pulmonary fibrosis (CAPACITY): Two randomised trials. *Lancet* **2011**, *377*, 1760–1769. [CrossRef]
18. Richeldi, L.; Cottin, V.; du Bois, R.M.; Selman, M.; Kimura, T.; Bailes, Z.; Schlenker-Herceg, R.; Stowasser, S.; Brown, K.K. Nintedanib in patients with idiopathic pulmonary fibrosis: Combined evidence from the TOMORROW and INPULSIS(®) trials. *Respir. Med.* **2016**, *113*, 74–79. [CrossRef]
19. Kamiya, H.; Panlaqui, O.M. Systematic review and meta-analysis of prognostic factors of acute exacerbation of idiopathic pulmonary fibrosis. *BMJ Open* **2020**, *10*, e035420. [CrossRef]
20. Gad, E.S.; Salama, A.A.A.; El-Shafie, M.F.; Arafa, H.M.M.; Abdelsalam, R.M.; Khattab, M. The anti-fibrotic and anti-inflammatory potential of bone marrow-derived mesenchymal stem cells and Nintedanib in bleomycin-induced lung fibrosis in rats. *Inflammation* **2020**, *43*, 123–134. [CrossRef]

21. Chen, W.-C.; Chen, N.-J.; Chen, H.-P.; Yu, W.-K.; Yi-Fong Su, V.; Chen, H.; Wu, H.-H.; Yang, K.-Y. Nintedanib reduces neutrophil chemotaxis via activating GRK2 in bleomycin-induced pulmonary fibrosis. *Int. J. Mol. Sci.* **2020**, *21*, 4735. [CrossRef]
22. Bray, C.; Bell, L.N.; Liang, H.; Haykal, R.; Kaiksow, F.; Mazza, J.J.; Yale, S.H. Erythrocyte Sedimentation Rate and C-reactive Protein measurements and their relevance in clinical medicine. *WMJ* **2016**, *115*, 317–321.
23. Papiris, S.A.; Kagouridis, K.; Kolilekas, L.; Papaioannou, A.I.; Roussou, A.; Triantafillidou, C.; Baou, K.; Malagari, K.; Argentos, S.; Kotanidou, A.; et al. Survival in Idiopathic Pulmonary Fibrosis acute exacerbations: The non-steroid approach. *BMC Pulm. Med.* **2015**, *15*, 162. [CrossRef]
24. Kishaba, T.; Tamaki, H.; Shimaoka, Y.; Fukuyama, H.; Yamashiro, S. Staging of acute exacerbation in patients with idiopathic pulmonary fibrosis. *Lung* **2014**, *192*, 141–149. [CrossRef]
25. Omote, N.; Matsuda, N.; Hashimoto, N.; Nishida, K.; Sakamoto, K.; Ando, A.; Nakahara, Y.; Nishikimi, M.; Higashi, M.; Matsu, S.; et al. High-Flow Nasal Cannula therapy for acute respiratory failure in patients with interstitial pneumonia: A retrospective observational study. *Nagoya J. Med. Sci.* **2020**, *82*, 301–313. [CrossRef]
26. Vianello, A.; Arcaro, G.; Paladini, L.; Iovino, S. Successful management of acute respiratory failure in an Idiopathic Pulmonary Fibrosis patient using an extracorporeal carbon dioxide removal system. *Sarcoidosis Vasc. Diffuse Lung Dis.* **2016**, *33*, 186–190.
27. Rush, B.; Wiskar, K.; Berger, L.; Griesdale, D. The use of mechanical ventilation in patients with idiopathic pulmonary fibrosis in the United States: A nationwide retrospective cohort analysis. *Respir. Med.* **2016**, *111*, 72–76. [CrossRef]

Journal of
Clinical Medicine

MDPI

Review

Review of the Diagnosis and Management of Pulmonary Hypertension Associated with Interstitial Lung Disease (ILD-PH)

Zein Kattih [1], Ho Cheol Kim [2], Shambhu Aryal [1] and Steven D. Nathan [1,*]

1 Advanced Lung Disease and Transplant Program, Inova Heart and Vascular Institute, Inova Fairfax Hospital, Falls Church, VA 22042, USA; zein.kattih@inova.org (Z.K.); shambhu.aryal@inova.org (S.A.)
2 Department of Pulmonary and Critical Care Medicine, Asan Medical Center, University of Ulsan College of Medicine, Seoul 05505, Republic of Korea; hocheol.kim@inova.org
* Correspondence: steven.nathan@inova.org

Abstract: Pulmonary hypertension associated with interstitial lung disease (ILD-PH) frequently complicates the course of patients with fibrotic ILD. In this narrative review, the authors assess current diagnostic tools and management considerations in ILD-PH patients. ILD-PH is associated with increased morbidity and mortality and may be suggested by the presence of symptoms out of proportion to the extent of the ILD. There are other clues to the presence of PH in the context of ILD including the need for supplemental oxygen, a reduced DLCO especially if accompanied by a disproportionately higher forced vital capacity, imaging demonstrating an enlarged pulmonary artery or a dilated right ventricle, or objective evidence of a reduced exercise capacity. While echocardiography is one screening tool, right heart catheterization remains the gold standard for the diagnosis of PH. When appropriate, treatment with inhaled treprostinil, or possibly other pulmonary vasodilators, may be indicated.

Keywords: ILD-PH; PH-ILD; interstitial lung disease; pulmonary hypertension; advanced lung disease

1. Introduction

Interstitial lung disease (ILD) encompasses a broad group of diseases affecting the pulmonary interstitium that are characterized by varying amounts of inflammation and/or fibrosis. When accompanied by fibrosis, any of these ILDs may result in associated pulmonary hypertension (PH) which is classified by the World Symposium for Pulmonary Hypertension (WSPH) under the World Health Organization (WHO) group 3 category [1–3]. Patients with group 1 pulmonary arterial hypertension (PAH) may have evidence of some mild ILD, and how much ILD is needed to be regarded as group 3 PH is controversial and should be determined on a case-by-case basis. Categorization as group 1 PAH or group 3 ILD-PH is important to discern, as this may have implications for prognosis, management, and especially treatment [4]. In this narrative review, we present definitions of PH as they pertain to patients with ILD-PH, explore the pathogenesis of PH in ILD, evaluate diagnostic findings that may be suggestive of ILD-PH, and examine pharmacologic therapies and management strategies for ILD-PH patients. A focused literature search was performed to identify initial key references by utilizing the PubMed database with the following keywords: "interstitial lung disease-associated pulmonary hypertension", "interstitial lung disease-associated AND pulmonary hypertension", and "pulmonary hypertension related to interstitial lung disease". Relevant systematic reviews and reviews from 2020 until 2024 were reviewed for inclusion. References from these manuscripts were also evaluated for inclusion if they provided unique information. The literature search was augmented by the authors' own knowledge. Where relevant, references were included for original studies and prediction model studies.

2. Definitions

PH is currently defined by a mean pulmonary artery pressure (mPAP) > 20 mmHg. Precapillary PH is accompanied by a pulmonary vascular resistance (PVR) > 2 Woods units (WU) and a pulmonary capillary wedge pressure (PCWP) of ≤15 mmHg [3]. This latter definition was initially proposed by the 2022 European Society of Cardiology/European Respiratory Society consensus statement and recently endorsed by the 7th WSPH [1]. Many of the prior estimates of disease prevalence were based on the older definitions of PH, specifically a mPAP ≥ 25 mmHg. Severe PH in the context of lung disease has been defined as a PVR >5 WU [2]. As yet, there is no definition of mild or moderate PH in the context of ILD (ILD-PH), although it is noteworthy that "mild" or borderline PH has been shown to carry a prognosis similar to patients with more severe PH [5].

3. Epidemiology

3.1. Prevalence and Incidence of ILD-PH

Estimates of the incidence and prevalence of ILD-PH depend first on the incidence and prevalence of the underlying ILDs. The incidence of PH associated with the respective ILDs depends on the cohort studied, their disease severity, and how the PH was defined. The prevalence of ILDs in the United States in 2019 was estimated to be 654,841 cases (95% confidence interval 566,536–745,855) [6], while the estimated prevalence of associated PH ranges from as low as 15% to as high as 86% [4]. Most estimates of PH associated with ILD originate from the idiopathic pulmonary fibrosis (IPF) literature. This broad range not only reflects the variability in the timing of the identification of PH in ILD patients but also the discrepancy in diagnostic threshold and modalities used for the diagnosis. Indeed, many of these estimates were obtained prior to 2018, and are therefore under the umbrella of the older definition; specifically, a mPAP ≥ 25 mmHg and precapillary PH further defined by a PVR of ≥3 WU and a PCWP ≤ 15 mmHg [3]. One study of IPF patients listed for lung transplantation demonstrated that the prevalence of PH using the pre-2018 definition was 47.6% but increased to 73.6% under the new definition [7]. There is a paucity of literature pertaining to the prevalence of PH in non-IPF ILDs with available estimates shown in Table 1 [8–19]. Most patients with ILD will have mild-to-moderate PH, and there is a subgroup of patients who are found to have severe PH at the time of their initial right heart catheterization (RHC) [2].

Table 1. Estimated prevalence of pulmonary hypertension according to interstitial lung disease subtype.

Subtype	Reference	PH Out of Total Cohort	Prevalence	Location	Diagnostic Modality of ILD	Diagnostic Modality of PH
Pooled Prevalence of ILD	Ang et al., 2024 (pre-6th WSPH definition) [8]		36%	International	Variable	RHC
	Ang et al., 2024 (6th WSPH definition) [8]		40%	International	Variable	RHC

Table 1. *Cont.*

Subtype	Reference	PH Out of Total Cohort	Prevalence	Location	Diagnostic Modality of ILD	Diagnostic Modality of PH
Idiopathic pulmonary fibrosis	Shorr et al., 2007 [10]	1163/2525	46%	UNOS Database	Variable	RHC
	Nathan et al., 2008 [11]	17/44	39%	United States	HRCT +/− pathology	RHC
	Todd et al., 2010 [12]	12/41	29%	United States	Clinical + CT +/− pathology	RHC
	Raghu et al., 2015 [13]	68/488	14%	Multicenter	Either surgical lung biopsy showing UIP or HRCT with definite UIP	RHC
	Tyagi et al., 2021 [14]	18/38	47%	India	Clinical + HRCT +/− pathology	TTE
Systemic sclerosis-ILD (SSc-ILD)	Young et al., 2019 [15]	29/93	31%	United States	ACR/EULAR classification criteria for SSc + HRCT showing ILD	RHC
CTD-ILD other than systemic sclerosis	Todd et al., 2010 [12]	9/14	64%	United States	Clinical + CT +/− pathology	RHC
	Cottin et al., 2011 [16]	28/61	47%	France	HRCT + PFT +/− clinical +/− exclusion of ILD with known etiology and exclusion of CTD	TTE
	Tyagi et al., 2021 (Autoimmune ILD) [14]	33/75	44%	India	Clinical + HRCT +/− pathology	TTE
Combined pulmonary fibrosis and emphysema	Cottin et al., 2005 [18]	61	47%	France	Emphysema on HRCT + diffuse parenchymal lung disease on HRCT	TTE
Nonspecific interstitial pneumonia (NSIP)	King et al., 2018 [17]	11/35	31%	United States	Biopsy-proven NSIP	RHC
Chronic hypersensitivity pneumonitis	Oliveira et al., 2014 [19]	22/50	44%	Brazil	Clinical + HRCT +/− pathology	RHC
	Tyagi et al., 2021 [14]	40/77	52%	India	Clinical + HRCT +/− pathology	TTE

Abbreviations: ACR/EULAR—American College of Rheumatology/European League of Rheumatology; CT—computed tomography of the chest; CTD-ILD—connective tissue disease-related ILD; HRCT—high resolution computed tomography of the chest; ILD—interstitial lung disease; PFT—pulmonary function test; pre-6th WSPH definition—pre-6th World Symposium on Pulmonary Hypertension Definition of PH; PH—pulmonary hypertension; RHC—right heart catheterization; TTE—transthoracic echocardiogram; UIP—usual interstitial pneumonia; UNOS—United Network for Organ Sharing.

3.2. PH in CTD-ILD

Patients with Connective Tissue Disease (CTD)-related ILD (CTD-ILD), such as scleroderma and rheumatoid arthritis, may have WHO Group 3 PH secondary to underlying lung disease, or they may have WHO Group 1 disease due to vascular involvement of their underlying CTD [1]. Therefore, defining the prevalence of WHO Group 3 PH in this group of patients remains challenging. In the Pulmonary Hypertension Assessment and Recognition of Outcomes in Scleroderma (PHAROS) study, 49 of 237 patients (20.6%) with scleroderma had PH [20]. In total, 15 of those 49 with PH had ILD-PH, which represents 6.3% of the total cohort [20]. These patients were primarily New York Heart Association (NYHA) functional class 2 (54%) and 3 (23%) [20]. In the DETECT study, 31% of patients with systemic sclerosis had PH with a mPAP $\geq$ 25 mmHg [21]. In a scleroderma-ILD cohort, 31% of patients had PH confirmed by RHC [15]. In rheumatoid arthritis-related patients, PH typically occurs in the setting of parenchymal lung involvement, though vascular involvement and chronic thromboembolic disease may also lead to PH [22,23]. One study estimated the prevalence of PH in patients with rheumatoid arthritis to be 14% using a resting PASP cutoff of >35 mmHg [24]. The incidence of PH by echocardiography in rheumatoid arthritis patients was 26.7% compared with 4.5% in controls, and there was a strong correlation between pulmonary artery pressure and the disease duration [22].

3.3. *PH in Combined Pulmonary Fibrosis and Emphysema*

Patients with combined pulmonary fibrosis and emphysema (CPFE) have a reported prevalence of PH 15 to 55% [25]. These patients tend to have relatively well-preserved forced vital capacities (FVC) due to the presence of concomitant hyperinflation from their emphysema [26]. Some studies have suggested that the severity of PH is worse among those with CPFE compared with both IPF and chronic obstructive pulmonary disease or emphysema alone [2,25]. Estimated systolic pulmonary artery pressures are higher in patients with CPFE than in those with isolated IPF [25]. The additional burden of emphysema, over and above a given extent of fibrosis, increases the risk of PH [25]. However, the likelihood of PH does not differ for matched extents of disease (combined fibrosis and emphysema) on HRCT (or when adjusted for DLCO) between patients with CPFE and those with fibrosis alone [25].

3.4. *Outcomes in ILD-PH*

ILD patients with PH have worse outcomes compared to those without PH [27,28]. Notably, patients with ILD-PH have higher one-year and three-year mortalities compared to those without PH [2,27,29]. One study suggested an estimated survival probability of 84%, 71%, and 66% at 1, 3, and 5 years, respectively, in patients with ILD without PH compared with 75%, 59%, and 47%, respectively, in patients with ILD-PH [29]. Patients with mild PH (mPAP 20–24 mmHg) appear to have prognoses that are not dissimilar to those with more severe PH [30]. Therefore, "mild" PH does not connote "mild" disease. Indeed, any PH in the context of ILD connotes "severe" disease given the accompanying dismal prognosis. A PVR > 5 Wood Units has been associated with a significantly worse survival compared to a PVR $\leq$ 5 Wood Units, resulting in this being the cut point for what is regarded as severe PH [2]. However, rather than one distinct PVR cut point, it is likely that the PVR impacts prognosis on a continuum rather than by distinct categories. Indeed, there is even data demonstrating that patients with mPAP < 20 mmHg (hence no PH by definition), but with PVRs $\geq$ 3, have a worse prognosis than those with lower PVRs [7,31]. The presence of PH is not only associated with greater mortality, but also with significant morbidity including a greater need for supplemental oxygen, decreased exercise tolerance, more frequent acute exacerbations, and greater health-care resource utilization [32].

4. Pathogenesis

The mechanisms underlying the development of PH and the progression of ILD are not yet fully understood and require further investigation. Although there is an association between the extent of parenchymal involvement and pulmonary hypertension, patients with mild parenchymal involvement can still develop severe PH [33]. The pathogenesis of PH in the context of ILD is complex and multifactorial. It is not only fibrosis and vascular ablation, but other factors are involved as well [2,4,34]. Hypoxemia may cause vasoconstriction thereby contributing to the development of PH [4]. Pulmonary vascular remodeling in PH is characterized by degenerative changes and pulmonary vascular cell proliferation [35]. Pulmonary vasculopathy also features vascular pruning with loss of small pulmonary vessels [36]. The influence of comorbidities is important to recognize as these may potentially be modifiable. Specifically, heart failure, sleep-disordered breathing, and thromboembolic disease may all be contributory [2,4]. The architectural distortion that accompanies fibrosis can lead to shear stress, which can perpetuate the PH. Some of the same cytokines that are upregulated as part of the fibrotic process have also been associated with the development of PH, including endothelin, thromboxane, and transforming growth factor alpha. These may lead to vasoconstriction and vascular smooth muscle proliferation, thereby contributing to the development or worsening of PH [34,37]. There are also reports suggesting that certain genetic pathways are associated with ILD-PH [38,39]. A cartoon depiction of the factors involved in the development of PH in ILD is shown in Figure 1.

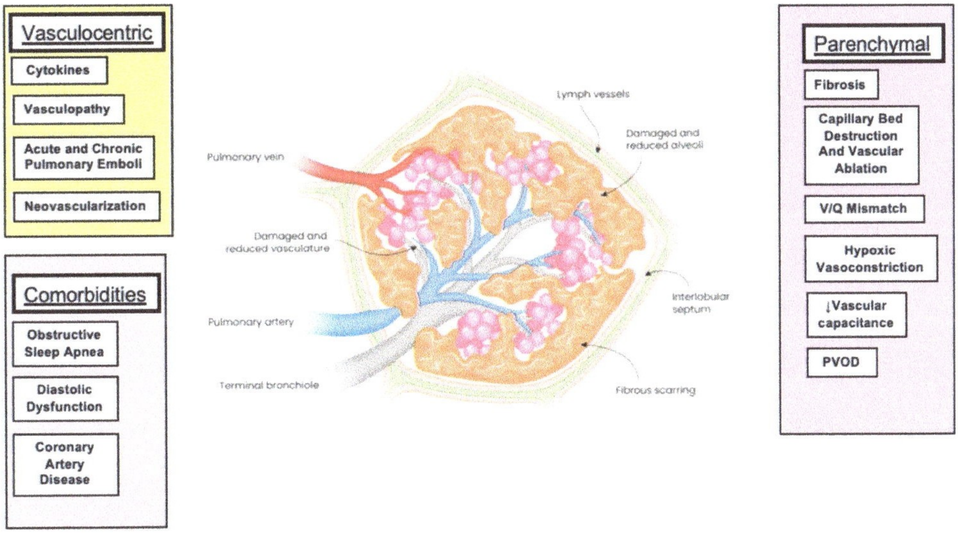

Figure 1. Pathogenic factors associated with the development of PH in ILD. Schematic diagram detailing the vasculocentric, parenchymal, and comorbid risk factors associated with the development of PH in ILD. ↓vascular capacitance = decreased vascular capacitance Adapted from Image © 2023 United Therapeutics Corporation. All rights reserved. Used with permission.

5. Diagnostics Suggestive of ILD-PH

The presence of PH in the setting of ILD may be suspected based on symptoms, physiologic testing, and abnormalities present on imaging. These findings include abnormalities on pulmonary function tests (PFT), six-minute walk test (6MWT), biomarkers, computed tomography (CT) imaging, and echocardiogram, as suggested in a multidisciplinary Delphi study of 16 pulmonologists with ILD and PH expertise [40]. The variables and tests that may raise the index of suspicion for PH complicating ILD are shown in Figure 2.

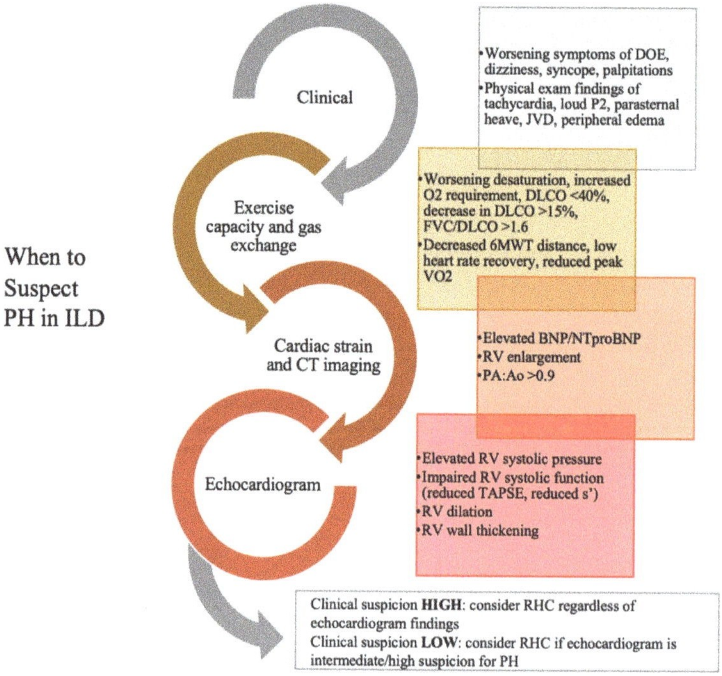

Figure 2. Features suggestive of PH in ILD patients. Abbreviations: 6MWT—six-minute walk test; BNP—brain natriuretic peptide; DLCO—diffusion capacity of carbon monoxide; DOE—dyspnea on exertion; FVC/DLCO—forced vital capacity/DLCO ratio; JVD—jugular venous distention; NT-proBNP—N-terminal pro b-type natriuretic peptide; PA:Ao—pulmonary artery to aorta ratio; PH—pulmonary hypertension; RHC—right heart catheterization; RV—right ventricle; TAPSE—tricuspid annular plane systolic excursion; VO2—maximum oxygen consumption.

5.1. Clinical Features

The symptoms of ILD-PH may be difficult to distinguish from the symptoms of the underlying ILD. These may include worsening shortness of breath that appears to be out of proportion to the severity of the underlying lung disease, especially if such worsening occurs in the context of an unchanged FVC [2]. Symptoms of syncope or pre-syncope are late signs that occur more commonly in group 1 PAH. Clinical features may be subtle, such as an increased P2 heart sound. A murmur of tricuspid regurgitation may be appreciated while more overt evidence of right heart failure may be seen in the later stages of disease progression [41].

5.2. Biomarkers

Patients with ILD-PH may have elevated brain natriuretic peptide (BNP) or N-terminal pro b-type natriuretic peptide (NT-proBNP) levels or elevated troponin levels suggestive of right ventricular dysfunction [42]. Elevated BNP levels have been shown to predict outcomes in patients with ILD. In a retrospective review of 131 patients with IPF, BNP was an independent predictor of prognosis, and patients with elevated BNP had a shorter survival time compared to those with normal BNP levels (70.5% vs. 23.7% 1-year mortality) [43]. In a review of 90 ILD patients, BNP level ≥ 20 pmol/L was correlated with increased mortality independent of age, sex, and pulmonary function (hazard ratio 2.93), and these patients had a 14-fold increase in mortality compared with patients with BNP < 4 pmol/L [44]. How much of this elevation in BNP was from underlying PH versus concurrent heart failure was uncertain. Importantly, a normal BNP or NT-proBNP does not rule out underlying PH in ILD patients. The specific role of biomarkers in ILD-PH is not as well defined as in WHO Group 1 disease, particularly in patients with concurrent renal dysfunction, obesity, or left heart disease.

5.3. Physiologic Testing

Pulmonary function testing is obtained as the standard of care in patients with ILD. Variables from these can provide clues to the presence of PH. It is important to note that there is a poor correlation between the extent of the restrictive physiology and the presence and severity of any underlying PH. The single-breath diffusing capacity for carbon monoxide (DLCO) is the one PFT variable that is associated with the presence of PH. A reduced DLCO (e.g., <40%) or an elevated FVC% predicted/diffusion lung capacity for carbon monoxide percent predicted (FVC%/DLCO%) ratio might indicate underlying PH. In one cohort of systemic sclerosis patients, 22% of patients with an FVC%/DLCO% greater than 1.4 had concurrent PH compared to only 2% of patients with a ratio < 1.4 [45]. While various thresholds have been suggested in the literature, these variables should rather be viewed on a continuum. Specifically, the lower the DLCO% and the higher the FVC%/DLCO% ratio, the greater the likelihood of underlying PH.

5.4. Functional Testing

The 6MWT is commonly used in the standard of care management of ILD patients. There are multiple clues from variables captured during the 6MWT which can indicate underlying PH. Generally, patients with ILD-PH walk less, require more oxygen, desaturate more, and have a lower heart rate recovery than non-PH ILD patients. Heart rate recovery is the difference between the heart rate at the end of the walk and the heart rate one minute into recovery. A lower heart rate recovery has been shown to correlate with worse outcomes in IPF patients and a heart rate recovery rate of <13 has been associated with the presence of PH [46].

Although not routinely obtained, cardiopulmonary exercise testing can be a useful test in patients with ILD to identify an exhausted circulatory reserve which might be suggestive of PH. Findings such as a reduced oxygen pulse, a low maximal oxygen consumption, an unchanged or decreased partial pressure of carbon dioxide during exercise, and a preserved breathing reserve can all suggest a contribution to exercise limitation from PH [47].

5.5. CT Imaging

Imaging of the lungs via high-resolution CT is another test that is obtained in the routine diagnosis and follow-up of patients with ILD. Radiographic evidence of an enlarged pulmonary artery (PA) diameter, which is best evaluated through the PA to aorta diameter ratio (>1), or the right ventricle to left ventricle ratio on axial CT images (Figure 3) of the chest should raise suspicion for underlying PH [41].

5.6. Echocardiography

Echocardiographic evidence of PH may include an elevated estimated right ventricular systolic pressure, impaired right ventricular systolic function as suggested by a reduced tricuspid annual plane systolic excursion or S′, and evidence of right ventricular hypertrophy and remodeling such as with right ventricular dilation or wall thickening [48]. PH may be present despite a normal right ventricular systolic pressure on an echocardiogram, and echocardiography may be inaccurate in estimating pulmonary pressures [49]. Thus, while echocardiography is a good noninvasive screening tool for PH, results must be placed in a clinical context, and right heart catheterization may still be considered if clinical suspicion for PH remains high, despite an echocardiogram suggesting a low probability of PH [40,50].

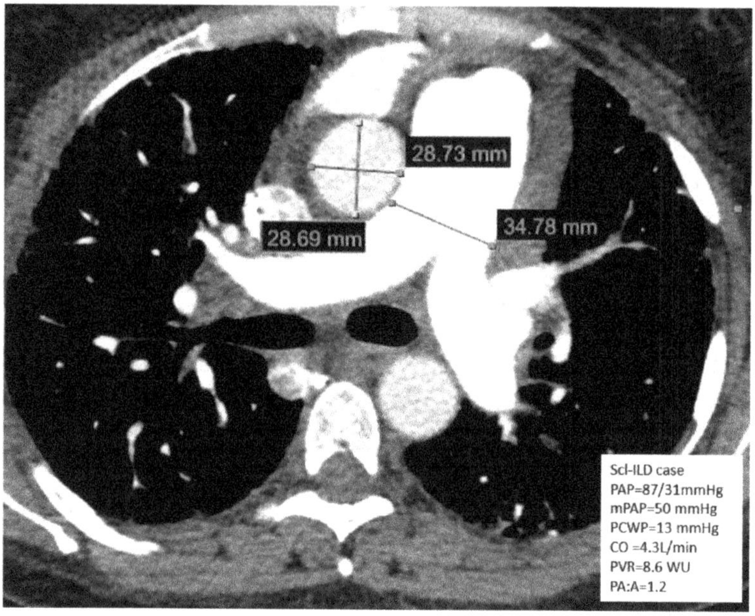

Figure 3. Axial view of CT angiogram of the chest with measurement of the pulmonary artery and aorta in a patient with ILD demonstrating a pulmonary artery to aorta ratio of 1.2. The patient's hemodynamics based on right heart catheterization are shown in the bottom right square. Abbreviations: mPAP—mean pulmonary artery pressure; PAP—pulmonary artery pressure; PA:A—pulmonary artery to aorta ratio; PVR—pulmonary vascular resistance; Scl-ILD—scleroderma-related interstitial lung disease; PCWP—pulmonary capillary wedge pressure.

5.7. Prediction Models

There have been a number of composite models proposed which incorporate elements of the modalities presented above. These have been developed to provide a more accurate prediction of PH in ILD patients. Select models are outlined in Table 2 [42,47,51–58], and a more comprehensive review of these predictive models is outlined in a narrative review by Arvanitaki and colleagues [59].

Table 2. Select prediction models for PH in ILD patients.

Reference	Population	Parameter	Prediction Equation	Outcome	*p*-Value (If Available)
Zisman et al., 2007 [51]	IPF	SpO2, FVC, DLCO	−11.9 + 0.272 × SpO2 + 0.0659 × (100−SpO2) 2 + 3.06 × (% FVC/% DLco)	mPAP	PPV 71% NPV 81%
Furukawa et al., 2018 [52]	IPF	DLCO, PA/Ao ratio on CT chest, PaO2	Simple scoring system assigning 1 point to each variable (DLCO < 50%, PA/Ao > 0.9, PaO2 < 80 Torr)	mPAP	C-index: 0.772, $p < 0.001$ OR of variables: DLCO 3.6, $p < 0.001$ PA/Ao 2.6, $p = 0.012$ PaO2 2.2, $p = 0.030$
Bax et al., 2018 [53]	ILD	PASP, right atrial area, early diastolic pulmonary regurgitant velocity, FAC, RV:LV ratio, eccentricity index	Stepwise echocardiographic algorithm	mPAP ≥ 35 mmHg	Score ≥ 7 predicting severe PH Sensitivity 89% Specificity 71% PPV 68% NPV 90%
Sonti et al., 2019 [54]	IPF	sPAP, FVC/DLco, PA/A ratio	mPAP = −14 + 20.3 × (PA:A ratio) + 2.6 × (FVC/DLCO) + 0.3 × (RVSP)	mPAP	Sensitivity 80% Specificity 68.6% PPV 56% NPV 87.2%

Table 2. *Cont.*

Reference	Population	Parameter	Prediction Equation	Outcome	*p*-Value (If Available)
Sobiecka et al., 2020 [55]	ILD	Age, TLC/DLCO, 6MWD, saturation at 6 min	Scoring system including age > 53 years, TLC/DLCO > 1.67, 6MWD < 507.5 m, saturation at 6 min < 93% (max score 10)	sPAP by echocardiography	AUC 0.867 Cutoff of 6 points yields: Sensitivity 66% Specificity 94% PPV 90% NPV 78%
Refini et al., 2021 [56]	IPF	sPAP, PA area by HRCT, and ratio of segmental artery to adjacent bronchus of L1/2	Composite index of these variables	mPAP	$R^2 = 0.53$, $p = 0.0009$ Sensitivity 100% Specificity 53% PPV 71% NPV 100%
Parikh et al., 2023 [58]	ILD	History, physical exam, 6MWD, DLCO, PA/A ratio, NT-proBNP	ILD-PH Detection tool (DLCO < 40%, 6MWD < 350 m, NTprBNP > 300 pg/mL, PA enlargement, physical exam for PH, supplemental O2, syncope/presyncope, CTD or sarcoid)	PH	Score of ≥7 predicting PH Sensitivity 87% Specificity 86%
Joseph et al., 2023 [47]	ILD	Gas exchange-derived pulmonary vascular capacitance (GXcap), RVSP, FVC/DLCO	GXcap < 416 mL*mmHg, FVC/DLCO > 1.7, RVSP > 73	ILD-PH	AUC 0.94 Sensitivity 86% Specificity 93%
Nathan et al., 2024 [57]	IPF	FVC/DLCO, oxygen saturation nadir, race, 6MWD	FORD calculator (continuous) and FORD index (simple point-score system)	PH (pre-6 WSPH definition)	Derivation cohort AUC 0.75 Validation cohort AUC 0.69

Abbreviations: 6MWD—six-minute walk test distance; AUC—area under the curve; CTD—connective tissue disease; DLCO—single breath diffusing capacity for carbon monoxide; FAC—fractional area change; FVC—forced vital capacity; ILD—interstitial lung disease; IPF—idiopathic pulmonary fibrosis; HRCT—high resolution computed tomography; mPAP—mean pulmonary artery pressure; NTproBNP—N-terminal pro b-type natriuretic peptide; NPV—negative predictive value; OR—odds ratio; PA/A ratio or PA/Ao ratio—pulmonary artery to aorta ratio; PaO2—partial pressure of oxygen; PASP—pulmonary artery systolic pressure; pre-6th WSPH definition—pre-6th World Symposium on Pulmonary Hypertension Definition of PH; PH—pulmonary hypertension; PPV—positive predictive value; RV:LV ratio—right ventricle to left ventricle ratio; RVSP—right ventricular systolic pressure; SPAP—systolic pulmonary artery pressure; SpO2—oxygen saturation; TLC—total lung capacity.

5.8. Hemodynamic Profile

RHC is the gold standard for the diagnosis of PH since this provides the direct measurement of the hemodynamic variables necessary to diagnose PH and pre-capillary PH [3]. Precapillary PH is defined by a mPAP > 20 mmHg, pulmonary artery wedge pressure ≤ 15 mmHg, and a PVR > 2 WU. IPF patients have an increased predisposition for comorbidities including heart failure and sleep-disordered breathing [2]. In patients suspected to have concurrent WHO group 2 disease, the use of volume challenge maneuvers or exercise during RHC may be considered [48]. Patients with ILD-PH tend to have mild to moderate PH, but any PH in the context of ILD is associated with a poor prognosis.

5.9. Distinguishing PAH from PH Due to Lung Disease

PH in patients with ILD can be considered on a continuum between WHO Group 1 and WHO Group 3 disease [4]. Evaluation of the extent of lung disease, hemodynamic profile, PFTs, and the presence of additional risk factors for PH can favor one category over the other [4].

Moderate-to-severe pulmonary hypertension is more suggestive of WHO group 1 disease, while more mild-to-moderate PH suggests WHO group 3 disease [4]. Patients with only mild impairment on their spirometry and a low or very low DLCO in comparison likely have a larger contribution from WHO group 1 disease, particularly when high-resolution CT of the chest demonstrates only mild or perhaps even moderate parenchymal lung disease [60]. Conversely, patients with moderate to extensive fibrosis and PFTs with moderate or severe restriction are best categorized as WHO group 3 disease [60].

6. Management of ILD-PH

The management of ILD-PH should always consider the management of the underlying ILD as one of the first steps. Immunosuppression may be indicated in patients with an underlying inflammatory component to their ILD (e.g., CTD-ILD). However, it is noteworthy that in ILDs which are purely inflammatory, there is very little data attesting to the prevalence and impact of PH. If the inflammatory component is reversible, then it makes intuitive sense that any accompanying PH will be reversible too. Fibrotic lung disease should be addressed with consideration for the institution of an antifibrotic therapy [61,62]. There are no data demonstrating that antifibrotic therapy will reverse or slow the development of PH. The need for supplemental oxygen, including sleep and exertion, should be assessed serially. There should also be a heightened index of suspicion and screening for any comorbid conditions which might be contributory. If present, management of sleep apnea, thromboembolic disease, or heart failure should be optimized [48]. Referral to pulmonary rehabilitation and early consideration for a lung transplantation evaluation in appropriate candidates is strongly encouraged. An algorithm for the management of patients with ILD-PH is shown in Figure 4.

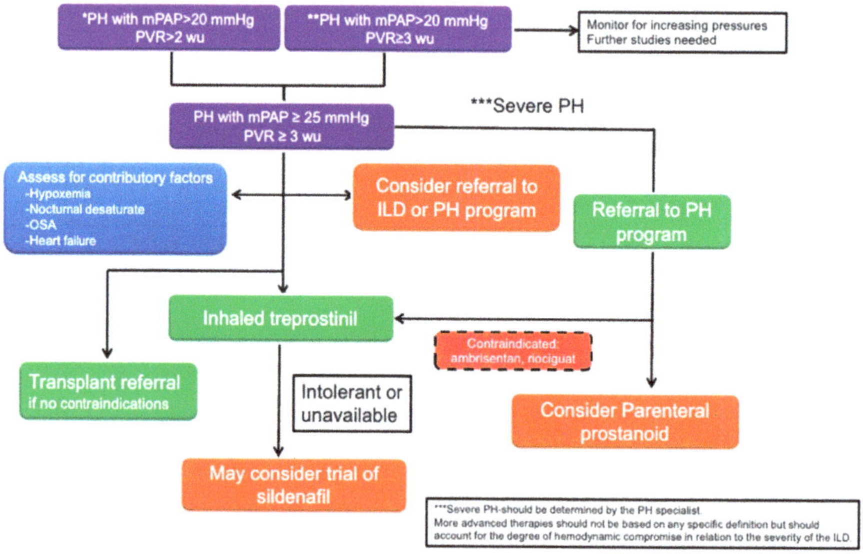

Figure 4. Algorithm for the management of patients with pulmonary hypertension associated with interstitial lung disease. * 2022 European Society of Cardiology and the European Respiratory Society definition of pulmonary hypertension ** 6th World Symposium on Pulmonary Hypertension Definition of Pulmonary Hypertension. *** Severe PH should be determined by the PH specialist. ILD = interstitial lung disease; mPAP = mean pulmonary artery pressure; OSA = obstructive sleep apnea; PH = pulmonary hypertension; PVR = pulmonary vascular resistance; wu = Wood units. Reprinted with permission of the American Thoracic Society. Copyright © 2024 American Thoracic Society. All rights reserved. Nathan SD. 2023. Progress in the Treatment of Pulmonary Hypertension Associated with Interstitial Lung Disease. Am J Respir Crit Care Med. 208(3):238–246. [63] The American Journal of Respiratory and Critical Care Medicine is an official journal of the American Thoracic Society.

7. Pharmacological Management of ILD-PH

7.1. Endothelin Receptor Antagonists (ERAs)

The ERAs are the oldest form of oral therapy approved for the treatment of PAH. There are currently three agents that are available, including bosentan, ambrisentan, and macitentan. These have all been subjected to clinical trials in IPF for their purported antifibrotic properties, but unfortunately, all three of these studies were negative [64–66]. Raghu and colleagues in the Randomized Placebo-Controlled Study to Evaluate Safety and Effectiveness of Ambrisentan in IPF (ARTEMIS-IPF) evaluated ambrisentan in IPF patients, 32 of whom had PH; however, the study was terminated early due to lack of efficacy in time to clinical worsening [64]. The later ARIES-3 open-label trial of ambrisentan in adult patients with PH due to Group 1, 3, 4, and 5 PH found no improvement in 6MWT distance in the subpopulation of patients with ILD, and, in fact, demonstrated a mean decline of 23 m on 6MWT [67].

The most robust of the ERA studies specifically targeting ILD-PH was the bosentan in pulmonary hypertension with fibrotic idiopathic interstitial pneumonia (BPHIT study) [66]. This study was a prospective, double-blind, controlled study of fibrotic ILD patients randomized in a 2:1 fashion to bosentan or placebo [66]. This study was negative based on the primary endpoint of reduction in the PVR index at 16 weeks. There were also 20 negative secondary endpoints with none showing even a trend to benefit [66].

7.2. Riociguat

Riociguat is a soluble guanylate stimulator approved for both PAH and chronic thromboembolic PH. It was shown in an open-label trial to be associated with improved cardiac output, PVR, and 6MWT distance at 12 weeks [68]. This was the basis for a subsequent phase 3 study (the Safety of Riociguat in Patients with Symptomatic Pulmonary Hypertension Associated with Idiopathic Interstitial Pneumonias- RISE-IIP), which was a double-blind, randomized, placebo-controlled study of 147 patients with RHC confirmed PH and an FVC of at least 45% of predicted [69]. Unfortunately, the study was terminated early due to increased adverse events in the riociguat group and increased mortality in patients treated with riociguat [69]. As a result of this trial, riociguat is contraindicated in patients with ILD-PH.

7.3. Phosphodiesterase 5 (PDE5) Inhibitors

There have been a number of retrospective and open-label trials that have evaluated the role of sildenafil [70–74], and at least one of tadalafil [71,75] in ILD-PH patients. Evidence from these retrospective studies has suggested the potential for improvement in the 6MWT [70,73,74], BNP [44], ventilation–perfusion matching, and oxygenation [72] with sildenafil. However, two prospective randomized controlled studies of sildenafil did not show a benefit in the 6MWT distance and Borg score [76,77]. Notably, sildenafil did improve oxygen saturation and quality of life as secondary endpoints in this study [77]. There have also been a number of studies of sildenafil in IPF populations enriched for the presence of PH by the inclusion criterion of a DLCO < 35% of predicted. The Sildenafil Trial of Exercise Performance in IPF (STEP-IPF) study, while a negative study based on the primary endpoint of a 20% improvement in the 6MWT distance, did have a number of secondary endpoints that were positive, including arterial oxygenation, DLCO, degree of dyspnea, and quality of life in favor of sildenafil [77]. In addition, a recent study reported that the use of PDE5 inhibitors was associated with favorable outcomes in severe PH associated with ILD [78].

7.4. Prostanoids

The prostanoids were the first class of agents approved for the treatment of PAH. In 1999, inhaled and intravenous prostanoids together with inhaled nitric oxide were studied in ILD patients and were shown to be associated with an improvement in gas exchange [79]. In 2007, Krowka and colleagues evaluated inhaled iloprost in 51 patients with IPF and demonstrated no difference in 6MWT, NYHA functional class, dyspnea score, or oxygen saturation with the drug [80]. Both epoprostinil [81] and treprostinil [82] have been evaluated in patients with ILD-PH. Saggar and associates reported improvements in multiple echocardiographic domains, 6MWT, and patient-reported outcomes in a prospective open-label study of parenteral treprostinil in patients with severe ILD-PH (mPAP $\geq$ 35 mmHg) [82]. One case series described the use of intravenous prostacyclins followed by maintenance inhaled prostacyclins for three patients with ILD-PH presenting as RV failure [38]. However, the most robust data pertaining to prostanoid therapy resulted from the INCREASE study of inhaled Treprostinil [83].

The INCREASE trial was a double-blind, randomized, multi-center, placebo-controlled trial of inhaled Treprostinil in patients with ILD-PH, including those with CPFE [83]. The trial enrolled 326 patients and demonstrated a 31.12 m placebo-corrected improvement in the 6MWT distance at 16 weeks with the use of inhaled Treprostinil [83]. There was also a 15% reduction in NT-proBNP levels in the treatment arm compared to a 46% increase in the placebo group, while clinical worsening occurred in 22.7% of the active treatment group vs. 33.1% of placebo patients ($p = 0.04$) [83]. Based on these results, inhaled Treprostinil became the first FDA-approved drug specifically for the treatment of ILD-PH.

There have been a number of post hoc analyses of the INCREASE trial, which have further explored the benefits of inhaled Treprostinil [84–86]. Less clinical worsening events with inhaled Treprostinil have been further validated in two of these analyses that have evaluated multiple progression events and employed a win ratio approach [85,86]. A potential direct antifibrotic effect of inhaled Treprostinil also emerged from the INCREASE trial [85]. Spirometry was performed in all participants as a safety endpoint, but what was noted was an apparent benefit in FVC with inhaled Trepostinil. Specifically, there was a placebo-corrected difference in the FVC of 28.5 mL at week 8 and 44.4 mL at week 16 favoring inhaled Treprostinil. This finding was most evident in patients with idiopathic interstitial pneumonia, especially IPF [85]. Another post hoc analysis of the INCREASE trial also suggested a long-term survival benefit of inhaled Treprostinil using models of survival that are commonly employed in the oncology literature [87].

A subsequent multicenter, non-randomized, open-label trial of ILD-PH patients was conducted in a Japanese population to evaluate change in pulmonary vascular resistance (PVR) index and peak 6MWT distance [88]. This trial of 20 patients demonstrated a PVR index decrease of 40.1% and a peak 6MWT distance increase of 13 m, reinforcing the efficacy shown in the INCREASE trial [88]. Interestingly, there also appeared to be a small improvement in the FVC in this population as well as a decrease in Krebs von den Lungen-6 levels, a fibrotic biomarker [88].

Based on these results, inhaled Treprostinil has emerged as the first-line treatment for ILD-PH. Inhaled Treprostinil allows for direct delivery of medications to the lungs, reducing the risk of systemic symptoms such as systemic vasodilation. Side effects that may limit the use of inhaled Treprostinil include cough, and modification of route of administration (via nebulizer or dry powder inhalation) may mitigate some side effects. PDE5 inhibitors such as sildenafil and tadalafil are also utilized, as are prostanoids on a case-by-case basis. ERAs and riociguat are generally contraindicated in these patients. As further evidence emerges, the management of these patients will continue to evolve. A suggested treatment approach is shown in Figure 4 [63].

7.5. Clinical Trials in ILD-PH

The prevalence of ILD and the risk of PH developing in many of these patients amplifies the need for further therapies to address this largely unmet need. There are many medications approved for PAH and only one therapy approved for ILD-PH, despite its much greater prevalence and more dire prognosis. There are numerous considerations in the design of ILD-PH trials including but not limited to the patient phenotype most likely to respond, the optimal duration of the study, and the best endpoint(s) to employ. A conceptual framework of these is outlined in Figure 5 [2,89].

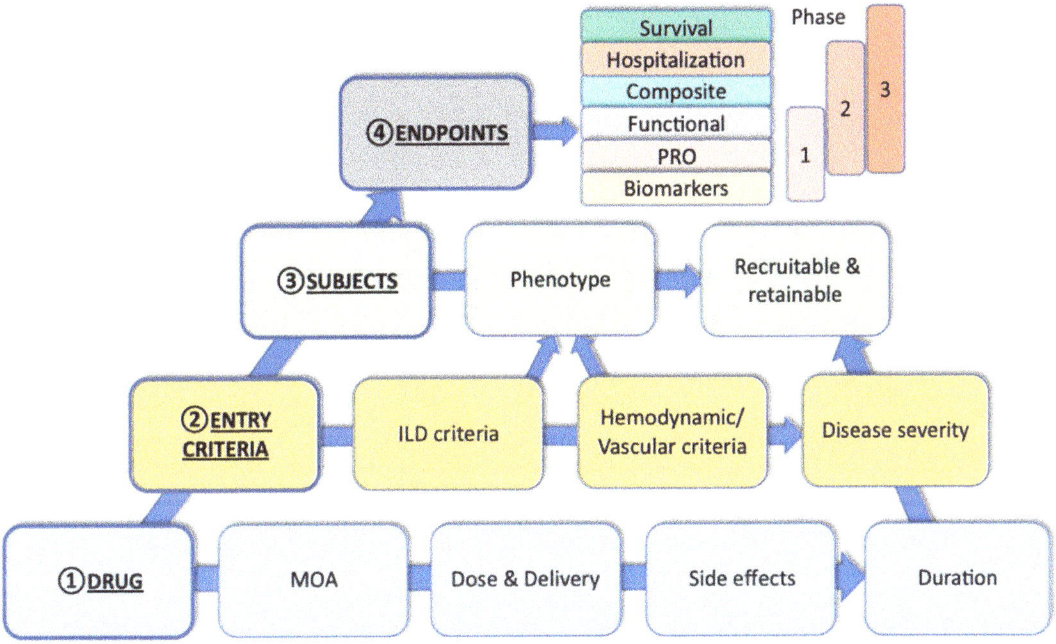

Figure 5. Conceptual framework for clinical trials in ILD-PH. Factors to consider in the design of future clinical trials for pulmonary hypertension associated with interstitial lung disease (ILD-PH). The diagram depicts four different pillars and how their respective variables interrelate and may be considered to optimize ILD-PH trial feasibility. MOA = mechanism of action; PRO = patient-reported outcome. Reprinted with permission of the American Thoracic Society. Copyright © 2024 American Thoracic Society. All rights reserved. Nathan SD. 2023. Progress in the Treatment of Pulmonary Hypertension Associated with Interstitial Lung Disease. Am J Respir Crit Care Med. 208(3):238–246. [63] The American Journal of Respiratory and Critical Care Medicine is an official journal of the American Thoracic Society.

Although there are well-established patient-reported outcome (PRO) questionnaires for both PAH and IPF, there are as yet no PROs specific to ILD-PH; hence this is another area for future research. Finally, further clinical data are required in patients meeting the updated definition of PH to determine the role of treatment in this subgroup. Trials are ongoing to evaluate the safety and efficacy of new therapies (Table 3).

Table 3. Ongoing pharmacologic clinical trials in ILD-PH.

Clinicaltrials.gov Number	Drug	Administration	Mechanism of Action	Phase of Study	Design	Treatment Period (Weeks)	Primary End Point
NCT05176951	Treprostinil palmitil	80 µg daily DPI titrated up to 640 µg	Inhaled prostanoid	2	RCT, double-blind, multicenter, placebo-controlled	16	Safety/tolerability; Change from baseline in 6MWT SpO2
NCT06129240	LIQ861 (treprostinil)	Variable QID DPI dosing	Inhaled prostanoid	3	Open-label ASCENT extension, multicenter	52	Safety/tolerability
NCT04691154	L606 (liposomal treprostini)	Twice daily aerosolized	Aerosolized liposomal prostanoid	3	Open-label extension	48	Safety/tolerability
NCT05128929	H01 (Hymecromone)	80 µg daily DPI titrated up to 640 µg	Inhibitor of hyaluronan synthesis	2	SATURN- RCT, double-blind, placebo-controlled	24	Change in PVR by RHC; safety/tolerability
NCT02036970	Bardoxolone methyl	Variable QID DPI dosing	Inducer of Nrf2 and suppressor of NF-kB	2	RCT, double-blind, placebo-controlled	16	Mean change in 6MWD
NCT06475781	Murivadelgat	Twice daily aerosolized	Aldehyde de-hydrogenase 2 activator	2	WINDWARD- RCT, double, blind, multinational, placebo-controlled	12	Mean change in PVR by RHC at week 12
NCT06635850	Mosliciguat	80 µg daily DPI titrated up to 640 µg	Soluble guanylate cyclase (sGC) activator	2	PHocus- RCT, double-blind, multicenter, placebo-controlled	24	Change in PVR by RHC at 26 weeks

8. Future Directions

There is a large unmet need for the treatment of ILD-PH and a significant knowledge gap in how best to phenotype these patients [50]. How best to integrate and evaluate the extent of the parenchymal lung disease, and the hemodynamics is also uncertain. Whereas there has been reliance on lung function testing to evaluate the former, there is increasing evidence that lung imaging has a critical role. In this regard, functional respiratory imaging has promise as an avenue to explore the extent of the fibrosis as well as details of the associated vascular involvement. The optimal screening strategies with further development and validation of risk assessment tools for PH in ILD patients require further study. This is the subject of an ongoing prospective study (PHinder study NCT05776225). At what point in a patient's clinical course should an RHC be obtained also remains uncertain. The level of suspicion juxtaposed to the likelihood of demonstrating PH is depicted in a concept figure (Figure 6). In addition, if ILD patients do not have PH on RHC, when is the optimal time to repeat their RHC, if ever? While the thresholds defining PH have been lowered, there is no data on what to do with patients who previously would not have been categorized as having PH (i.e., those with PVR 2–3 WU). In addition, controversy remains as to whether to treat ILD-PH patients with PVR of 3–4 WU. While most of the epidemiologic and prognostic data pertaining to ILD-PH is derived from IPF patients, further data on the prevalence and progression of disease within the other ILD subtypes is currently lacking. In summary, there are abundant opportunities and a need for further research into many aspects of ILD-PH [2].

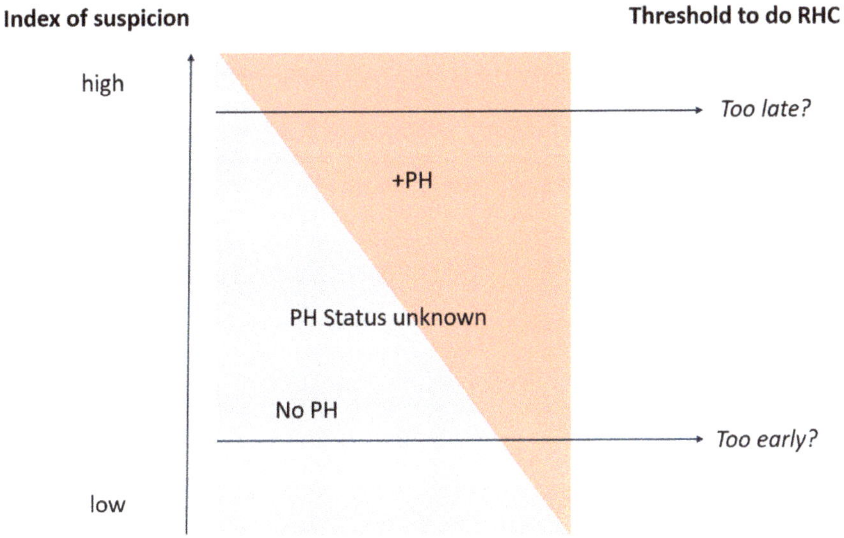

Figure 6. Conceptual depiction of the threshold to perform an RHC and the likelihood of demonstrating its presence. The "Sweet spot" to recommend an RHC remains uncertain.

9. Conclusions

PH in the presence of ILD is associated with significant morbidity and mortality, and early recognition is crucial for the management of these patients. Clinical, biomarker, and physiologic data, may suggest the presence of PH in ILD patients while echocardiography provides further supportive evidence, but right heart catheterization remains the gold standard for the diagnosis of precapillary PH. There is now an available treatment option for ILD-PH which is currently only approved in a few countries, namely, inhaled Treprostinil. Other off-label therapies such as intravenous and/or subcutaneous prostanoids may be considered on a case-by-case basis, but these should only be implemented at expert centers. Further research is needed in phenotyping patients with ILD-PH and in evaluating screening tools and novel treatment modalities.

Funding: This research received no external funding.

Conflicts of Interest: SDN is a consultant for United Therapeutics and is on the Board of Directors for Gossamer Bio. The other authors have no disclosures as they pertain to this manuscript.

Abbreviations

6MWT—six-minute walk test; BNP—brain natriuretic peptide; CPET—cardiopulmonary exercise test; CT—computed tomography; DLCO—diffusion capacity for carbon monoxide; ERA—endothelin receptor antagonists; FEV1—forced expiratory volume in one second; FVC—forced vital capacity; ILD—interstitial lung disease; ILD-PH—pulmonary hypertension associated with ILD; IPF—idiopathic pulmonary fibrosis; mPAP—mean pulmonary arterial pressure; NT-proBNP—N-terminal pro b-type natriuretic peptide; NYHA—New York Heart Association; PA—pulmonary artery; PAH—pulmonary arterial hypertension; PDE5—Phosphodiesterase 5; PFT—pulmonary function test; PH—pulmonary hypertension; PRO—patient-reported outcomes; PVR—pulmonary vascular resistance; RHC—right heart catheterization; WHO—World Health Organization; WU—Wood Units

References

1. Kovacs, G.; Bartolome, S.; Denton, C.P.; Gatzoulis, M.A.; Gu, S.; Khanna, D.; Badesch, D.; Montani, D. Definition, classification and diagnosis of pulmonary hypertension. *Eur. Respir. J.* **2024**, *64*, 2401324. [CrossRef] [PubMed]
2. Shlobin, O.A.; Adir, Y.; Barbera, J.A.; Cottin, V.; Harari, S.; Jutant, E.M.; Pepke-Zaba, J.; Ghofrani, H.A.; Channick, R. Pulmonary hypertension associated with lung diseases. *Eur. Respir. J.* **2024**, *64*, 820–835. [CrossRef] [PubMed]
3. Humbert, M.; Kovacs, G.; Hoeper, M.M.; Badagliacca, R.; Berger, R.M.F.; Brida, M.; Carlsen, J.; Coats, A.J.S.; Escribano-Subias, P.; Ferrari, P.; et al. 2022 ESC/ERS Guidelines for the diagnosis and treatment of pulmonary hypertension. *Eur. Heart J.* **2022**, *43*, 3618–3731. [CrossRef]
4. Nathan, S.D.; Barbera, J.A.; Gaine, S.P.; Harari, S.; Martinez, F.J.; Olschewski, H.; Olsson, K.M.; Peacock, A.J.; Pepke-Zaba, J.; Provencher, S.; et al. Pulmonary hypertension in chronic lung disease and hypoxia. *Eur. Respir. J.* **2019**, *53*, 1801914. [CrossRef] [PubMed]
5. Sato, T.; Furukawa, T.; Teramachi, R.; Fukihara, J.; Yamano, Y.; Yokoyama, T.; Matsuda, T.; Kataoka, K.; Kimura, T.; Sakamoto, K.; et al. Mild elevation of pulmonary vascular resistance predicts mortality regardless of mean pulmonary artery pressure in mild interstitial lung disease. *Thorax* **2024**, *79*, 422–429. [CrossRef]
6. Jeganathan, N.; Sathananthan, M. The prevalence and burden of interstitial lung diseases in the USA. *ERJ Open Res.* **2022**, *8*, 00630-2021. [CrossRef]
7. Nathan, S.D.; Barnett, S.D.; King, C.S.; Provencher, S.; Barbera, J.A.; Pastre, J.; Shlobin, O.A.; Seeger, W. Impact of the new definition for pulmonary hypertension in patients with lung disease: An analysis of the United Network for Organ Sharing database. *Pulm. Circ.* **2021**, *11*, 2045894021999960. [CrossRef] [PubMed]
8. Ang, H.L.; Schulte, M.; Chan, R.K.; Tan, H.H.; Harrison, A.; Ryerson, C.J.; Khor, Y.H. Pulmonary Hypertension in Interstitial Lung Disease: A Systematic Review and Meta-Analysis. *Chest* **2024**, *166*, 778–792. [CrossRef]
9. Nikkho, S.M.; Richter, M.J.; Shen, E.; Abman, S.H.; Antoniou, K.; Chung, J.; Fernandes, P.; Hassoun, P.; Lazarus, H.M.; Olschewski, H.; et al. Clinical significance of pulmonary hypertension in interstitial lung disease: A consensus statement from the Pulmonary Vascular Research Institute's innovative drug development initiative-Group 3 pulmonary hypertension. *Pulm. Circ.* **2022**, *12*, e12127. [CrossRef]
10. Shorr, A.F.; Wainright, J.L.; Cors, C.S.; Lettieri, C.J.; Nathan, S.D. Pulmonary hypertension in patients with pulmonary fibrosis awaiting lung transplant. *Eur. Respir. J.* **2007**, *30*, 715–721. [CrossRef]
11. Nathan, S.D.; Shlobin, O.A.; Ahmad, S.; Koch, J.; Barnett, S.D.; Ad, N.; Burton, N.; Leslie, K. Serial development of pulmonary hypertension in patients with idiopathic pulmonary fibrosis. *Respiration* **2008**, *76*, 288–294. [CrossRef] [PubMed]
12. Todd, N.W.; Lavania, S.; Park, M.H.; Iacono, A.T.; Franks, T.J.; Galvin, J.R.; Jeudy, J.; Britt, E.J.; Luzina, I.G.; Hasday, J.D.; et al. Variable prevalence of pulmonary hypertension in patients with advanced interstitial pneumonia. *J. Heart Lung Transplant.* **2010**, *29*, 188–194. [CrossRef]
13. Raghu, G.; Nathan, S.D.; Behr, J.; Brown, K.K.; Egan, J.J.; Kawut, S.M.; Flaherty, K.R.; Martinez, F.J.; Wells, A.U.; Shao, L.; et al. Pulmonary hypertension in idiopathic pulmonary fibrosis with mild-to-moderate restriction. *Eur. Respir. J.* **2015**, *46*, 1370–1377. [CrossRef] [PubMed]
14. Tyagi, R.; Kant, S.; Verma, S.K.; Kushwaha, R.A.S.; Kumar, S.; Garg, R.; Verma, A.K.; Srivastava, A.; Bajaj, D.K.; Wakhlu, A.; et al. Spectrum of interstitial lung diseases and their association with pulmonary hypertension. *Monaldi Arch. Chest Dis.* **2021**, *92*, 2027. [CrossRef]
15. Young, A.; Vummidi, D.; Visovatti, S.; Homer, K.; Wilhalme, H.; White, E.S.; Flaherty, K.; McLaughlin, V.; Khanna, D. Prevalence, Treatment, and Outcomes of Coexistent Pulmonary Hypertension and Interstitial Lung Disease in Systemic Sclerosis. *Arthritis Rheumatol.* **2019**, *71*, 1339–1349. [CrossRef]
16. Cottin, V.; Nunes, H.; Mouthon, L.; Gamondes, D.; Lazor, R.; Hachulla, E.; Revel, D.; Valeyre, D.; Cordier, J.F.; Groupe d'Etudes et de Recherche sur les Maladies "Orphelines, P. Combined pulmonary fibrosis and emphysema syndrome in connective tissue disease. *Arthritis Rheum.* **2011**, *63*, 295–304. [CrossRef]
17. King, C.S.; Brown, A.W.; Shlobin, O.A.; Weir, N.; Libre, M.; Franco-Palacios, D.; Ahmad, S.; Nathan, S.D. Prevalence and impact of WHO group 3 pulmonary hypertension in advanced idiopathic nonspecific interstitial pneumonia. *Eur. Respir. J.* **2018**, *52*, 1800545. [CrossRef] [PubMed]
18. Cottin, V.; Nunes, H.; Brillet, P.Y.; Delaval, P.; Devouassoux, G.; Tillie-Leblond, I.; Israel-Biet, D.; Court-Fortune, I.; Valeyre, D.; Cordier, J.F.; et al. Combined pulmonary fibrosis and emphysema: A distinct underrecognised entity. *Eur. Respir. J.* **2005**, *26*, 586–593. [CrossRef]
19. Oliveira, R.K.; Pereira, C.A.; Ramos, R.P.; Ferreira, E.V.; Messina, C.M.; Kuranishi, L.T.; Gimenez, A.; Campos, O.; Silva, C.M.; Ota-Arakaki, J.S. A haemodynamic study of pulmonary hypertension in chronic hypersensitivity pneumonitis. *Eur. Respir. J.* **2014**, *44*, 415–424. [CrossRef]

20. Hinchcliff, M.; Fischer, A.; Schiopu, E.; Steen, V.D.; Investigators, P. Pulmonary Hypertension Assessment and Recognition of Outcomes in Scleroderma (PHAROS): Baseline characteristics and description of study population. *J. Rheumatol.* **2011**, *38*, 2172–2179. [CrossRef]
21. Coghlan, J.G.; Denton, C.P.; Grunig, E.; Bonderman, D.; Distler, O.; Khanna, D.; Muller-Ladner, U.; Pope, J.E.; Vonk, M.C.; Doelberg, M.; et al. Evidence-based detection of pulmonary arterial hypertension in systemic sclerosis: The DETECT study. *Ann. Rheum. Dis.* **2014**, *73*, 1340–1349. [CrossRef] [PubMed]
22. Udayakumar, N.; Venkatesan, S.; Rajendiran, C. Pulmonary hypertension in rheumatoid arthritis-relation with the duration of the disease. *Int. J. Cardiol.* **2008**, *127*, 410–412. [CrossRef]
23. Shahane, A. Pulmonary hypertension in rheumatic diseases: Epidemiology and pathogenesis. *Rheumatol. Int.* **2013**, *33*, 1655–1667. [CrossRef] [PubMed]
24. Reeves, G.E.; Collins, N.; Hayes, P.; Knapp, J.; Squance, M.; Tran, H.; Bastian, B. SAPHIRE: Stress and Pulmonary Hypertension in Rheumatoid Evaluation-A Prevalence Study. *Int. J. Rheumatol.* **2016**, *2016*, 4564531. [CrossRef] [PubMed]
25. Cottin, V.; Selman, M.; Inoue, Y.; Wong, A.W.; Corte, T.J.; Flaherty, K.R.; Han, M.K.; Jacob, J.; Johannson, K.A.; Kitaichi, M.; et al. Syndrome of Combined Pulmonary Fibrosis and Emphysema: An Official ATS/ERS/JRS/ALAT Research Statement. *Am. J. Respir. Crit. Care Med.* **2022**, *206*, e7–e41. [CrossRef]
26. Zhao, A.; Gudmundsson, E.; Mogulkoc, N.; van Moorsel, C.; Corte, T.J.; Vasudev, P.; Romei, C.; Chapman, R.; Wallis, T.J.M.; Denneny, E.; et al. Mortality surrogates in combined pulmonary fibrosis and emphysema. *Eur. Respir. J.* **2024**, *63*, 2300127. [CrossRef]
27. Lettieri, C.J.; Nathan, S.D.; Barnett, S.D.; Ahmad, S.; Shorr, A.F. Prevalence and outcomes of pulmonary arterial hypertension in advanced idiopathic pulmonary fibrosis. *Chest* **2006**, *129*, 746–752. [CrossRef]
28. Chebib, N.; Mornex, J.F.; Traclet, J.; Philit, F.; Khouatra, C.; Zeghmar, S.; Turquier, S.; Cottin, V. Pulmonary hypertension in chronic lung diseases: Comparison to other pulmonary hypertension groups. *Pulm. Circ.* **2018**, *8*, 2045894018775056. [CrossRef]
29. Alhamad, E.H.; Cal, J.G.; Alrajhi, N.N.; Alharbi, W.M. Predictors of Mortality in Patients with Interstitial Lung Disease-Associated Pulmonary Hypertension. *J. Clin. Med.* **2020**, *9*, 3828. [CrossRef]
30. Piccari, L.; Allwood, B.; Antoniou, K.; Chung, J.H.; Hassoun, P.M.; Nikkho, S.M.; Saggar, R.; Shlobin, O.A.; Vitulo, P.; Nathan, S.D.; et al. Pathogenesis, clinical features, and phenotypes of pulmonary hypertension associated with interstitial lung disease: A consensus statement from the Pulmonary Vascular Research Institute's Innovative Drug Development Initiative—Group 3 Pulmonary Hypertension. *Pulm. Circ.* **2023**, *13*, e12213.
31. Douschan, P.; Kovacs, G.; Avian, A.; Foris, V.; Gruber, F.; Olschewski, A.; Olschewski, H. Mild Elevation of Pulmonary Arterial Pressure as a Predictor of Mortality. *Am. J. Respir. Crit. Care Med.* **2018**, *197*, 509–516. [CrossRef]
32. Behr, J.; Nathan, S.D. Pulmonary hypertension in interstitial lung disease: Screening, diagnosis and treatment. *Curr. Opin. Pulm. Med.* **2021**, *27*, 396–404. [CrossRef]
33. Olsson, K.M.; Corte, T.J.; Kamp, J.C.; Montani, D.; Nathan, S.D.; Neubert, L.; Price, L.C.; Kiely, D.G. Pulmonary hypertension associated with lung disease: New insights into pathomechanisms, diagnosis, and management. *Lancet Respir. Med.* **2023**, *11*, 820–835. [CrossRef]
34. Singh, I.; Ma, K.C.; Berlin, D.A. Pathophysiology of Pulmonary Hypertension in Chronic Parenchymal Lung Disease. *Am. J. Med.* **2016**, *129*, 366–371. [CrossRef] [PubMed]
35. Budhiraja, R.; Tuder, R.M.; Hassoun, P.M. Endothelial dysfunction in pulmonary hypertension. *Circulation* **2004**, *109*, 159–165. [CrossRef] [PubMed]
36. Alkhanfar, D.; Shahin, Y.; Alandejani, F.; Dwivedi, K.; Alabed, S.; Johns, C.; Lawrie, A.; Thompson, A.A.R.; Rothman, A.M.K.; Tschirren, J.; et al. Severe pulmonary hypertension associated with lung disease is characterised by a loss of small pulmonary vessels on quantitative computed tomography. *ERJ Open Res.* **2022**, *8*, 00503-2021. [CrossRef]
37. Guignabert, C.; Aman, J.; Bonnet, S.; Dorfmuller, P.; Olschewski, A.J.; Pullamsetti, S.; Rabinovitch, M.; Schermuly, R.T.; Humbert, M.; Stenmark, K.R. Pathology and pathobiology of pulmonary hypertension: Current insights and future directions. *Eur. Respir. J.* **2024**, *64*, 2401095. [CrossRef] [PubMed]
38. Jiang, Q.; Liu, C.; Liu, S.; Lu, W.; Li, Y.; Luo, X.; Ma, R.; Zhang, C.; Chen, H.; Chen, Y.; et al. Dysregulation of BMP9/BMPR2/SMAD signalling pathway contributes to pulmonary fibrosis and pulmonary hypertension induced by bleomycin in rats. *Br. J. Pharmacol.* **2021**, *178*, 203–216. [CrossRef]
39. Chen, N.Y.; Collum, S.D.; Luo, F.; Weng, T.; Le, T.T.; Hernandez, A.M.; Philip, K.; Molina, J.G.; Garcia-Morales, L.J.; Cao, Y.; et al. Macrophage bone morphogenic protein receptor 2 depletion in idiopathic pulmonary fibrosis and Group III pulmonary hypertension. *Am. J. Physiol. Lung Cell Mol. Physiol.* **2016**, *311*, L238–L254. [CrossRef]
40. Rahaghi, F.F.; Kolaitis, N.A.; Adegunsoye, A.; de Andrade, J.A.; Flaherty, K.R.; Lancaster, L.H.; Lee, J.S.; Levine, D.J.; Preston, I.R.; Safdar, Z.; et al. Screening Strategies for Pulmonary Hypertension in Patients With Interstitial Lung Disease: A Multidisciplinary Delphi Study. *Chest* **2022**, *162*, 145–155. [CrossRef]

41. Waxman, A.B.; Elia, D.; Adir, Y.; Humbert, M.; Harari, S. Recent advances in the management of pulmonary hypertension with interstitial lung disease. *Eur. Respir. Rev.* **2022**, *31*, 210220. [CrossRef]
42. Parikh, R.; Thomas, A.; Sharofi, A.; Moallem, N.; Fiscus, G.; Farber, H.W. Severe pulmonary hypertension-interstitial lung disease presenting as right ventricular failure: Stabilisation with intravenous prostacyclin and maintenance with inhaled prostacyclin. *ERJ Open Res.* **2024**, *10*, 00659-2023. [CrossRef] [PubMed]
43. Song, J.W.; Song, J.K.; Kim, D.S. Echocardiography and brain natriuretic peptide as prognostic indicators in idiopathic pulmonary fibrosis. *Respir. Med.* **2009**, *103*, 180–186. [CrossRef] [PubMed]
44. Corte, T.J.; Wort, S.J.; Gatzoulis, M.A.; Engel, R.; Giannakoulas, G.; Macdonald, P.M.; Wells, A.U. Elevated brain natriuretic peptide predicts mortality in interstitial lung disease. *Eur. Respir. J.* **2010**, *36*, 819–825. [CrossRef]
45. Steen, V.D.; Graham, G.; Conte, C.; Owens, G.; Medsger, T.A., Jr. Isolated diffusing capacity reduction in systemic sclerosis. *Arthritis Rheum.* **1992**, *35*, 765–770. [CrossRef]
46. Swigris, J.; Nathan, S.; Tighe, R.; Nagra, S.; Rabe, C.; Kelkhoff, D.; Switzer, T.; Kolatkar, N.; Belloni, P.; Golden, J. STARMAP: An observational study to assess disease-relevant outcomes using home-monitoring devices in patients with idiopathic pulmonary fibrosis (IPF). *Eur. Respir. J.* **2019**, *54* (Suppl. S63), PA1333.
47. Joseph, P.; Savarimuthu, S.; Zhao, J.; Yan, X.; Oakland, H.T.; Cullinan, M.; Heerdt, P.M.; Singh, I. Noninvasive determinants of pulmonary hypertension in interstitial lung disease. *Pulm. Circ.* **2023**, *13*, e12197. [CrossRef]
48. King, C.S.; Shlobin, O.A. The Trouble With Group 3 Pulmonary Hypertension in Interstitial Lung Disease: Dilemmas in Diagnosis and the Conundrum of Treatment. *Chest* **2020**, *158*, 1651–1664. [CrossRef] [PubMed]
49. Fisher, M.R.; Forfia, P.R.; Chamera, E.; Housten-Harris, T.; Champion, H.C.; Girgis, R.E.; Corretti, M.C.; Hassoun, P.M. Accuracy of Doppler echocardiography in the hemodynamic assessment of pulmonary hypertension. *Am. J. Respir. Crit. Care Med.* **2009**, *179*, 615–621. [CrossRef] [PubMed]
50. Arslan, A.; Smith, J.; Qureshi, M.R.; Uysal, A.; Patel, K.K.; Herazo-Maya, J.D.; Bandyopadhyay, D. Evolution of pulmonary hypertension in interstitial lung disease: A journey through past, present, and future. *Front. Med.* **2023**, *10*, 1306032. [CrossRef]
51. Zisman, D.A.; Ross, D.J.; Belperio, J.A.; Saggar, R.; Lynch, J.P., 3rd; Ardehali, A.; Karlamangla, A.S. Prediction of pulmonary hypertension in idiopathic pulmonary fibrosis. *Respir. Med.* **2007**, *101*, 2153–2159. [CrossRef] [PubMed]
52. Furukawa, T.; Kondoh, Y.; Taniguchi, H.; Yagi, M.; Matsuda, T.; Kimura, T.; Kataoka, K.; Johkoh, T.; Ando, M.; Hashimoto, N.; et al. A scoring system to predict the elevation of mean pulmonary arterial pressure in idiopathic pulmonary fibrosis. *Eur. Respir. J.* **2018**, *51*, 1701311. [CrossRef]
53. Bax, S.; Bredy, C.; Kempny, A.; Dimopoulos, K.; Devaraj, A.; Walsh, S.; Jacob, J.; Nair, A.; Kokosi, M.; Keir, G.; et al. A stepwise composite echocardiographic score predicts severe pulmonary hypertension in patients with interstitial lung disease. *ERJ Open Res.* **2018**, *4*, 00124-2017. [CrossRef]
54. Sonti, R.; Gersten, R.A.; Barnett, S.; Brown, A.W.; Nathan, S.D. Multimodal noninvasive prediction of pulmonary hypertension in IPF. *Clin. Respir. J.* **2019**, *13*, 567–573. [CrossRef]
55. Sobiecka, M.; Lewandowska, K.; Kober, J.; Franczuk, M.; Skoczylas, A.; Tomkowski, W.; Kus, J.; Szturmowicz, M. Can a New Scoring System Improve Prediction of Pulmonary Hypertension in Newly Recognised Interstitial Lung Diseases? *Lung* **2020**, *198*, 547–554. [CrossRef]
56. Refini, R.M.; Bettini, G.; Kacerja, E.; Cameli, P.; d'Alessandro, M.; Bergantini, L.; De Negri, F.; Rottoli, P.; Sestini, P.; Bargagli, E.; et al. The role of the combination of echo-HRCT score as a tool to evaluate the presence of pulmonary hypertension in idiopathic pulmonary fibrosis. *Intern. Emerg. Med.* **2021**, *16*, 941–947. [CrossRef]
57. Nathan, S.D.; Chandel, A.; Wang, Y.; Xu, J.; Shao, L.; Watkins, T.R.; Diviney, J.; King, C.S.; Han, L. Derivation and validation of a noninvasive prediction tool to identify pulmonary hypertension in patients with IPF: Evolution of the model FORD. *J. Heart Lung Transplant.* **2024**, *43*, 547–553. [CrossRef]
58. Parikh, R.; Konstantinidis, I.; O'Sullivan, D.M.; Farber, H.W. Pulmonary hypertension in patients with interstitial lung disease: A tool for early detection. *Pulm. Circ.* **2022**, *12*, e12141. [CrossRef]
59. Arvanitaki, A.; Diller, G.P.; Gatzoulis, M.A.; McCabe, C.; Price, L.C.; Wort, S.J. Noninvasive diagnostic modalities and prediction models for detecting pulmonary hypertension associated with interstitial lung disease: A narrative review. *Eur. Respir. Rev.* **2024**, *33*, 240092. [CrossRef]
60. Singh, N.; Dorfmuller, P.; Shlobin, O.A.; Ventetuolo, C.E. Group 3 Pulmonary Hypertension: From Bench to Bedside. *Circ. Res.* **2022**, *130*, 1404–1422. [CrossRef]
61. Flaherty, K.R.; Wells, A.U.; Cottin, V.; Devaraj, A.; Walsh, S.L.F.; Inoue, Y.; Richeldi, L.; Kolb, M.; Tetzlaff, K.; Stowasser, S.; et al. Nintedanib in Progressive Fibrosing Interstitial Lung Diseases. *N. Engl. J. Med.* **2019**, *381*, 1718–1727. [CrossRef] [PubMed]
62. King, T.E., Jr.; Bradford, W.Z.; Castro-Bernardini, S.; Fagan, E.A.; Glaspole, I.; Glassberg, M.K.; Gorina, E.; Hopkins, P.M.; Kardatzke, D.; Lancaster, L.; et al. A phase 3 trial of pirfenidone in patients with idiopathic pulmonary fibrosis. *N. Engl. J. Med.* **2014**, *370*, 2083–2092. [CrossRef]

63. Nathan, S.D. Progress in the Treatment of Pulmonary Hypertension Associated with Interstitial Lung Disease. *Am. J. Respir. Crit. Care Med.* **2023**, *208*, 238–246. [CrossRef]
64. Raghu, G.; Behr, J.; Brown, K.K.; Egan, J.J.; Kawut, S.M.; Flaherty, K.R.; Martinez, F.J.; Nathan, S.D.; Wells, A.U.; Collard, H.R.; et al. Treatment of idiopathic pulmonary fibrosis with ambrisentan: A parallel, randomized trial. *Ann. Intern. Med.* **2013**, *158*, 641–649. [CrossRef] [PubMed]
65. Raghu, G.; Million-Rousseau, R.; Morganti, A.; Perchenet, L.; Behr, J.; Group, M.S. Macitentan for the treatment of idiopathic pulmonary fibrosis: The randomised controlled MUSIC trial. *Eur. Respir. J.* **2013**, *42*, 1622–1632. [CrossRef] [PubMed]
66. Corte, T.J.; Keir, G.J.; Dimopoulos, K.; Howard, L.; Corris, P.A.; Parfitt, L.; Foley, C.; Yanez-Lopez, M.; Babalis, D.; Marino, P.; et al. Bosentan in pulmonary hypertension associated with fibrotic idiopathic interstitial pneumonia. *Am. J. Respir. Crit. Care Med.* **2014**, *190*, 208–217. [CrossRef]
67. Badesch, D.B.; Feldman, J.; Keogh, A.; Mathier, M.A.; Oudiz, R.J.; Shapiro, S.; Farber, H.W.; McGoon, M.; Frost, A.; Allard, M.; et al. ARIES-3: Ambrisentan therapy in a diverse population of patients with pulmonary hypertension. *Cardiovasc. Ther.* **2012**, *30*, 93–99. [CrossRef]
68. Hoeper, M.M.; Halank, M.; Wilkens, H.; Gunther, A.; Weimann, G.; Gebert, I.; Leuchte, H.H.; Behr, J. Riociguat for interstitial lung disease and pulmonary hypertension: A pilot trial. *Eur. Respir. J.* **2013**, *41*, 853–860. [CrossRef]
69. Nathan, S.D.; Behr, J.; Collard, H.R.; Cottin, V.; Hoeper, M.M.; Martinez, F.J.; Corte, T.J.; Keogh, A.M.; Leuchte, H.; Mogulkoc, N.; et al. Riociguat for idiopathic interstitial pneumonia-associated pulmonary hypertension (RISE-IIP): A randomised, placebo-controlled phase 2b study. *Lancet Respir. Med.* **2019**, *7*, 780–790. [CrossRef]
70. Corte, T.J.; Gatzoulis, M.A.; Parfitt, L.; Harries, C.; Wells, A.U.; Wort, S.J. The use of sildenafil to treat pulmonary hypertension associated with interstitial lung disease. *Respirology* **2010**, *15*, 1226–1232. [CrossRef]
71. Zimmermann, G.S.; von Wulffen, W.; Huppmann, P.; Meis, T.; Ihle, F.; Geiseler, J.; Leuchte, H.H.; Tufman, A.; Behr, J.; Neurohr, C. Haemodynamic changes in pulmonary hypertension in patients with interstitial lung disease treated with PDE-5 inhibitors. *Respirology* **2014**, *19*, 700–706. [CrossRef]
72. Ghofrani, H.A.; Wiedemann, R.; Rose, F.; Schermuly, R.T.; Olschewski, H.; Weissmann, N.; Gunther, A.; Walmrath, D.; Seeger, W.; Grimminger, F. Sildenafil for treatment of lung fibrosis and pulmonary hypertension: A randomised controlled trial. *Lancet* **2002**, *360*, 895–900. [CrossRef]
73. Collard, H.R.; Anstrom, K.J.; Schwarz, M.I.; Zisman, D.A. Sildenafil improves walk distance in idiopathic pulmonary fibrosis. *Chest* **2007**, *131*, 897–899. [CrossRef] [PubMed]
74. Chapman, T.H.; Wilde, M.; Sheth, A.; Madden, B.P. Sildenafil therapy in secondary pulmonary hypertension: Is there benefit in prolonged use? *Vascul Pharmacol.* **2009**, *51*, 90–95. [CrossRef] [PubMed]
75. Brewis, M.J.; Church, A.C.; Johnson, M.K.; Peacock, A.J. Severe pulmonary hypertension in lung disease: Phenotypes and response to treatment. *Eur. Respir. J.* **2015**, *46*, 1378–1389. [CrossRef]
76. Jackson, R.M.; Glassberg, M.K.; Ramos, C.F.; Bejarano, P.A.; Butrous, G.; Gomez-Marin, O. Sildenafil therapy and exercise tolerance in idiopathic pulmonary fibrosis. *Lung* **2010**, *188*, 115–123. [CrossRef] [PubMed]
77. Idiopathic Pulmonary Fibrosis Clinical Research, N.; Zisman, D.A.; Schwarz, M.; Anstrom, K.J.; Collard, H.R.; Flaherty, K.R.; Hunninghake, G.W. A controlled trial of sildenafil in advanced idiopathic pulmonary fibrosis. *N. Engl. J. Med.* **2010**, *363*, 620–628.
78. Dawes, T.J.W.; McCabe, C.; Dimopoulos, K.; Stewart, I.; Bax, S.; Harries, C.; Samaranayake, C.B.; Kempny, A.; Molyneaux, P.L.; Seitler, S.; et al. Phosphodiesterase 5 inhibitor treatment and survival in interstitial lung disease pulmonary hypertension: A Bayesian retrospective observational cohort study. *Respirology* **2023**, *28*, 262–272. [CrossRef]
79. Olschewski, H.; Ghofrani, H.A.; Walmrath, D.; Schermuly, R.; Temmesfeld-Wollbruck, B.; Grimminger, F.; Seeger, W. Inhaled prostacyclin and iloprost in severe pulmonary hypertension secondary to lung fibrosis. *Am. J. Respir. Crit. Care Med.* **1999**, *160*, 600–607. [CrossRef]
80. Krowka, M.J.; Ahmad, S.; de Andrade, J.A.; Frost, A.; Glassberg, M.K.; Lancaster, L.H.; Lasky, J.; Mathier, M.A.; Stocks, J. A randomized, double-blind, placebo-controlled study to evaluate the safety and efficacy of iloprost inhalation in adults with abnormal pulmonary arterial pressure and exercise limitation associated with idiopathic pulmonary fibrosis. *Chest* **2007**, *132*, 633A. [CrossRef]
81. Minai, O.A.; Sahoo, D.; Chapman, J.T.; Mehta, A.C. Vaso-active therapy can improve 6-min walk distance in patients with pulmonary hypertension and fibrotic interstitial lung disease. *Respir. Med.* **2008**, *102*, 1015–1020. [CrossRef] [PubMed]
82. Saggar, R.; Khanna, D.; Vaidya, A.; Derhovanessian, A.; Maranian, P.; Duffy, E.; Belperio, J.A.; Weigt, S.S.; Dua, S.; Shapiro, S.S.; et al. Changes in right heart haemodynamics and echocardiographic function in an advanced phenotype of pulmonary hypertension and right heart dysfunction associated with pulmonary fibrosis. *Thorax* **2014**, *69*, 123–129. [CrossRef] [PubMed]
83. Waxman, A.; Restrepo-Jaramillo, R.; Thenappan, T.; Ravichandran, A.; Engel, P.; Bajwa, A.; Allen, R.; Feldman, J.; Argula, R.; Smith, P.; et al. Inhaled Treprostinil in Pulmonary Hypertension Due to Interstitial Lung Disease. *N. Engl. J. Med.* **2021**, *384*, 325–334. [CrossRef] [PubMed]

84. Nathan, S.D.; Tapson, V.F.; Elwing, J.; Rischard, F.; Mehta, J.; Shapiro, S.; Shen, E.; Deng, C.; Smith, P.; Waxman, A. Efficacy of Inhaled Treprostinil on Multiple Disease Progression Events in Patients with Pulmonary Hypertension due to Parenchymal Lung Disease in the INCREASE Trial. *Am. J. Respir. Crit. Care Med.* **2022**, *205*, 198–207. [CrossRef]
85. Nathan, S.D.; Waxman, A.; Rajagopal, S.; Case, A.; Johri, S.; DuBrock, H.; De La Zerda, D.J.; Sahay, S.; King, C.; Melendres-Groves, L.; et al. Inhaled treprostinil and forced vital capacity in patients with interstitial lung disease and associated pulmonary hypertension: A post-hoc analysis of the INCREASE study. *Lancet Respir. Med.* **2021**, *9*, 1266–1274. [CrossRef]
86. Nathan, S.D.; Medarov, B.; Ho, L.; Kingrey, J.; Hong, T.; Rao, Y.; Shen, E.; Smith, P.; Deng, C.; Waxman, A. A Novel Approach to Clinical Change Endpoints: A Win Ratio Analysis of the INCREASE Trial. *Ann. Am. Thorac. Soc.* **2023**, *20*, 1537–1540. [CrossRef]
87. Nathan, S.D.; Johri, S.; Joly, J.M.; King, C.S.; Raina, A.; McEvoy, C.A.; Lee, D.; Shen, E.; Smith, P.; Deng, C.; et al. Survival analysis from the INCREASE study in PH-ILD: Evaluating the impact of treatment crossover on overall mortality. *Thorax* **2024**, *79*, 301–306. [CrossRef]
88. Sakao, S.; Kondoh, Y.; Kinoshita, H.; Nishiyama, O.; Ogo, T.; Tanabe, N.; Minatsuki, S.; Nakayama, K.; Taniguchi, Y.; Takahashi, K.; et al. Efficacy, safety, and pharmacokinetics of inhaled treprostinil in Japanese patients with pulmonary hypertension associated with interstitial lung disease. *Respir. Investig.* **2024**, *62*, 980–986. [CrossRef]
89. Nathan, S.D.; Fernandes, P.; Psotka, M.; Vitulo, P.; Piccari, L.; Antoniou, K.; Nikkho, S.M.; Stockbridge, N. Pulmonary hypertension in interstitial lung disease: Clinical trial design and endpoints: A consensus statement from the Pulmonary Vascular Research Institute's Innovative Drug Development Initiative-Group 3 Pulmonary Hypertension. *Pulm. Circ.* **2022**, *12*, e12178. [CrossRef]

Journal of
Clinical Medicine

MDPI

Review

Updates in Diagnostic Tools for ILD

Arsal Tharwani and Manuel L. Ribeiro Neto *

Department of Pulmonary Medicine, Integrated Hospital Care Institute, Cleveland Clinic,
Cleveland, OH 44195, USA; tharwaa@ccf.org
* Correspondence: ribeirm@ccf.org

Abstract: Interstitial lung disease (ILD) is a group of diffuse parenchymal disorders, which are diagnosed in many cases by multidisciplinary discussion (MDD). In some cases, diagnosis can be challenging, and the addition of histopathology can increase diagnostic confidence. The tools to obtain a histopathological sample to diagnose ILD are expanding. In this review, we will discuss the various modalities, their sensitivities and specificities, and procedural complication rates. In this review, we conducted a comprehensive review of literature focusing on emerging and established diagnostic tools for ILD. A systematic search of peer-reviewed publications was performed using PubMed with a focus on clinical trials, retrospective and prospective cohort studies, and systematic reviews. The key diagnostic modalities in focus were genomic classifier (GC), transbronchial cryobiopsy (TBLC), surgical lung biopsy (SLB), endobronchial ultrasound cryobiopsy (EBUS-C), genetic testing, and speckled transthoracic echocardiography (STE). Data extracted from these studies focused on diagnostic yield, specificity, sensitivity, and procedural complication rate. Genomic classifier, a gene-based molecular diagnostic tool, has a high specificity for histological usual interstitial pneumonia (UIP). However, in cases of a negative result, it often results in a need for further invasive sampling by TBLC or SLB. TBLC results in a larger histological sample, which can increase diagnostic yield and increase diagnostic confidence at MDD. Recent prospective trials have compared this modality with SLB and found 63–77% interobserver agreement between pathologists. SLB remains the gold standard with diagnostic yields reported to be more than 90%. EBUS-C has shown promising results increasing diagnostic yield in patients with suspected sarcoidosis or lymphoma. All diagnostic modalities have procedural complications with most common being pneumothorax, bleeding and, rarely, death. Advancements in diagnostic tools for interstitial lung disease (ILD) have significantly improved accuracy. Even though surgical lung biopsy remains the gold standard, the alternative modalities are promising and provide a promising yield with a lower procedural risk.

Keywords: interstitial lung diseases; biopsy; diagnosis

1. Introduction

Interstitial lung disease (ILD) is a heterogenous group of diffuse parenchymal lung disorders with varying treatment responses and survival rates [1]. In most cases, the diagnosis is idiopathic pulmonary fibrosis (IPF), for which the mainstay of treatment is anti-fibrotic therapy [1–3]. Immunosuppression in IPF can lead to harm [4]. In other cases, such as hypersensitivity pneumonitis (HP) and sarcoidosis, removal of the offending agent (in HP) and immunosuppression are helpful [5,6]. Similarly, in connective tissue disease-associated ILD (CTD-ILD), the primary treatment is immunosuppression with or without anti-fibrotic therapy [2,3,7,8]. Therefore, an accurate diagnosis is key because it can have treatment and prognostic implications.

Most cases of ILD can be diagnosed with high confidence by a multidisciplinary discussion (MDD), involving clinical and radiological data [1,9]. When discussing a case with other pulmonologists and thoracic radiologists at the MDD before a lung biopsy is performed, for example, a consensus of a probable usual interstitial pneumonia (UIP) pattern and IPF could be reached with high confidence, avoiding unnecessary procedures [10]. However, in 10–40% of newly diagnosed ILD, the addition of histopathology, by a lung biopsy, may be needed to establish a diagnosis and/or improve diagnostic confidence [9]. In those cases, the MDD could assist in choosing the best diagnostic modality. For example, if non-specific interstitial pneumonia (NSIP) is in the differential, the MDD may recommend a surgical lung biopsy (SLB) over a transbronchial lung cryobiopsy (TBLC).

In IPF, a clinical likelihood assessment can be made based on certain risk factors, such as older age (>60 years of age), male sex, current or former tobacco smoking history, or Velcro crackles on auscultation (Figure 1) [11]. If these risk factors are present, it increases the pre-test clinical probability of IPF. On the other hand, exposure to antigens implicated with HP, the presence of autoimmune features, and acute/sub-acute onset decreases the pre-test clinical probability of IPF [11]. Clinicians can use these data to classify patients into a high (70–100%), intermediate (30–70%), or low (0–30%) pre-test clinical probability of IPF [11]. However, these clinical probability models have to be used with caution, since some features could be present in many different ILDs. For example, an UIP pattern can be seen in CTD patients. Prospective studies are needed to validate these models.

	Clinical likelihood of IPF		
	Likelihood decreased if present		Likelihood increased if present
Sex	Female sex	←→	Male sex
Age	< 50 years	←→	> 60 years
Tobacco history	Never smoker	←→	Ex-smoker (or current smoker)
Auscultation	Absence of crackles Presence of squeaks or wheezing	←→	Velcro crackles
Clubbing	Absent	←→	Present
Exposure to significant antigens that may cause hypersensitivity pneumonitis	Present	←→	Absent
Autoimmune features	Present	←→	Absent
Plausible differential diagnosis	Yes	←→	No
Familial aggregation of fibrotic ILD	No	←→	Yes
Lung function	Airflow obstruction or mixed physiology not ascribable to emphysema	←→	Restrictive physiology
Onset	Acute or subacute onset	←→	Chronic onset

Figure 1. Clinical likelihood of IPF based on demographics and clinical features [11]. Legend. IPF, idiopathic pulmonary fibrosis; ILD, interstitial lung disease. Reprinted with permission of the American Thoracic Society,

The radiographic assessment of UIP in high-resolution computed tomography (HRCT) should classify patients into one of the four categories: UIP (presence of basilar and peripheral reticulations, honeycombing with or without traction bronchiectasis), probable UIP (presence of basilar and peripheral reticulations, traction bronchiectasis without honeycombing), indeterminate for UIP (diffuse fibrosis distribution that do not suggest any specific etiology), or HRCT suggesting an alternative diagnosis (with features including presence of ground glass changes, cysts, consolidations, nodules). In a high pre-test clinical probability of UIP, radiographic patterns consistent with UIP or probable UIP are suggestive of IPF without a need for biopsy (Figure 2). In an intermediate pre-test clinical probability of IPF, an HRCT pattern consistent with UIP can be used to confirm a diagnosis of IPF without a need for biopsy. In all other cases, a biopsy may be needed for better assessment.

		HRCT pattern			
		UIP	Probable UIP	Indeterminate for UIP	Alternative diagnosis
Clinical likelihood	High (70% or more)	Definite diagnosis of IPF (biopsy not indicated)	Definite diagnosis of IPF (biopsy not indicated)	Low-confidence provisional diagnosis of IPF (biopsy is likely to inform diagnosis)	Probability of IPF comparable to that of other ILD diagnosis (biopsy, if performed, is highly likely to inform diagnosis)
	Intermediate for IPF (30–70%)	High-confidence provisional diagnosis of IPF (biopsy generally not indicated)	Low-confidence provisional diagnosis of IPF (biopsy is likely to inform diagnosis)	Probability of IPF comparable to that of other ILD diagnosis (biopsy, if performed, is highly likely to inform diagnosis)	Probability of ILD other than IPF greater than IPF (biopsy, if performed, is highly likely to inform diagnosis)
	Low (30% or less)	Low-confidence provisional diagnosis of IPF (further evaluation needed to make a diagnosis)	Probability of IPF comparable to that of other ILD diagnosis (biopsy, if performed, is highly likely to inform diagnosis)	Probability of ILD other than IPF greater than IPF (biopsy, if performed, is highly likely to inform diagnosis)	Probability of ILD other than IPF greater than IPF (biopsy, if performed, is highly likely to inform diagnosis)

Figure 2. Probability of non-invasive diagnosis of IPF based on clinical diagnosis and radiographic data [11]. Legend. HRCT, high-resolution computed tomography; UIP, usual interstitial pneumonia; IPF, idiopathic pulmonary fibrosis. Reprinted with permission of the American Thoracic Society.

The decision to pursue biopsy in these undifferentiated cases of ILD should be weighed against the patient's risk of procedural complications and should be considered if the biopsy is going to result in a change in clinical management: for example, differentiating fibrotic-HP from IPF or CTD-ILD from IPF [12]. These forms of fibrotic ILDs can present with a progressive fibrosis phenotype, for which a biopsy is essential to exclude IPF from the other types (such as HP or CTD-ILD) because treatment is going to be vastly different [12,13], In other cases of undifferentiated ILD, atypical radiological patterns, such as extensive consolidation, ground glass changes, cysts, and nodules may require a histopathological assessment if no clear etiology has been identified on clinical or radiological evaluation [14]. Furthermore, the presence of histological UIP on histopathology has been shown to have a progressive phenotype and is likely to result in adverse outcomes [15]. Hence, in these scenarios, having histopathology can also help in the prognostication of ILD. In the past, SLB was the preferred method for histopathological diagnosis [16–18]. With the advent of newer and less invasive methods, such as genomic classifier (GC) and TBLC, pulmonologists have a wide range of newer tools available. Despite the availability of newer modalities, there is a lack of guidance on what modality to use for clinical situations. In this chapter, we will discuss the tools available for diagnosing ILD, their use in clinical practice, their sensitivity, specificity, and procedural complication rates. Table 1 shows a summary of the pros and cons of the modalities discussed herein.

Table 1. Pros and cons of diagnostic tools.

Diagnostic Tool	Pros	Cons
GC	• Good specificity for UIP (around 90%) • Lower risk compared to TBLC or SLB	• Availability indefinitely on hold by manufacturer • Poor sensitivity for UIP, so many false-negative tests • It cannot differentiate different causes of UIP (e.g., IPF versus HP versus CTD-ILD)
TBLC	• Good diagnostic yield (around 80%) • Lower risk compared to SLB	• Learning curve exists • Higher risk compared to TBB/GC • Conflicting data in its ability to differentiate UIP from fibrotic HP • Conflicting data in its ability to diagnose NSIP • Patient may still require an SLB if TBLC is nondiagnostic
SLB	• Highest diagnostic yield (>90%)	• Highest risk
Genetic testing	• May help diagnose FPF • Noninvasive test • May help identify patients who should not be on immunosuppression	• Variable coverage by insurance companies • It cannot diagnose specific patterns, since both TRG and SRG mutations can cause different patterns
EBUS-C	• Diagnostic yield for sarcoidosis probably higher than with EBUS-TBNA • Diagnostic yield for lymphoma or uncommon tumors is higher than with EBUS-TBNA	• Learning curve exists • Increase in procedure time • Futile in most patients with suspected sarcoidosis

Legend. GC, genomic classifier; TBLC, transbronchial lung cryobiopsy; SLB, surgical lung biopsy; EBUS-C, endobronchial ultrasound-guided cryobiopsy; UIP, usual interstitial pneumonia; FPF, familial pulmonary fibrosis; TBNA, transbronchial needle aspiration; IPF, idiopathic pulmonary fibrosis; HP, hypersensitivity pneumonitis; CTD-ILD, connective tissue disease-related interstitial lung disease; TBB, transbronchial biopsy; NSIP, non-specific interstitial pneumonia; TRG, telomere-related genes; SRG, surfactant-related genes.

2. Genomic Classifier

The reliable identification of UIP in conventional transbronchial forceps biopsies (TBB) has been challenging due to an inadequate sampling of alveoli and lung parenchyma [19]. In retrospective studies, the overall yield has been variable and reported to be less than 10% by some, while others have reported a yield of 30–43% [20–22]. Given the poor yield of conventional TBB, Parkantz et al. described the addition of a machine-learning methodology with TBB to train an algorithm to differentiate UIP from non-UIP [23]. This was the Envisia Genomic Classifier (Veracyte, San Francisco, CA, USA), which is a gene expression based molecular diagnostic tool, which utilizes RNA sequencing to detect molecular UIP gene expression signature [23,24]. The output is a binary result, UIP or non-UIP.

The initial study by Parkantz et al. described a test specificity of 86% and sensitivity of 63% [23]. In a prospective study by Raghu et al., the classifier identified UIP in TBB samples in 49 patients with 88% specificity and 70% sensitivity [24]. Among these patients, 42 had possible or indeterminate UIP patterns on HRCT. The GC also increased diagnostic confidence, especially in cases where the histopathology was non-diagnostic [24]. Similarly, Richeldi et al. showed a sensitivity and specificity of 60% and 92%, respectively [25]. When used in conjunction with HRCT patterns of UIP, the sensitivity of the test improved to 79% [25]. Pooling data from all prior studies on genomic classifier, a meta-analysis reported a combined sensitivity of 68% and specificity of 92% [26].

Given the high specificity of the test, the results can be useful in cases of probable and/or indeterminate UIP pattern by HRCT, where the diagnostic confidence of IPF is low in MDD settings. In a study, the addition of GC increased diagnostic confidence for IPF from 30% to 69% [27,28]. The concurrent increase in IPF diagnosis led to an increase in recommendation of antifibrotic from 10% to 46% in this cohort [27,28]. Therefore, it reduces the need for further invasive sampling by TBLC or SLB. The use of a genomic classifier can also enhance understanding regarding prognostication and disease progression for ILD, as shown by Chaudhry et al. [13]. A positive GC result of UIP was significantly associated with a higher risk of progression and annual FVC decline [13]. This finding may influence the decision to pursue antifibrotics as a management strategy. Hence, the role of GC is expandable beyond diagnostic data and applicable to management as well. Furthermore, it can also be utilized in limited resource centers without access to ILD experts.

However, the test has a low sensitivity, and false negatives are common. Hence, in cases where the GC results are a non-UIP result, it will likely result in a need for a more invasive sampling by TBLC or SLB.

The complication rate from GC is related to the risk of conventional TBB. The main complications are bleeding and pneumothorax. In general, the risk of pneumothorax is 5% [12,29]. However, in pulmonary fibrosis with resting hypoxia and severe reduction in DLCO, the risk can be increased to 7% [30]. The risk of major bleeding requiring a balloon placement, causing hemodynamic or respiratory disturbance, or termination of the procedure, is between 1 and 3% [29,31]. The rates of these complications are still considerably lower than those of TBLC and SLB.

In summary, the GC has a high specificity for histological UIP, which has a high predictive value for IPF. However, caution must be exercised in interpretation of a GC positive UIP result because non-IPF ILDs, such as fibrotic HP and CTD-ILD, can have a histological UIP pattern. Most importantly, a GC negative UIP result does not rule out UIP due to its low sensitivity and high chance of a false negative test result.

3. Transbronchial Cryobiopsy

Transbronchial cryobiopsy has been increasingly utilized as an alternative diagnostic technique across many centers. Cryoprobes utilize cooling agents (e.g., carbon dioxide or nitric oxide) under high pressure, which leads to gaseous expansion and to the pulmonary tissue adhering to the cold probe tip. This results in a larger sample available for histopathological analysis than the one obtained through conventional TBB. The initial meta-analysis reported a diagnostic yield of TBLC ranging from 70% to 84% as compared to SLB's yield of >90% [32–34]. However, these studies were mainly retrospective, and some were prospective cohort studies without a direct comparison to SLB. Romagnoli et al. attempted a direct comparison study between TBLC and SLB in the CryoPID study and showed a poor interobserver agreement of 38% (kappa 0.22) [35]. However, this study was underpowered with a small sample size (N = 21) and utilized only one pathologist for histopathology review.

The COLDICE study was a prospective cohort study with sequential TBLC and SLB for histopathological and MDD agreement [36]. The pathologists were blinded to the clinical and radiographic data, which was followed by discussion at MDD regarding the final diagnosis. Histopathological agreement was 71% (kappa 0.7) and diagnostic agreement at MDD was 77% (kappa 0.62) with a high degree of concordance [36]. For TBLC with high or definitive confidence at MDD, there was a 95% concordance with SLB [36]. In cases with low confidence or non-diagnostic TBLC, SLB helped inform decisions in 23% of cases [36]. The predominant diagnosis at MDD was IPF, which was followed by HP [36].

The COLD study was the first randomized-controlled trial comparing TBLC and SLB. It compared a step-up strategy, TBLC followed by SLB, with an immediate SLB for diagnosis of ILD after MDD discussion [37]. The diagnostic yield of TBLC was 82% [37]. TBLC was inconclusive in 11% (3/28) of cases, necessitating SLB for diagnosis [37]. The overall histopathological agreement between pathologists for the lung biopsies was 63% (kappa 0.53), being 61% in the step-up strategy (kappa 0·53) and 65% in the immediate SLB group (kappa 0.51) [37]. Predominant diagnoses were HP and idiopathic non-specific interstitial pneumonia (NSIP) [37].

The CAN-ICE study looked at the interobserver agreement between TBLC and SLB within and between academic centers in The Netherlands [38]. They showed a moderate agreement between TBLC-MDD and SLB-MDD with 62% of concordance (kappa 0.46). Discordance in MDD was related to the TBLC diagnosis of IPF, which was classified as HP on SLB. TBLC was also likely to yield more unclassifiable ILD. Between-center agreement was better for SLB (kappa 0.71) than TBLC (kappa 0.29).

The use of TBLC and GC has been investigated by a prospective study, which showed that the addition of GC to TBLC increased diagnostic confidence in MDD for probable UIP pattern and diagnosis of IPF [39]. The diagnostic confidence of IPF increased from 31% to 92% after the addition of GC to TBLC [39]. However, for indeterminate patterns of UIP, the addition of GC to TBLC made no significant difference in diagnostic confidence. In these cases, TBLC by itself helped increase diagnostic confidence in MDD [39]. Hence, in cases with a radiographic patten of probable UIP, the addition of GC to TBLC can help increase diagnostic confidence, especially in cases of non-diagnostic histopathology.

The decision to pursue a TBLC depends on a variety of factors. First, is the institution comfortable with the procedure both from procedural (given potential complications) and pathology expertise (due to its lower sample size compared to SLB) standpoints? Second, can it be determined based on the differential diagnoses being considered, such as NSIP, HP, cystic lung diseases or an indeterminate pattern for UIP [14]? Third, patients who are likely to be poor SLB candidates (due to respiratory disease or comorbidities) can benefit from TBLC [14]. The European respiratory society recommends TBLC as the first step for obtaining a histopathological sample in undifferentiated ILD [14].

Major complications associated with TBLC are major airway bleeding and pneumothorax. Based on pooled data from meta-analyses, the risk of pneumothorax from the procedure requiring a chest tube is 5.6% [10,36–38,40]. In cases requiring chest tube drainage for pneumothorax, the chest tube is usually removed within 24 h. Compared to SLB, the duration of chest tube placement is shorter, the hospital stay is shorter, and the infection risk is lower in TBLC [10,37,38].

Unfortunately, due to the lack of standardization of grades of airway bleeding during and post-procedure, the complication rates are variable for airway bleeding. Moderate bleeding requiring bronchoscopic intervention with the instillation of cold saline and/or reinflation of balloon is reported to be between 22 and 36% [36–38]. Severe airway bleeding requiring reintubation, bronchial blocker, angioembolization or procedural abortion was a rare event in these studies and has been reported to be 1.6% based on meta-analyses [36–38,40]. However, in one study, severe airway bleeding requiring reintubation and bronchial blocker placement was reported to be around 12% [10]. Mortality from TBLC has been estimated to be 0.4% [39].

4. Surgical Lung Biopsy

Surgical lung biopsy remains the reference standard for the diagnosis of ILD. The most common technique is video-assisted thoracoscopy (VATS) with diagnostic yields reported to be around 95% [41]. However, the decision to pursue a VATS for a diagnosis is a complicated one, considering the morbidity and mortality of the procedure.

In-hospital mortality after SLB has been reported to be 1.7% for elective procedures across 10-year studies (from 1990s to 2000s) in the United States and United Kingdom [16,42]. The 30-day and 90-day mortality for the procedure can approach 2.4% and 3.9%, respectively [16,43]. For non-elective procedures, the in-hospital mortality rates are considerably higher with estimates of around 16% [42]. Certain patient factors, such as advanced age, higher Charleston comorbidity scores and pre-operative respiratory failure, have been associated with increased risk of mortality after VATS [16,42–44].

A recent study from the United States looked at cases between 2012 and 2019, and it did not report any mortality for elective procedures after VATS [45]. For patients who were hospitalized, post-operative mortality was 10% [45]. Similarly, a prospective study from France did not report any post-operative mortality for patients undergoing elective VATS [18]. The lower rates of mortality, as compared to earlier studies, can be attributed toward refined surgical techniques and patient selection criteria [18].

The clinical decision to pursue an SLB should be based on patient risk factors, such as age, comorbidities, the physiological severity of ILD, and baseline hypoxemia. It is also dependent on a clinical center's diagnostic yield from TBLC. The decision to pursue an SLB may further be enforced if a TBLC is inconclusive and the addition of histopathology to a case will influence management decisions. Morbidity after VATS is common and has been reported as bleeding, pneumothorax, infection and prolonged hospitalization [17,42,45,46]. The rate of recurrent or persistent pneumothorax is 5.5% [40]. The risk of empyema or pneumothorax is 2.1% [40]. The risk of 30-day mortality is 1.7% [40]. Morbidity is lower for elective procedures as opposed to the hospitalized cohort. However, morbidity rates, such as acute exacerbation of ILD (6.1%), persistent air leak (5.9%), respiratory infection (6.5%), and delayed wound healing (3.3%) are higher than those for transbronchial cryobiopsy [12,47].

In summary, SLB remains the reference standard for ILD diagnosis. Given the relatively high risk of complications from the procedure, a thorough review of patient factors, such as age, comorbidities, along with the nature of the procedure (elective vs. emergent) and use of an MDD discussion, should be considered.

5. Genetic Testing

Genetic predisposition to pulmonary fibrosis has been confirmed by the discovery of several key gene mutations [48–50]. Monogenic mutations, such as genes involved in telomere or surfactant hemostasis, namely telomere-related genes (TRGs) or surfactant-related genes (SRGs), have been identified in familial pulmonary fibrosis (FPF) [48,50].

Mutations in TRG are associated with pathological chromosomal shortening, which results in pulmonary and extra-pulmonary manifestations. The prototypical manifestation of a homozygous TRG mutation is dyskeratosis congenita, which is associated with abnormal skin pigmentation, oral leukoplakia, nail dystrophy and bone marrow failure [51]. In heterozygous TRG mutations, predominantly found in adults, extra-pulmonary abnormalities involving the hematological and hepatic systems are common [48–50]. It can also be associated with the premature graying of hair. Pulmonary fibrosis subtypes in TRG mutations include IPF, NSIP, fibrotic HP, and CTD-ILD [52]. Mutations in TRG are associated with poor outcomes in IPF and in lung transplantation. Apart from prognosis, treatment with immunosuppression for pulmonary fibrosis in TRG is associated with adverse outcomes [49].

Mutations in SRG are associated with various radiographic and histological variants, namely UIP, NSIP and desquamative interstitial pneumonia [50]. Since surfactant production is limited to the lungs, these mutations do not cause extra-pulmonary manifestations; however, they are associated with increased risk of lung cancer, especially adenocarcinoma [53].

Genomics-based testing options include genetic testing and telomere length measurement. Testing for the telomere length of peripheral leukocytes and reporting as age-adjusted values is one of the tools available [49]. Mutations in TRG may present with short telomere length, which is usually less than that in the 25th percentile [54]. However, some mutation variants in TRG present with normal telomere length, which does not rule out the disorder [54]. In these cases, genomic sequencing, by whole genome, whole exon or panel sequencing, for previously recognized high-risk genes can give valuable information [50]. For SRG mutations, genomic sequencing is the only way to test [55].

Single nucleotide polymorphisms (SNPs) have also been identified in fibrotic ILD patients. The most studied is the MUC5B promoter gene rs35705950, which has been found in patients with IPF, FPF, rheumatoid arthritis (RA)-ILD, and fibrotic HP [48]. MUC5B promoter variant identified in IPF is associated with better survival and slower progression [56]. It is not associated with better survival in familial or early-onset fibrosis [49,56].

Unfortunately, there is no consensus on when to test individuals for TRG and SRG mutations. In patients with a clinical suspicion, the European Respiratory Society recommends testing if fibrosing ILD is detected before the age of 50, when a first- or second degree relative has fibrotic ILD, or in any patient with a relative carrying a known pathogenic variant [49]. Treatment of these pathogenic variants includes anti-fibrotic therapy and/or early referral for lung transplantation [50].

6. Endobronchial Ultrasound-Guided Cryobiopsy

In one specific ILD, sarcoidosis, a biopsy of thoracic lymph nodes may be enough to confirm its diagnosis. Endobronchial ultrasound-guided cryobiopsy (EBUS-C) is a recent innovation that can potentially increase the diagnostic yield of lymph node biopsies in suspected sarcoidosis patients.

This has been demonstrated by a retrospective Italian cohort that included 48 patients who had both EBUS-C and EBUS-transbronchial needle aspiration (TBNA) in the same procedure for mediastinal or hilar lesions. For sarcoidosis, the diagnostic yield of EBUS-C was higher than that of EBUS-TBNA (93% versus 79%, respectively) [57]. Those findings were corroborated by a larger prospective European cohort that included 137 patients with mediastinal or hilar lesions. In that study, the diagnostic yield for sarcoidosis of EBUS-C was also higher than that of EBUS-TBNA (93% versus 41%, respectively). Importantly, EBUS-C also had a higher diagnostic yield for "uncommon tumors" including lymphoma [58].

In a separate prospective Spanish cohort, however, different results were demonstrated. Fifty patients with mediastinal and hilar lesions were included in that study, and both EBUS-C and EBUS-TBNA identified all six patients with sarcoidosis. The overall diagnostic yield, however, was higher for EBUS-C compared to EBUS-TBNA (96% versus 82%, respectively), which was driven by lymphoma and other malignancies [59].

When applying these data to patient care, we also suggest that clinicians consider the pre-test probability of sarcoidosis before the bronchoscopy. If the pre-test probability is high, with a typical pattern of thoracic adenopathy, EBUS-TBNA is probably enough to achieve an accurate diagnosis of sarcoidosis. In atypical cases, especially when lymphoma is being suspected, EBUS-C is a reasonable option and should be considered.

7. Speckled Transthoracic Echocardiography

The right ventricle (RV) can face an increase in afterload in patients with fibrotic ILD due to hypoxemic vasoconstriction and architectural destruction, which can lead to reduction in RV function and lead to RV–arterial uncoupling [60]. The use of speckle tracking echocardiography (STE) to analyze global myocardial strain has been studied to prognosticate patients with fibrotic ILD [61–63].

Using parameters, such as RV global longitudinal strain (RV GLS) and lateral wall longitudinal strain (LWLS), earlier signs of RV dysfunction can be detected in patients with early IPF [62]. These parameters are available using speckle tracking echocardiography (STE). The change in these parameters becomes pronounced on exercise in patients with IPF as compared to patients without fibrotic interstitial lung disease [62]. Parameters of standard echocardiography, such as tricuspid annular plane systolic excursion (TAPSE) and RV tissue doppler velocity (TD), are not sensitive enough to detect signs of early RV dysfunction [62].

Another study used RV function metrics, such as the ratio of tricuspid annular plane systolic excursion (TAPSE) or RV global longitudinal strain (GLS) to the systolic pulmonary arterial pressure (sPAP), to assess RV–arterial coupling. The study found that the RV GLS/sPAP is a reliable non-invasive parameter of RV–arterial uncoupling and is associated with worse outcomes in patients with fibrotic ILD [61]. Among patients with fibrotic ILD with RV–arterial uncoupling, patients with IPF tend to have the poorest prognosis. Among patients with IPF, left ventricular (LV) diastolic dysfunction was common, which was commonly assessed by using LV global longitudinal strain [63].

Hence, STE has a role in patients with fibrotic ILD, particularly IPF, in looking for signs of RV–arterial uncoupling, which can help prognosticate these patients for the clinicians.

8. Putting Everything Together

With so many tools available to diagnose ILD, the decision-making process may be overwhelming for both clinicians and patients. A simple approach is to decide how high the pre-test probability of the leading diagnosis is, and what are the differential diagnoses in each case. Depending on those two variables, the diagnostic pathway will lead clinicians and patients to different decisions. For example, in a patient with a high pre-test probability of IPF (no clinical features of alternative diseases) and a UIP pattern on HRCT, no biopsy is needed. In a patient with highly suspected fibrotic HP and an obvious antigen exposure, either imaging alone or a bronchoalveolar lavage with lymphocytosis may be enough to establish a confident diagnosis. In a patient with suspected organizing pneumonia, a conventional forceps TBB may easily yield the correct diagnosis. The fact that we can use all of those tools does not mean that we have to. However, if the pre-test probably is not high enough for any disease, and the differential diagnoses are many, the use of the diagnostic tools discussed above are certainly welcome (Figure 3).

Another important aspect is to consider patient's values and preferences during this process. If a patient's goal is to achieve an accurate diagnosis as fast as possible, with a single procedure, and he or she is willing to accept the risks, an SLB may be the best option for that patient in most situations. On the other hand, if a patient's goal is to avoid procedural risks, and he or she is willing to undergo two separate procedures if needed, a TBLC may be the best option for that patient before an SLB.

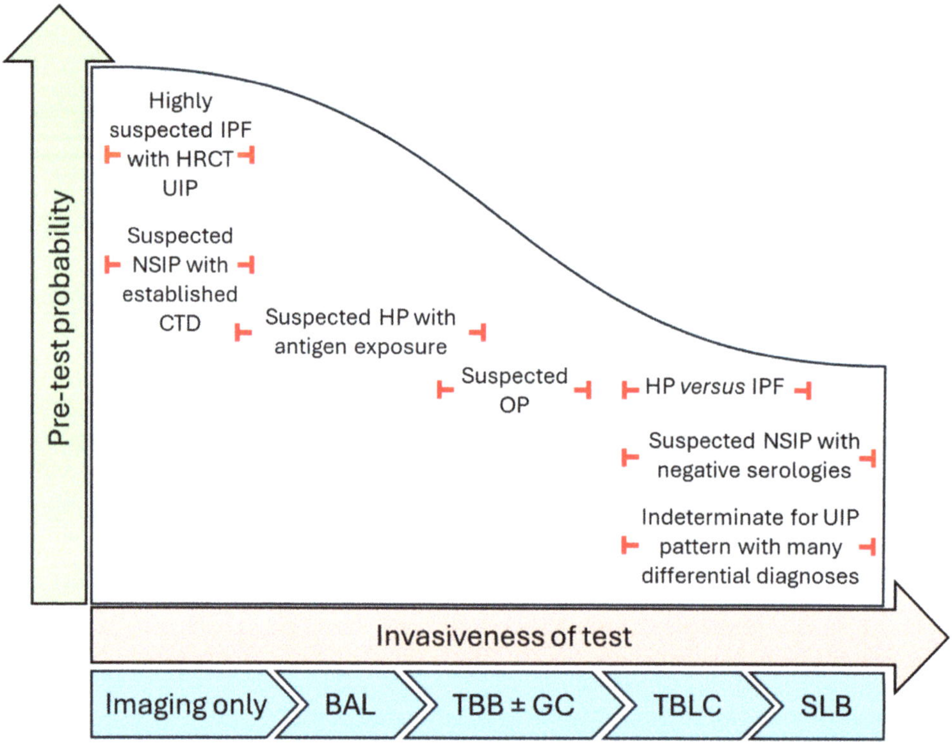

Figure 3. Relationship between pre-test probability and invasiveness of tests. Legend. NSIP, non-specific interstitial pneumonia; HP, hypersensitivity pneumonitis; IPF, idiopathic pulmonary fibrosis; UIP, usual interstitial pneumonia; OP, organizing pneumonia; HRCT, high-resolution computed tomography; CTD, connective tissue disease; SLB, surgical lung biopsy; TBLC, transbronchial lung cryobiopsy; TBB, transbronchial biopsy; GC, genomic classifier; BAL, bronchoalveolar lavage.

In this review, we have a generalized assumption that GC, TBLC and SLB expertise is available to the clinical centers. These procedures are governed by the technique of the bronchoscopist and thoracic surgeon, which influences diagnostic yield. Hence, this is subject to bias and may introduce variability in diagnostic results.

Finally, we must keep in mind that some degree of uncertainty may always exist in some ILD cases, as it is inherently part of the process. Neither is the interobserver agreement between thoracic radiologists perfect, nor is the interobserver agreement between pathologists perfect as shown above. Therefore, ILD patients and caregivers need to be comfortable with the imperfect characteristics of these tests.

9. Future Directions

There are multiple tools available for the diagnosis of ILD. Unfortunately, given the large number of different ILDs and the recency of some of the diagnostic tools, there is no clear or simple algorithm for which technique to perform in every diagnosis. Even though the histological yield is higher with surgical lung biopsy, the availability of alternative tools is promising. Further research is needed to continue to improve the way patients with ILD are diagnosed. For example, more research is needed clarifying the use of TBLC in NSIP or to differentiate fibrotic HP versus UIP. Additional studies are also needed to determine the clinical utility of the GC, and more studies are needed to help clinicians decide which suspected sarcoidosis patients need an EBUS-C versus an EBUS-TBNA. As those and other questions are answered with future studies, we will be able to better use these important diagnostic tools.

Funding: This research received no external funding.

Conflicts of Interest: The authors declare no conflict of interest.

References

1. Raghu, G.; Remy-Jardin, M.; Richeldi, L.; Thomson, C.C.; Antoniou, K.M.; Bissell, B.D.; Bouros, D.; Buendia-Roldan, I.; Caro, F.; Crestani, B.; et al. Idiopathic Pulmonary Fibrosis (an Update) and Progressive Pulmonary Fibrosis in Adults: An Official ATS/ERS/JRS/ALAT Clinical Practice Guideline. *Am. J. Respir. Crit. Care Med.* **2022**, *205*, E18–E47. [CrossRef] [PubMed]
2. Flaherty, K.R.; Wells, A.U.; Cottin, V.; Devaraj, A.; Walsh, S.L.F.; Inoue, Y.; Richeldi, L.; Kolb, M.; Tetzlaff, K.; Stowasser, S.; et al. Nintedanib in Progressive Fibrosing Interstitial Lung Diseases. *N. Engl. J. Med.* **2019**, *381*, 1718–1727. [CrossRef]
3. Maher, T.M.; Corte, T.J.; Fischer, A.; Kreuter, M.; Lederer, D.J.; Molina-Molina, M.; Axmann, J.; Kirchgaessler, K.U.; Samara, K.; Gilberg, F.; et al. Pirfenidone in patients with unclassifiable progressive fibrosing interstitial lung disease: A double-blind, randomised, placebo-controlled, phase 2 trial. *Lancet Respir. Med.* **2020**, *8*, 147–157. [CrossRef] [PubMed]
4. Idiopathic Pulmonary Fibrosis Clinical Research Network; Raghu, G.; Anstrom, K.J.; King, T.E., Jr.; Lasky, J.A.; Martinez, F.J. Prednisone, Azathioprine, and N-Acetylcysteine for Pulmonary Fibrosis. *N. Engl. J. Med.* **2012**, *366*, 1968–1977. [PubMed]
5. Spagnolo, P.; Rossi, G.; Trisolini, R.; Sverzellati, N.; Baughman, R.P.; Wells, A.U. Pulmonary sarcoidosis. *Lancet Respir. Med.* **2018**, *6*, 389–402. [CrossRef]
6. Salisbury, M.L.; Myers, J.L.; Belloli, E.A.; Kazerooni, E.A.; Martinez, F.J.; Flaherty, K.R. Diagnosis and treatment of fibrotic hypersensitivity pneumonia: Where we stand and where we need to go. *Am. J. Respir. Crit. Care Med.* **2017**, *196*, 690–699. [CrossRef]
7. Distler, O.; Highland, K.B.; Gahlemann, M.; Azuma, A.; Fischer, A.; Mayes, M.D.; Raghu, G.; Sauter, W.; Girard, M.; Alves, M.; et al. Nintedanib for Systemic Sclerosis–Associated Interstitial Lung Disease. *N. Engl. J. Med.* **2019**, *380*, 2518–2528. [CrossRef]
8. Mathai, S.C.; Danoff, S.K. Management of interstitial lung disease associated with connective tissue disease. *BMJ* **2016**, *352*, h6819. [CrossRef] [PubMed]
9. Tomassetti, S.; Ravaglia, C.; Puglisi, S.; Ryu, J.H.; Colby, T.V.; Cavazza, A.; Wells, A.U.; Pavone, M.; Vancheri, C.; Lavorini, F.; et al. Impact of Lung Biopsy Information on Treatment Strategy of Patients with Interstitial Lung Diseases. *Ann. Am. Thorac. Soc.* **2022**, *19*, 737–745. [CrossRef]
10. Ribeiro Neto, M.L.; Arrossi, A.V.; Yadav, R.; Culver, D.A.; Mukhopadhyay, S., Parambil, J.G.; Southern, B.D.; Tolle, L.; Pande, A.; Almeida, F.A.; et al. Prospective cohort of cryobiopsy in interstitial lung diseases: A single center experience. *BMC Pulm. Med.* **2022**, *22*, 215. [CrossRef]
11. Cottin, V.; Tomassetti, S.; Valenzuela, C.; Walsh, S.L.F.; Antoniou, K.M.; Bonella, F.; Brown, K.K.; Collard, H.R.; Corte, T.J.; Flaherty, K.R.; et al. Integrating Clinical Probability into the Diagnostic Approach to Idiopathic Pulmonary Fibrosis An International Working Group Perspective. *Am. J. Respir. Crit. Care Med.* **2022**, *206*, 247–259. [CrossRef]
12. Hariri, L.P.; Roden, A.C.; Chung, J.H.; Danoff, S.K.; Manjarres, D.C.G.; Hartwig, M.; Kheir, F.; King, C.; Kreider, M.; Lynch, D.A.; et al. The Role of Surgical Lung Biopsy in the Diagnosis of Perspective from the Pulmonary Fibrosis Foundation. *Ann. Am. Thorac. Soc.* **2021**, *18*, 1601–1609. [CrossRef]
13. Ravaglia, C.; Nicholson, A.G. Biopsy in interstitial lung disease: Specific diagnosis and the identification of the progressive fibrotic phenotype. *Curr. Opin. Pulm. Med.* **2021**, *27*, 355–362. [CrossRef]

14. Korevaar, D.A.; Colella, S.; Fally, M.; Camuset, J.; Colby, T.V.; Hagmeyer, L.; Hetzel, J.; Maldonado, F.; Morais, A.; Ravaglia, C.; et al. European Respiratory Society guidelines on transbronchial lung cryobiopsy in the diagnosis of interstitial lung diseases. *Eur. Respir. J.* **2022**, *60*, 2200425. [CrossRef] [PubMed]
15. Goobie, G.C.; Guler, S.A. The alternative approach: Genomic classifiers for prognostication in interstitial lung disease. *Eur. Respir. J.* **2023**, *61*, 2300033. [CrossRef] [PubMed]
16. Hutchinson, J.P.; McKeever, T.M.; Fogarty, A.W.; Navaratnam, V.; Hubbard, R.B. Surgical lung biopsy for the diagnosis of interstitial lung disease in England: 1997–2008. *Eur. Respir. J.* **2016**, *48*, 1453–1461. [CrossRef] [PubMed]
17. Fisher, J.H.; Shapera, S.; To, T.; Marras, T.K.; Gershon, A.; Dell, S. Procedure volume and mortality after surgical lung biopsy in interstitial lung disease. *Eur. Respir. J.* **2019**, *53*, 1801164. [CrossRef]
18. Radu, D.; Freynet, O.; Kambouchner, M.; Boubaya, M.; Nunes, H.; Uzunhan, Y.; Brillet, P.Y.; Guiraudet, P.; Noorah, M.Z.; Israël-Biet, D.; et al. Diagnosis Yield and Safety of Surgical Biopsy in Interstitial Lung Diseases: A Prospective Study. *Ann. Thorac. Surg.* **2022**, *114*, 1911–1917. [CrossRef]
19. Katzenstein, A.A.; Mukhopadhyay, S.; Myers, J.L. Erratum to "Diagnosis of usual interstitial pneumonia and distinction from other fibrosing interstitial lung diseases" [Hum Pathol 39 (2008) 1275-1294]. *Hum. Pathol.* **2008**, *39*, 1562–1581. [CrossRef]
20. Tomassetti, S.; Cavazza, A.; Colby, T.V.; Ryu, J.H.; Nanni, O.; Scarpi, E.; Tantalocco, P.; Buccioli, M.; Dubini, A.; Piciucchi, S.; et al. Transbronchial biopsy is useful in predicting UIP pattern. *Respir. Res.* **2012**, *13*, 96. [CrossRef]
21. Shim, H.S.; Park, M.S.; Park, I.K. Histopathologic findings of transbronchial biopsy in usual interstitial pneumonia.pdf. *Pathol. Int.* **2010**, *60*, 373–377. [CrossRef] [PubMed]
22. Berbescu, E.A.; Katzenstein, A.-L.A.; Snow, J.L.; Zisman, D.A. Transbronchial Biopsy in Usual Interstitial Pneumonia. *Chest* **2006**, *129*, 1126–1131. [CrossRef]
23. Pankratz, D.G.; Choi, Y.; Imtiaz, U.; Fedorowicz, M.; Anderson, J.D.; Colby, T.V.; Myers, J.L.; Lynch, D.A.; Brown, K.K.; Flaherty, K.R.; et al. Usual Interstitial Pneumonia Can Be Detected in Transbronchial Biopsies Using Machine Learning. *Ann. Am. Thorac. Soc.* **2017**, *14*, 1646–1654. [CrossRef]
24. Raghu, G.; Flaherty, K.R.; Lederer, D.J.; Lynch, D.A.; Colby, T.V.; Myers, J.L.; Groshong, S.D.; Larsen, B.T.; Chung, J.H.; Steele, M.P.; et al. Use of a molecular classifier to identify usual interstitial pneumonia in conventional transbronchial lung biopsy samples: A prospective validation study. *Lancet Respir.* **2024**, *7*, 487–496. [CrossRef]
25. Richeldi, L.; Scholand, M.B.; Lynch, D.A.; Colby, T.V.; Myers, J.L.; Groshong, S.D.; Chung, J.H.; Benzaquen, S.; Nathan, S.D.; Davis, J.R.; et al. Utility of a Molecular Classifier as a Complement to High-Resolution Computed Tomography to Identify Usual Interstitial Pneumonia. *Am. J. Respir. Crit. Care Med.* **2021**, *203*, 211–220. [CrossRef] [PubMed]
26. Kheir, F.; Becerra, J.P.U.; Bissell, B.; Ghazipura, M.; Herman, D.; Hon, S.M.; Hossain, T.; Khor, Y.H.; Knight, S.L.; Kreuter, M.; et al. Use of a Genomic Classifier in Patients with Interstitial Lung Disease A Systematic Review and Meta-Analysis. *Ann. Am. Thorac. Soc.* **2022**, *19*, 827–832. [CrossRef] [PubMed]
27. Lasky, J.A.; Case, A.; Unterman, A.; Kreuter, M.; Scholand, M.B.; Chaudhary, S.; Lofaro, L.R.; Johnson, M.; Huang, J.; Bhorade, S.M.; et al. The Impact of the Envisia Genomic Classifier in the Diagnosis and Management of Patients with Idiopathic Pulmonary Fibrosis. *Ann. Am. Thorac. Soc.* **2022**, *19*, 916–924. [CrossRef]
28. Goobie, G.C.; Kass, D.J. Genomic Classifiers in Diagnosing Interstitial Lung Disease: Finding the Right Place at the Right Time. *Ann. Am. Thorac. Soc.* **2022**, *19*, 895–897. [CrossRef] [PubMed]
29. Arya, R.; Boujaoude, Z.; Rafferty, W.J.; Abouzgheib, W. Usefulness and safety of transbronchial biopsy with large forceps during flexible bronchoscopy. *Baylor Univ. Med. Cent. Proc.* **2020**, *34*, 232–236. [CrossRef]
30. Galli, J.A.; Panetta, N.L.; Gaeckle, N.; Martinez, F.J.; Moore, B.; Moore, T.; Courey, A.; Flaherty, K.; Criner, G.J. Pneumothorax After Transbronchial Biopsy in Pulmonary Fibrosis: Lessons from the Multicenter COMET Trial. *Lung* **2017**, *195*, 537–543. [CrossRef]
31. Pajares, V.; Núñez-Delgado, M.; Bonet, G.; Pérez-Pallarés, J.; Martínez, R.; Cubero, N.; Zabala, T.; Cordovilla, R.; Flandes, J.; Disdier, C.; et al. Transbronchial biopsy results according to diffuse interstitial lung disease classification. Cryobiopsy versus forceps: MULTICRIO study. *PLoS ONE* **2020**, *15*, e0239114. [CrossRef] [PubMed]
32. Sethi, J.; Ali, M.S.; Mohananey, D.; Nanchal, R.; Maldonado, F.; Musani, A. Are Transbronchial Cryobiopsies Ready for Prime Time? *J. Bronchol. Interv. Pulmonol.* **2019**, *26*, 22–32. [CrossRef]
33. Iftikhar, I.H.; Alghothani, L.; Sardi, A.; Berkowitz, D.; Musani, A.I. Transbronchial Lung Cryobiopsy and Video-assisted Thoracoscopic Lung Biopsy in the Diagnosis of Diffuse Parenchymal Lung Disease A Meta-analysis of Diagnostic Test Accuracy. *Ann. Am. Thorac. Soc.* **2017**, *14*, 1197–1211. [CrossRef]
34. Johannson, K.A.; Marcoux, V.S.; Ronksley, P.E.; Ryerson, C.J. Diagnostic Yield and Complications of Transbronchial Lung Cryobiopsy for Interstitial Lung Disease. *Ann. Am. Thorac. Soc.* **2016**, *13*, 1828–1838. [CrossRef] [PubMed]

35. Romagnoli, M.; Colby, T.V.; Berthet, J.; Gamez, A.S.; Mallet, J.; Serre, I.; Cancellieri, A.; Cavazza, A.; Solovei, L.; Amore, A.D.; et al. Poor Concordance between Sequential Transbronchial Lung Cryobiopsy and Surgical Lung Biopsy in the Diagnosis of Diffuse Interstitial Lung Diseases. *Am. J. Respir. Crit. Care Med.* **2019**, *199*, 1249–1256. [CrossRef]
36. Troy, L.K.; Grainge, C.; Corte, T.J.; Williamson, J.P.; Vallely, M.P.; Cooper, W.A.; Mahar, A.; Myers, J.L.; Lai, S.; Mulyadi, E.; et al. Diagnostic accuracy of transbronchial lung cryobiopsy for interstitial lung disease diagnosis (COLDICE): A prospective, comparative study. *Lancet Respir. Med.* **2020**, *8*, 171–181. [CrossRef]
37. Kalverda, K.A.; Ninaber, M.K.; Wijmans, L.; von der Thüsen, J.; Jonkers, R.E.; Daniels, J.M.; Miedema, J.R.; Dickhoff, C.; Hölters, J.; Heineman, D.; et al. Transbronchial cryobiopsy followed by as-needed surgical lung biopsy versus immediate surgical lung biopsy for diagnosing interstitial lung disease (the COLD study): A randomised controlled trial. *Lancet Respir. Med.* **2024**, *12*, 513–522. [CrossRef]
38. Fortin, M.; Liberman, M.; Delage, A.; Dion, G.; Martel, S.; Rolland, F.; Soumagne, T.; Trahan, S.; Assayag, D.; Albert, E.; et al. Transbronchial Lung Cryobiopsy and Surgical LungBiopsy: A Prospective Multi-Centre Agreement Clinical Trial(CAN-ICE). *Am. J. Respir. Crit. Care Med.* **2023**, *207*, 1612–1619. [CrossRef] [PubMed]
39. Kheir, F.; Alkhatib, A.; Berry, G.J.; Daroca, P.; Diethelm, L.; Rampolla, R.; Saito, S.; Smith, D.L.; Weill, D.; Bateman, M.; et al. Using Bronchoscopic Lung Cryobiopsy and a Genomic Classifier in the Multidisciplinary Diagnosis of Diffuse Interstitial Lung Diseases. *Chest* **2020**, *158*, 2015–2025. [CrossRef]
40. Rodrigues, I.; Gomes, R.E.; Coutinho, L.M.; Rego, M.T.; Machado, F.; Morais, A.; Bastos, H.N. Diagnostic yield and safety of transbronchial lung cryobiopsy and surgical lung biopsy in interstitial lung diseases: A systematic review and meta-analysis. *Eur. Respir. Rev.* **2022**, *31*, 210280. [CrossRef]
41. Han, Q.; Luo, Q.; Xie, J.; Wu, L.; Liao, L. Diagnostic yield and postoperative mortality associated with surgical lung biopsy for evaluation of interstitial lung diseases: A systematic review and meta-analysis. *J. Thorac. Cardiovasc. Surg.* **2015**, *149*, 1394–1401. [CrossRef] [PubMed]
42. Hutchinson, J.P.; Fogarty, A.W.; Mckeever, T.M.; Hubbard, R.B. In-Hospital Mortality after Surgical Lung Biopsy for Interstitial Lung Disease in the United States 2000 to 2011. *Am. J. Respir. Crit. Care Med.* **2016**, *193*, 1161–1167. [CrossRef] [PubMed]
43. Sigurdsson, M.I.; Isaksson, H.J.; Gudmundsson, G.; Gudbjartsson, T. Diagnostic Surgical Lung Biopsies for Suspected Interstitial Lung Diseases: A Retrospective Study. *Ann. Thorac. Surg.* **2009**, *88*, 227–232. [CrossRef] [PubMed]
44. Carrillo, G.; Estrada, A.; Pedroza, J.; Aragón, B.; Mejía, M.; Navarro, C.; Selman, M. Preoperative Risk Factors Associated With Mortality in Lung Biopsy Patients With Interstitial Lung Disease. *J. Investig. Surg.* **2005**, *18*, 39–45. [CrossRef]
45. Pastre, J.; Khandhar, S.; Barnett, S.; Ksovreli, I.; Mani, H.; Brown, A.W.; Shlobin, O.A.; Ahmad, K.; Khangoora, V.; Aryal, S.; et al. Surgical Lung Biopsy for Interstitial Lung Disease. *Ann. Am. Thorac. Soc.* **2021**, *18*, 460–467. [CrossRef]
46. Hutchinson, J.; Hubbard, R.; Raghu, G. Surgical lung biopsy for interstitial lung disease: When considered necessary, should these be done in larger and experienced centres only? *Eur. Respir. J.* **2019**, *53*, 1900023. [CrossRef]
47. Ravaglia, C.; Bonifazi, M.; Wells, A.U.; Tomassetti, S.; Gurioli, C.; Piciucchi, S.; Dubini, A.; Tantalocco, P.; Sanna, S.; Negri, E.; et al. Safety and Diagnostic Yield of Transbronchial Lung Cryobiopsy in Diffuse Parenchymal Lung Diseases: A Comparative Study versus Video-Assisted Thoracoscopic Lung Biopsy and a Systematic Review of the Literature. *Respiration* **2016**, *91*, 215–227. [CrossRef]
48. Adegunsoye, A.; Kropski, J.A.; Behr, J.; Blackwell, T.S.; Corte, T.J. Genetics and Genomics of Pulmonary Fibrosis Charting the Molecular Landscape and Shaping Precision Medicine. *Am. J. Respir. Crit. Care Med.* **2024**, *210*, 401–423. [CrossRef]
49. Al, R.B.E.T.; Borie, R.; Kannengiesser, C.; Antoniou, K.; Bonella, F.; Crestani, B.; Fabre, A.; Froidure, A.; Galvin, L.; Griese, M.; et al. European Respiratory Society statement on familial pulmonary fibrosis. *Eur. Respir. J.* **2023**, *61*, 2201383. [CrossRef]
50. Zhang, D.; Newton, C.A. Familial Pulmonary Fibrosis Genetic Features and Clinical Implications. *Chest* **2021**, *160*, 1764–1773. [CrossRef]
51. Savage, S.A.; Alter, B.P. Dyskeratosis Congenita. *Hematol. Oncol. Clin. N. Am.* **2009**, *23*, 215–231. [CrossRef] [PubMed]
52. Borie, R.; Kannengiesser, C.; De Fontbrune, F.S.; Gouya, L.; Nathan, N.; Crestani, B. Management of suspected monogenic lung fibrosis in a specialised centre. *Eur. Respir. Rev.* **2017**, *26*, 160122. [CrossRef] [PubMed]
53. Wang, Y.; Kuan, P.J.; Xing, C.; Cronkhite, J.T.; Torres, F.; Rosenblatt, R.L.; DiMaio, J.M.; Kinch, L.N.; Grishin, N.V.; Garcia, C.K. Genetic Defects in Surfactant Protein A2 Are Associated with Pulmonary Fibrosis and Lung Cancer. *Am. J. Hum. Genet.* **2009**, *84*, 52–59. [CrossRef]
54. Alder, J.K.; Hanumanthu, V.S.; Strong, M.A.; DeZern, A.E.; Stanley, S.E.; Takemoto, C.M.; Danilova, L.; Applegate, C.D.; Bolton, S.G.; Mohr, D.W.; et al. Diagnostic utility of telomere length testing in a hospital-based setting. *Proc. Natl. Acad. Sci. USA* **2018**, *115*, E2358–E2365. [CrossRef]

55. Van Moorsel, C.H.M.; Van Oosterhout, M.F.M.; Barlo, N.P.; De Jong, P.A.; Van Der Vis, J.J.; Ruven, H.J.T.; Van Es, H.W.; Van Den Bosch, J.M.; Grutters, J.C. Surfactant Protein C Mutations Are the Basis ofa Significant Portion of Adult Familial PulmonaryFibrosis in a Dutch Cohort. *Am. J. Respir. Crit. Care Med.* **2010**, *182*, 1419–1425. [CrossRef] [PubMed]
56. Peljto, A.L.; Zhang, Y.; Fingerlin, T.E.; Shwu-Fan, M.; Garcia, J.G.N.; Richards, T.J.; Silveira, L.J.; Lindell, K.O.; Steele, M.P.; Loyd, J.E.; et al. Association between the MUC5B promoter polymorphism and survival in patients with idiopathic pulmonary fibrosis. *JAMA* **2013**, *309*, 2232–2239. [CrossRef]
57. Poletti, V.; Petrarulo, S.; Piciucchi, S.; Dubini, A.; De Grauw, A.J.; Sultani, F.; Martinello, S.; Gonunguntla, H.K.; Ravaglia, C. EBUS-guided cryobiopsy in the diagnosis of thoracic disorders. *Pulmonology* **2024**, *30*, 459–465. [CrossRef]
58. Mangold, M.S.; Franzen, D.P.; Hetzel, J.; Latshang, T.D.; Roeder, M.; Vesenbeckh, S.M.; Ulrich, S.; Gaisl, T.; Steinack, C. Ultrasound-guided transbronchial cryobiopsy of mediastinal and hilar lesions: A multicenter pragmatic cohort study with real-world evidence. *BMJ Open Respir. Res.* **2024**, *11*, e002617. [CrossRef]
59. Ariza-Prota, M.; Pérez-Pallarés, J.; Fernández-Fernández, A.; García-Alfonso, L.; Cascón, J.A.; Torres-Rivas, H.; Fernández-Fernández, L.; Sánchez, I.; Gil, M.; García-Clemente, M.; et al. Endobronchial ultrasound-guided transbronchial mediastinal cryobiopsy in the diagnosis of mediastinal lesions: Safety, feasibility and diagnostic yield—Experience in 50 cases. *ERJ Open Res.* **2023**, *9*, 00448–2022. [CrossRef]
60. Chemla, D.; Castelain, V.; Hoette, S.; Creuzé, N.; Provencher, S.; Zhu, K.; Humbert, M.; Herve, P. Strong linear relationship between heart rate and mean pulmonary artery pressure in exercising patients with severe precapillary pulmonary hypertension. *Am. J. Physiol. Hear. Circ. Physiol.* **2013**, *305*, 769–777. [CrossRef]
61. Santoro, C.; Buonauro, A.; Canora, A.; Rea, G.; Canonico, M.E.; Esposito, R.; Sanduzzi, A.; Esposito, G.; Bocchino, M. Non-Invasive Assessment of Right Ventricle to Arterial Coupling for Prognosis Stratification of Fibrotic Interstitial Lung Diseases. *J. Clin. Med.* **2022**, *11*, 6115. [CrossRef] [PubMed]
62. D'Andrea, A.; Stanziola, A.A.; Saggar, R.; Saggar, R.; Sperlongano, S.; Conte, M.; D'Alto, M.; Ferrara, F.; Gargani, L.; Lancellotti, P.; et al. Right Ventricular Functional Reserve in Early-Stage Idiopathic Pulmonary Fibrosis: An Exercise Two-Dimensional Speckle Tracking Doppler Echocardiography Study. *Chest* **2019**, *155*, 297–306. [CrossRef] [PubMed]
63. Buonauro, A.; Santoro, C.; Galderisi, M.; Canora, A.; Sorrentino, R.; Esposito, R.; Lembo, M.; Canonico, M.E.; Ilardi, F.; Fazio, V.; et al. Impaired right and left ventricular longitudinal function in patients with fibrotic interstitial lung diseases. *J. Clin. Med.* **2020**, *9*, 587. [CrossRef]

MDPI AG
Grosspeteranlage 5
4052 Basel
Switzerland
Tel.: +41 61 683 77 34

Journal of Clinical Medicine Editorial Office
E-mail: jcm@mdpi.com
www.mdpi.com/journal/jcm

www.ingramcontent.com/pod-product-compliance
Lightning Source LLC
Chambersburg PA
CBHW061519210926
51850CB00008B/1975
9783725868469